Teen Health Series

DATE

APR 08

APR 22 2019

PRINTED IN U.S.A.

DATE DUE

Drug Abuse

SOURCEBOOK

Fourth Edition

Health Reference Series

Fourth Edition

Drug Abuse
SOURCEBOOK

*Basic Consumer Health Information about the
Abuse of Cocaine, Club Drugs, Marijuana, Inhalants,
Heroin, Hallucinogens, and Other Illicit Substances
and the Misuse of Prescription and
Over-the-Counter Medications*

*Along with Facts and Statistics about Drug Use and
Addiction, Treatment and Recovery, Drug Testing, Drug
Abuse Prevention and Intervention, Glossaries of Related
Terms, and Directories of Resources for Additional Help
and Information*

Edited by
Laura Larsen

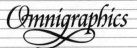

155 W. Congress, Suite 200, Detroit, MI 48226

10-31-14
LN
$95.00

Bibliographic Note

Because this page cannot legibly accommodate all the copyright notices, the Bibliographic Note portion of the Preface constitutes an extension of the copyright notice.

Edited by Laura Larsen

Health Reference Series
Karen Bellenir, *Managing Editor*
David A. Cooke, MD, FACP, *Medical Consultant*
Elizabeth Collins, *Research and Permissions Coordinator*
EdIndex, Services for Publishers, *Indexers*

* * *

Omnigraphics, Inc.
Matthew P. Barbour, *Senior Vice President*
Kevin M. Hayes, *Operations Manager*

* * *

Peter E. Ruffner, *Publisher*
Copyright © 2014 Omnigraphics, Inc.
ISBN 978-0-7808-1307-6

E-ISBN 978-0-7808-1308-3

Library of Congress Cataloging-in-Publication Data

Drug abuse sourcebook : basic consumer health information about the abuse of cocaine, club drugs, marijuana, inhalants, heroin, hallucinogens, and other illicit substances and the misuse of prescription and over-the-counter medications; along with facts and statistics about drug use and addiction, treatment and recovery, drug testing, drug abuse prevention and intervention, glossaries of related terms, and directories of resources for additional help and information / edited by Laura Larsen. -- Fourth edition.
       pages cm
   Includes bibliographical references and index.
   Summary: "Provides basic consumer health information about the abuse of illegal drugs and misuse of prescription and over-the-counter medications, along with facts about prevention, treatment, and recovery. Includes index, glossary of related terms and directory of resources"-- Provided by publisher.
   ISBN 978-0-7808-1307-6 (hardcover : alk. paper) 1. Drug abuse--Prevention--Handbooks, manuals, etc. 2. Drug abuse--Treatment--Handbooks, manuals, etc. 3. Drug addiction--Treatment--Handbooks, manuals, etc. I. Larsen, Laura.
   HV5801.D724 2014
   362.29--dc23
                                                              2013037324

Table of Contents

Visit www.healthreferenceseries.com to view *A Contents Guide to the Health Reference Series*, a listing of more than 16,000 topics and the volumes in which they are covered.

Part II: Drug Abuse and Specific Populations

Part III: Drugs of Abuse

Part IV: The Causes and Consequences of Drug Abuse and Addiction

Part VI: Drug Abuse Testing and Prevention

Part VII: Additional Help and Information

Preface

About This Book

Drug abuse remains a growing problem in the United States. A survey conducted by the Substance Abuse and Mental Health Services Administration (SAMHSA) in 2010 found that 8.9% of the population had used an illicit drug or abused a prescription medication. This figure represented an increase from previous years mainly due to the widespread prevalence of marijuana use and increasing prescription drug misuse. There are spots of good news, however. The same survey also found that the abuse of other illicit drugs, such as heroin and cocaine, had decreased in recent years. Nevertheless, the medical, social, and familial costs of substance use are enormous—nearly $200 billion a year according to the U.S. Department of Justice.

Drug Abuse Sourcebook, Fourth Edition, provides updated information about the abuse of illegal drugs and the misuse of prescription and over-the-counter medications. It offers facts and statistics related to U.S. drug-using populations and presents details about specific drugs of abuse, including their health-related consequences, addiction potential, and other harms to individuals, their families, and communities. Drug treatment and recovery options are discussed, along with information on drug testing and drug-use prevention strategies for parents, employers, individuals, and others seeking help for themselves or a loved one. The book concludes with glossaries of terms related to drug abuse and directories of resources for additional help and information.

How to Use This Book

This book is divided into parts and chapters. Parts focus on broad areas of interest. Chapters are devoted to single topics within a part.

Part I: Facts and Statistics about Drug Abuse in the United States presents core data regarding the drug abuse problem, detailing the prevalence of drug abuse and the costs to society in terms of medical care, hospitalization, social consequences, and treatment outcomes. It also discusses federal regulation of prescriptions, laws pertaining to illegal and legal drugs, and the current debate over medical and legalized marijuana.

Part II: Drug Abuse and Specific Populations describes drug use initiation and the effects of drug abuse on various groups of people, including children, adolescents, and women. It also addresses different social factors affecting drug abuse, such as socioeconomic or employment status, and it considers drug use in inmate, veteran, senior, and disabled populations.

Part III: Drugs of Abuse provides facts about illicit and misused substances, such as performance enhancers, cannabinoids, inhalants, hallucinogens, narcotics, sedatives, and stimulants, including anabolic steroids, marijuana, Rohypnol, ecstasy (MDMA), LSD, heroin, hydrocodone, cocaine, methamphetamine, and many others. The part concludes with information about new and emerging drugs of abuse.

Part IV: The Causes and Consequences of Drug Abuse and Addiction explains the science behind addiction and what is known about the risk factors that can lead to drug dependancy. Concerns related to coexisting alcohol problems or multidrug use are addressed, and the medical, legal, financial, and social ramifications of drug abuse are discussed. The part also looks at the connection between substance abuse and infectious diseases, and it addresses related mental health issues, including suicide ideation.

Part V: Drug Abuse Treatment and Recovery offers suggestions for recognizing the existence of a drug problem and options for taking steps toward achieving and maintaining a healthy lifestyle, including first aid, intervention, and detoxification. It provides details about various treatment approaches and reports on strategies for sustaining recovery. The part also discusses the legal rights of those in recovery and concerns related to the criminal justice system.

Part VI: Drug Abuse Testing and Prevention lays the groundwork for responses to drug abuse—in society, in schools, and especially in the home. It discusses the influence of parents on their children's choices related to drug abuse, and it addresses concerns about preventing drug abuse in the workplace. Drug testing is discussed in detail, and federal drug abuse prevention campaigns are described.

Part VII: Additional Help and Information provides resources for readers seeking further assistance. It includes a glossary of terms related to drug abuse and a listing of street terms for common drugs of abuse. It concludes with directories of state substance abuse agencies and other organizations providing resources on drug abuse and addiction.

Bibliographic Note

This volume contains documents and excerpts from publications issued by the following U.S. government agencies: Centers for Disease Control and Prevention (CDC); Consumer Product Safety Commission (CPSC); Drug Enforcement Agency (DEA); Drug Enforcement Agency Office of Diversion Control; National Criminal Justice Reference Service (NCJRS); National Institute on Alcohol Abuse and Alcoholism (NIAAA); National Institute on Drug Abuse (NIDA); Small Business Administration (SBA); Substance Abuse and Mental Health Services Administration (SAMHSA); U.S. Department of Health and Human Services (HHS); U.S. Department of Labor (DOL); U.S. Federal Bureau of Investigation (FBI); U.S. Food and Drug Administration (FDA); and White House Office of National Drug Control Policy (ONDCP).

In addition, this volume contains copyrighted documents from the following organizations: A.D.A.M., Inc.; American Association for Clinical Chemistry; American Psychological Association; BioMed Central; DARSYS, Inc.; Drug Policy Alliance; Hormone Health Network; Illinois Attorney General; Integrated Research Services; March of Dimes; Mercyhurst Civic Institute; Narconon International; Narcotics Anonymous; National Center on Addiction and Substance Abuse at Columbia University (CASA Columbia); Nemours Foundation; New York State Office of Alcoholism and Substance Abuse Services; The Partnership at Drugfree.org; University of Cincinnati; and University of Missouri.

Full citation information is provided on the first page of each chapter or section. Every effort has been made to secure all necessary rights to reprint the copyrighted material. If any omissions have been made, please contact Omnigraphics to make corrections for future editions.

Acknowledgements

Thanks go to the many organizations, agencies, and individuals who have contributed materials for this *Sourcebook* and to medical consultant Dr. David Cooke and prepress services provider Whimsy-Ink. Special thanks go to managing editor Karen Bellenir and research and permissions coordinator Liz Collins for their help and support.

About the Health Reference Series

The *Health Reference Series* is designed to provide basic medical information for patients, families, caregivers, and the general public. Each volume takes a particular topic and provides comprehensive coverage. This is especially important for people who may be dealing with a newly diagnosed disease or a chronic disorder in themselves or in a family member. People looking for preventive guidance, information about disease warning signs, medical statistics, and risk factors for health problems will also find answers to their questions in the *Health Reference Series*. The *Series*, however, is not intended to serve as a tool for diagnosing illness, in prescribing treatments, or as a substitute for the physician/patient relationship. All people concerned about medical symptoms or the possibility of disease are encouraged to seek professional care from an appropriate health care provider.

A Note about Spelling and Style

Health Reference Series editors use *Stedman's Medical Dictionary* as an authority for questions related to the spelling of medical terms and the *Chicago Manual of Style* for questions related to grammatical structures, punctuation, and other editorial concerns. Consistent adherence is not always possible, however, because the individual volumes within the *Series* include many documents from a wide variety of different producers and copyright holders, and the editor's primary goal is to present material from each source as accurately as is possible following the terms specified by each document's producer. This sometimes means that information in different chapters or sections may follow other guidelines and alternate spelling authorities. For example, occasionally a copyright holder may require that eponymous terms be shown in possessive forms (Crohn's disease *vs.* Crohn disease) or that British spelling norms be retained (leukaemia *vs.* leukemia).

Locating Information within the Health Reference Series

The *Health Reference Series* contains a wealth of information about a wide variety of medical topics. Ensuring easy access to all the fact sheets, research reports, in-depth discussions, and other material contained within the individual books of the *Series* remains one of our highest priorities. As the *Series* continues to grow in size and scope, however, locating the precise information needed by a reader may become more challenging.

A Contents Guide to the Health Reference Series was developed to direct readers to the specific volumes that address their concerns. It presents an extensive list of diseases, treatments, and other topics of general interest compiled from the Tables of Contents and major index headings. To access *A Contents Guide to the Health Reference Series*, visit www.healthreferenceseries.com.

Medical Consultant

Medical consultation services are provided to the *Health Reference Series* editors by David A. Cooke, MD, FACP. Dr. Cooke is a graduate of Brandeis University, and he received his M.D. degree from the University of Michigan. He completed residency training at the University of Wisconsin Hospital and Clinics. He is board-certified in Internal Medicine. Dr. Cooke currently works as part of the University of Michigan Health System and practices in Ann Arbor, MI. In his free time, he enjoys writing, science fiction, and spending time with his family.

Our Advisory Board

We would like to thank the following board members for providing guidance to the development of this *Series*:

- Dr. Lynda Baker, Associate Professor of Library and Information Science, Wayne State University, Detroit, MI

- Nancy Bulgarelli, William Beaumont Hospital Library, Royal Oak, MI

- Karen Imarisio, Bloomfield Township Public Library, Bloomfield Township, MI

- Karen Morgan, Mardigian Library, University of Michigan-Dearborn, Dearborn, MI

xix

- Rosemary Orlando, St. Clair Shores Public Library, St. Clair Shores, MI

Health Reference Series Update Policy

The inaugural book in the *Health Reference Series* was the first edition of *Cancer Sourcebook* published in 1989. Since then, the *Series* has been enthusiastically received by librarians and in the medical community. In order to maintain the standard of providing high-quality health information for the layperson the editorial staff at Omnigraphics felt it was necessary to implement a policy of updating volumes when warranted.

Medical researchers have been making tremendous strides, and it is the purpose of the *Health Reference Series* to stay current with the most recent advances. Each decision to update a volume is made on an individual basis. Some of the considerations include how much new information is available and the feedback we receive from people who use the books. If there is a topic you would like to see added to the update list, or an area of medical concern you feel has not been adequately addressed, please write to:

Editor
Health Reference Series
Omnigraphics, Inc.
155 W. Congress, Suite 200
Detroit, MI 48226
E-mail: editorial@omnigraphics.com

Part One

Facts and Statistics about Drug Abuse in the United States

Chapter 1

Prevalence of Illicit Drug Use and Substance Abuse

Nationwide Trends

A major source of information on substance use, abuse, and dependence among Americans aged 12 and older is the annual National Survey on Drug Use and Health (NSDUH) conducted by the Substance Abuse and Mental Health Services Administration (SAMHSA). Following are facts and statistics on substance use in America from 2011, the most recent year for which NSDUH survey data have been analyzed.

Illicit Drug Use

Illicit drug use in America has been increasing. In 2011, an estimated 22.5 million Americans aged 12 or older—or 8.7% of the population—had used an illicit drug or abused a psychotherapeutic medication (such as a pain reliever, stimulant, or tranquilizer) in the past month. This is up from 8.3% in 2002. The increase mostly reflects a recent rise in the use of marijuana, the most commonly used illicit drug.

Past month use among 12 and older (in millions) is as follows:

- **All illicit drugs:** 22.5%

- **Marijuana:** 18.1%

"DrugFacts: Nationwide Trends," National Institute on Drug Abuse (www.drugabuse.gov), December 2012, and "Club Drugs—Facts and Figures," National Criminal Justice Reference Service, U.S. Department of Justice (www.ncjrs.gov), December 12, 2012.

- **Psychotherapeutics:** 6.1%
- **Cocaine:** 1.4%
- **Hallucinogens:** 1%
- **Inhalants:** 0.6%
- **Heroin:** 0.3%

Marijuana use has increased since 2007. In 2011, there were 18.1 million current (past-month) users—about 7.0% of people aged 12 or older—up from 14.4 million (5.8%) in 2007.

Use of most drugs other than marijuana has not changed appreciably over the past decade or has declined. In 2011, 6.1 million Americans aged 12 or older (or 2.4%) had used psychotherapeutic prescription drugs nonmedically (without a prescription or in a manner or for a purpose not prescribed) in the past month—a decrease from 2010. And 972,000 Americans (0.4%) had used hallucinogens (a category that includes ecstasy [MDMA] and LSD [lysergic acid diethylamide]) in the past month—a decline from 2010.

Cocaine use has gone down in the last few years; from 2006 to 2011, the number of current users aged 12 or older dropped from 2.4 million to 1.4 million. Methamphetamine use has also dropped, from 731,000 current users in 2006 to 439,000 in 2011.

Most people use drugs for the first time when they are teenagers. There were just over 3.0 million new users (initiates) of illicit drugs in 2011, or about 8,400 new users per day. Half (51%) were under 18.

More than half of new illicit drug users begin with marijuana. Next most common are prescription pain relievers, followed by inhalants (which is most common among younger teens).

First specific drug initiating drug use in past year are as follows:

- **Marijuana:** 67.5%
- **Pain relievers:** 14%
- **Inhalants:** 7.5%
- **Tranquilizers:** 4.2%
- **Hallucinogens:** 2.8%
- **Stimulants:** 2.6%
- **Sedatives:** 1.2%
- **Cocaine:** 0.2%
- **Heroin:** 0.1%

Drug use is highest among people in their late teens and twenties. In 2011, 23.8% of 18- to 20-year-olds reported using an illicit drug in the past month.

Drug use is increasing among people in their fifties. This is, at least in part, due to the aging of the baby boomers, whose rates of illicit drug use have historically been higher than those of previous cohorts.

Alcohol

Drinking by underage persons (ages 12–20) has declined. Current alcohol use by this age group declined from 28.8% to 25.1% between 2002 and 2011, while binge drinking declined from 19.3% to 15.8% and the rate of heavy drinking went from 6.2% to 4.4%.

Binge and heavy drinking are more prevalent among men than among women. In 2011, 30.0% of men 12 and older and 13.9% of women reported binge drinking (five or more drinks on the same occasion) in the past month; and 9.1% of men and 2.6% of women reported heavy alcohol use (binge drinking on at least five separate days in the past month).

Driving under the influence of alcohol has also declined slightly. In 2011, an estimated 28.6 million people, or 11.1% of persons aged 12 or older, had driven under the influence of alcohol at least once in the past year, down from 14.2% in 2002. Although this decline is encouraging, any driving under the influence remains a cause for concern.

Tobacco

Fewer Americans are smoking. In 2011, an estimated 56.8 million Americans aged 12 or older, or 22% of the population, were current (past-month) cigarette smokers. This reflects a continual but slow downward trend from 2002, when the rate was 26%.

Teen smoking is declining more rapidly. The rate of past-month cigarette use among 12- to 17-year-olds went from 13% in 2002 to 7.8% in 2011.

Substance Dependence/Abuse and Treatment

Rates of alcohol dependence/abuse declined from 2002 to 2011. In 2011, 16.7 million Americans (6.5% of the population) were dependent on alcohol or had problems related to their use of alcohol (abuse). This is a decline from 18.1 million (or 7.7%) in 2002.

After alcohol, marijuana has the highest rate of dependence or abuse among all drugs. In 2011, 4.2 million Americans met clinical criteria for dependence or abuse of marijuana in the past year—more

5

than twice the number for dependence/abuse of prescription pain relievers (1.8 million) and four times the number for dependence/abuse of cocaine (821,000).

Drug dependence or abuse in past year among 12 and older is as follows:

- **Marijuana:** 4,165,000

- **Pain relievers:** 1,768,000

- **Cocaine:** 821,000

- **Heroin:** 426,000

- **Tranquilizers:** 400,000

- **Hallucinogens:** 342,000

- **Stimulants:** 329,000

- **Inhalants:** 141,000

- **Sedatives:** 78,000

There continues to be a large "treatment gap" in this country. In 2011, an estimated 21.6 million Americans (8.4%) needed treatment for a problem related to drugs or alcohol, but only about 2.3 million people (less than 1%) received treatment at a specialty facility.

Learn More

Complete NSDUH findings are available at www.samhsa.gov/data/NSDUH/2k11Results/NSDUHresults2011.htm.

Club Drugs—Facts and Figures

Findings from the 2011 National Survey on Drug Use and Health (2012), which includes interviews with approximately 67,500 persons each year, include the following:

- An estimated 544,000 individuals aged 12 or older were current (past-month) users of ecstasy, representing 0.2% of the population.

- There were an estimated 439,000 current users of methamphetamine, aged 12 or older, representing 0.2% of the population.

Sponsored by the National Institute on Drug Abuse (NIDA), the Monitoring the Future program at the University of Michigan conducts annual anonymous written surveys of nationally representative samples of students in public and private secondary schools throughout the coterminous United States. Approximately 46,700 students in 400 secondary schools participated in the 2011 Monitoring the Future Survey. Results from the 2011 Monitoring the Future Survey (2012) include the following:

- Among high school seniors surveyed in 2011, 5.3% used MDMA, 1.4% used meth, 1.4% used GHB (gamma hydroxybutyrate), 1.7% used ketamine, and 1.3% used Rohypnol within the year prior to being surveyed.

- Approximately 2.6% of 8th graders, 6.6% of 10th graders, and 8% of 12th graders reported lifetime use of MDMA. Also, 1.3% of 8th graders, 2.1% of 10th graders, and 2.1% of 12th graders reported lifetime use of methamphetamine.

- Approximately 37.1% of 12th graders, 24.8% of 10th graders, and 12% of 8th graders reported that MDMA was "fairly easy" or "very easy" to obtain.

SAMHSA's Drug Abuse Warning Network (DAWN) provides data from a review of emergency department (ED) medical records nationwide. Estimates from the 2009 National Estimates of Drug-Related Emergency Department Visits (2011) are based on data submitted by 242 hospitals and apply to the entire United States. Findings from the ED record reviews during 2009 include the following:

- 973,591 total drug-related ED visits

- 64,117 of the drug-related ED visits involved methamphetamine

- 22,816 involved MDMA

- 1,758 involved GHB

- 800 involved Rohypnol

- 529 involved ketamine

The following statistics are according to National Seizure System (NSS) data as of July 7, 2011, presented in the National Drug Intelligence Center's National Drug Threat Assessment 2011 (2011):

- The number of reported domestic methamphetamine laboratory seizures in 2010 (6,768) represents a 12% increase over the total number of methamphetamine laboratories seized in 2009 (6,032).

- In the United States, 11 MDMA laboratories were seized in 2009; none were seized in 2008.

Additional NSS data from the National Drug Threat Assessment 2011 show the following:

- 6,601 kilograms of methamphetamine were seized in the United States during full year 2009. Data from January 1–November 5, 2010, indicate the seizure of 8,699 kilograms in the U.S.

- 2,479 kilograms of MDMA were seized in the United States during full year 2009. Data from January 1–November 5, 2010, indicate the seizure of 2,124 kilograms in the U.S.

Chapter 2

Injection Drug Use and Related Risk Behaviors

- Combined 2006 to 2008 data indicate that an annual average of 425,000 persons aged 12 or older (0.17%) used a needle to inject heroin, cocaine, methamphetamine, or other stimulants during the past year.

- One-eighth (13.0%) of past-year injection drug users had used a needle that they knew or suspected someone else had used before them the last time they used a needle to inject drugs.

- Less than one-third (29.0%) of past-year injection drug users cleaned the needle with bleach prior to their last injection.

- More than one-half (52.8%) of past-year injection drug users purchased the last needle they used from a pharmacy, and 12.4% obtained the needle through a needle exchange program.

Injection drug use is a high-risk behavior that can be further exacerbated by reusing or sharing needles and/or failing to clean the needle with bleach after each use. These actions can increase the user's risk for blood borne infections, such as the human immunodeficiency virus (HIV), hepatitis C, hepatitis B, and herpes simplex virus 2. In 2006, 16% of new HIV cases involved intravenous drug use as a mode of transmission, and 27.6% of persons living with HIV/AIDS in 2007,

Excerpted from "The NSDUH Report: Injection Drug Use and Related Risk Behaviors," Substance Abuse and Mental Health Services Administration, Office of Applied Studies (oas.samhsa.gov), October 29, 2009.

could have contracted the disease through intravenous drug use. Monitoring the prevalence of injection drug use and the associated risk behaviors is vital for making decisions about designing and implementing programs to address these behaviors.

The National Survey on Drug Use and Health (NSDUH) asks respondents aged 12 or older whether or not they have ever used a needle to inject heroin, cocaine, methamphetamine, other stimulants, other drugs that were not prescribed for them, or drugs that they took only for the feeling or experience they caused. Respondents who report needle use also are asked how recently they did so. In addition, for their last episode of needle use, they are asked if they had reused a needle that they used before; if they used a needle that they knew or suspected someone else had used before; if someone else used the needle after them, whether or not they used bleach to clean the needle before they used it; and how they got the needle. All findings presented in the report are annual averages based on combined data from 2006 to 2008.

Prevalence of Needle Use

An annual average of 425,000 persons aged 12 or older (0.17%) used a needle to inject heroin, cocaine, methamphetamine, or other stimulants during the past year. An estimated 241,000 persons injected heroin during the past year; 166,000 injected cocaine; 165,000 injected methamphetamines; and 95,000 injected other stimulants.

The rate of past-year injection drug use was higher among persons aged 18 to 25 and those aged 26 to 34 (0.28% and 0.26%, respectively) than among those aged 12 to 17 and those aged 50 or older (0.09% and 0.11%, respectively). Additionally, those aged 18 to 25 were more likely to have injected drugs than those aged 35 to 49 (0.28% vs. 0.19%). Males were twice as likely as females to have injected drugs (0.24% vs. 0.11%). Past-year injection drug use varied among racial/ethnic groups, with Asians and Native Hawaiians or Other Pacific Islanders having lower rates than other groups.

Drug Injection Risk Behaviors

The last time they injected drugs, more than one-half (51.0%) of past-year injection drug users indicated that they reused a needle that they had used before, approximately one in eight (13.0%) indicated that they used a needle that they knew or suspected someone else had used before them, and one in six (17.7%) indicated that they used a needle that someone used after them. Less than one-third (29.0%) of past-year injection drug users cleaned the needle with bleach the last time they used a needle to inject drugs.

Needle Sources

More than one-half (52.8%) of past-year injection drug users reported that the last time they injected drugs, the needle had been purchased from a pharmacy, and 12.4% had obtained the needle through a needle exchange program.

Discussion

HIV prevention and education programs targeted at out-of-treatment injection drug users have been in effect for nearly two decades. The findings from NSDUH, however, suggest that the need for such programs still remains. By identifying varying rates of injection drug use among demographic groups, they also help to delineate specific subpopulations for whom modifying current programs or developing new ones may prove to be most effective.

Chapter 3

Drug Abuse and Related Hospitalization Costs

Chapter Contents

Section 3.1

Substance Abuse Cost to Society

Excerpted from: The National Center on Addiction and Substance Abuse at Columbia University (CASAColumbia™). (2009). *Shoveling Up II: The Impact of Substance Abuse on Federal, State and Local Budgets.* New York: National Center on Addiction and Substance Abuse at Columbia University. © 2009. All rights reserved.

In 2005, federal, state, and local governments spent at least $467.7 billion on substance abuse and addiction. This report is the first comprehensive picture of substance related spending across all levels of government. Building on CASA's 2001 report, *Shoveling Up: The Impact of Substance Abuse on State Budgets*, this report reveals the pervasive and devastating burden of substance abuse and addiction to all government budgets.

Federal and state governments spent $3.3 trillion in 2005 to operate government and provide public services such as education, health care, income assistance, child welfare, mental health, law enforcement and justice services, transportation, and highway safety. Hidden in this spending was a stunning $373.9 billion—11.2%—that was spent on tobacco, alcohol, and other drug abuse and addiction. A conservative estimate of local government spending on substance abuse and addiction in 2005 is $93.8 billion.

The vast majority of federal and state substance related spending—95.6% or $357.4 billion—went to carry the burden to government programs of our failure to prevent and treat the problem while only 1.9% was spent on preventing or treating addiction. Another 0.4% was spent on research and the remaining 2% was spent on alcohol and tobacco tax collection, regulation and operation of state liquor stores (1.4%), and federal drug interdiction (0.7 %). For every dollar the federal and state governments spent on prevention and treatment, they spent $59.83 shoveling up the consequences.

A staggering 71.1% of total *federal and state* spending on the burden of addiction is in two areas: health and justice. Almost three-fifths (58.0 %) of federal and state spending on the burden of substance abuse and addiction (74.1% of the federal burden) is in the area of

14

health care where untreated addiction causes or contributes to over 70 other diseases requiring hospitalization. The second largest area of substance-related federal and state burden spending is the justice system (13.1%).

This report shows how governmental spending is skewed toward shoveling up the burden of our continued failure to prevent and treat the problem rather than toward investing in cost-effective approaches to prevent and minimize the disease and its consequences. Despite a significant and growing body of knowledge documenting that addiction is a preventable and treatable disease, and despite a growing array of prevention, treatment, and policy interventions of proven efficacy, our nation still looks the other way while substance abuse and addiction cause illness, injury, death, and crime, savage our children, overwhelm social service systems, impede education, and slap a heavy and growing tax on our citizens.

In the current fiscal climate of growing economic hardship, we no longer can afford costly and ineffective policies that sap on average $1,486 annually in government taxes and fees from each man, woman, and child in America—$5,944 each year for a family of four.

Shoveling Up establishes the categories of state spending that are tightly linked to tobacco, alcohol, and other drug abuse and addiction (including both illicit and controlled prescription drugs)—the targets for policy intervention. It uses existing research to establish the proportion of government spending in each of these target categories that is substance related, providing estimates of the total costs of substance abuse and addiction—the aggregate costs—which include both avoidable and unavoidable costs. The bottom line for government is identifying where substance abuse and addiction must be prevented or treated if public costs are to be reduced or avoided. We include examples of proven and promising ways to reduce those costs and examples of the potential for specific cost avoidance/savings.

Key findings of this report are that in 2005:

- The federal government spent $238.2 billion on substance abuse and addiction or 9.6% of the federal budget. If substance abuse and addiction were its own budget category, it would rank sixth in size—behind social security, national defense, income security, Medicare, and other health programs.

- State governments, including the District of Columbia and Puerto Rico, spent 15.7% of their budgets ($135.8 billion) to deal with substance abuse and addiction—up from 13.3% in 1998. If substance abuse and addiction were its own budget category, it would rank second behind elementary and secondary education. States spend more on substance abuse and addiction than they spend on Medicaid, higher education, transportation, or justice.

- Local governments spent conservatively $93.8 billion on substance abuse and addiction or 9.0% of local budgets, outstripping local spending for transportation and public welfare.

- Of every dollar federal and state governments spent on substance abuse and addiction:

  - 95.6 cents went to pay for the burden of this problem on public programs. Substance abuse and addiction increases, for example, the cost of America's prisons and jails; Medicaid and other health programs; elementary and secondary schools; child welfare, juvenile justice, and mental health systems; public safety; and government payrolls.

  - 1.9 cents went to fund prevention and treatment programs aimed at reducing the incidence and consequences of substance abuse and addiction.

  - 1.4 cents covered costs of collecting alcohol and tobacco taxes, regulating alcohol and tobacco products, and operating state liquor stores.

  - 0.4 cents was spent on addiction-related research.

  - 0.7 cents was spent by the federal government on drug interdiction.

- For every dollar federal and state governments spent to prevent and treat substance abuse and addiction, they spent $59.83 in public programs shoveling up its wreckage, despite a substantial and growing body of scientific evidence confirming the efficacy of science-based interventions and treatment and their cost-saving potential.

- The largest area of federal and state government spending on the burden of substance abuse and addiction was health care, totaling $207.2 billion (58.0%) in 2005. Federal substance-related health care spending totaled $170.3 billion, 74.1% of all federal burden spending.

- The second largest area of federal and state spending on the burden of substance abuse and addiction, and the largest area of state spending, is the justice system, including costs of incarceration, probation and parole, juvenile justice, and criminal and family court costs of substance-involved offenders. These costs totaled $47.0 billion (13.1%) in federal and state burden spending in 2005. State substance-related justice spending totaled $41.4 billion, 32.5% of all state burden spending.

- Other areas of significant federal and state spending on the burden to government of our failure to prevent or treat substance abuse and addiction include:

  - $33.9 billion on the burden to education programs,

  - $46.7 billion on the burden to child and family assistance programs, and

  - $11.8 billion on the burden to mental health and developmental disabilities programs.

- Almost half (47.3%) of government spending on substance abuse and addiction cannot be disaggregated by substance. In fact, research shows that most individuals with substance use disorders use more than one drug. Of the $248 billion in substance-related spending that can be linked to specific drugs of abuse, 92.3% is linked to the legal drugs of alcohol and tobacco.

- For every dollar federal and state governments spent on prevention or treatment for children, they spent $60.25 on the consequences of substance abuse and addiction to them. Combined federal and state government spending in 2005 on costs of substance abuse and addiction to children totaled $54.2 billion.

- Alcohol and tobacco taxes fail to pay their way. The public health goal for tobacco taxes is to help eliminate use. The public health goal for alcohol taxes is to curb underage and adult excessive drinking. For each dollar in alcohol and tobacco taxes and liquor store revenues that hit federal and state coffers, these governments spent $8.95 cleaning up the wreckage of substance abuse and addiction. Federal, state, and local governments collected $14.0 billion in alcohol and $21.2 billion in tobacco taxes in 2005 for a total of $35.2 billion; 18 states expended $4.4 billion in 2005 operating liquor stores and collected $5.6 billion in revenues. Few governments dedicate revenues to reducing the burden of substance abuse or addiction or use alcohol tax increases as a way to reduce use by teens.

- According to the National Institute on Drug Abuse, the return on investing in treatment alone may exceed 12:1; that is, every dollar spent on treatment can reduce future burden costs by $12 or more in reduced drug-related crime and criminal justice and health care costs.

Building on the methodology developed for our first analysis, this report is the result of an intensive three year analysis. As part of this unprecedented study, CASA convened an advisory panel of distinguished public officials, researchers, and representatives of federal, state, and local governments and interest groups.

Section 3.2

Drug-Related Hospital Emergency Room Visits

"DrugFacts: Drug-Related Hospital Emergency Room Visits,"
National Institute on Drug Abuse (www.drugabuse.gov), May 2011.

National estimates on drug-related visits to hospital emergency departments (ED) are obtained from the Drug Abuse Warning Network (DAWN), a public health surveillance system managed by the Substance Abuse and Mental Health Services Administration (SAMHSA). DAWN data are based on a national sample of general, non-federal hospitals operating 24-hour emergency departments (EDs). Information is collected for all types of drugs—including illegal drugs, inhalants, alcohol—and abuse (nonmedical use) of prescription and over-the-counter (OTC) medications and dietary supplements.

Highlights from the 2009 Drug Abuse Warning Network

In 2009, there were nearly 4.6 million drug-related ED visits nationwide. These visits included reports of drug abuse, adverse reactions to drugs, or other drug-related consequences. Almost 50% were attributed to adverse reactions to pharmaceuticals taken as prescribed, and 45% involved drug abuse. DAWN estimates show the following related to the 2.1 million drug abuse visits:

- 27.1% involved nonmedical use of pharmaceuticals (i.e., prescription or OTC medications, dietary supplements).

- 21.2% involved illicit drugs.

- 14.3% involved alcohol, in combination with other drugs.

ED visits involving nonmedical use of pharmaceuticals (either alone or in combination with another drug) increased 98.4% between 2004 and 2009, from 627,291 visits to 1,244,679, respectively. ED visits involving adverse reactions to pharmaceuticals increased 82.9% between 2005 and 2009, from 1,250,377 to 2,287,273 visits, respectively.

The majority of drug-related ED visits were made by patients 21 or older (80.9%, or 3,717,030 visits). Of these, slightly less than half involved drug abuse. Patients aged 20 or younger accounted for 19.1% (877,802 visits) of all drug-related visits in 2009; about half of these visits involved drug abuse.

Illicit Drugs

In 2009, almost one million visits involved an illicit drug, either alone or in combination with other types of drugs:

- Cocaine was involved in 422,896 ED visits.

- Marijuana was involved in 376,467 ED visits.

- Heroin was involved in 213,118 ED visits.

- Stimulants, including amphetamines and methamphetamine, were involved in 93,562 ED visits.

- Other illicit drugs—such as PCP (phencyclidine), ecstasy, and GHB (gamma hydroxybutyrate)—were involved much less frequently than any of the other drug types mentioned.

The rates of ED visits involving cocaine, marijuana, and heroin were higher for males than for females. Rates for cocaine were highest among individuals aged 35–44, rates for heroin were highest among individuals aged 21–24, stimulant use was highest among those 25–29, and marijuana use was highest for those aged 18–20.

Alcohol and Other Drugs

Approximately 32% (658,263) of all drug abuse ED visits in 2009 involved the use of alcohol, either alone or in combination with another drug. DAWN reports alcohol-related data when it is used alone among individuals under the age of 21 or in combination with other drugs among all groups, regardless of age. Because DAWN does not account for ED visits involving alcohol use alone in adults, the actual number of ED visits involving alcohol among the general population is thought to be significantly higher than what is reported in DAWN.

In 2009, DAWN estimated 519,650 ED visits related to the use of alcohol in combination with other drugs. Alcohol was most frequently combined with the following:

- Central nervous system agents (e.g., analgesics, stimulants, sedatives) (229,230 visits)
- Cocaine (152,631 visits)
- Marijuana (125,438 visits)
- Psychotherapeutic agents (e.g., antidepressants and antipsychotics) (44,217 visits)
- Heroin (43,110 visits)

While alcohol use is illegal for individuals under age 21, DAWN estimates that in 2009 there were 199,429 alcohol-related ED visits among individuals under age 21; 76,918 ED visits were reported among those aged 12 to 17, and 120,853 alcohol-related ED visits were reported among those aged 18 to 20.

Nonmedical Use of Pharmaceuticals

In 2009, 1.2 million ED visits involved the nonmedical use of pharmaceuticals or dietary supplements. The most frequently reported drugs in the nonmedical use category of ED visits were opiate/opioid analgesics, present in 50% of nonmedical-use ED visits; and psychotherapeutic agents (commonly used to treat anxiety and sleep disorders), present in more than one-third of nonmedical ED visits. Included among the most frequently reported opioids were single-ingredient formulations (e.g., oxycodone) and combination forms (e.g., hydrocodone with acetaminophen). Methadone, together with single-ingredient and combination forms of oxycodone and hydrocodone, was also included under the most frequently reported opioids classification:

- Hydrocodone (alone or in combination) in 104,490 ED visits
- Oxycodone (alone or in combination) in 175,949 ED visits
- Methadone in 70,637 ED visits

Increases in Drug-Related ED Visits Over Time

The total number of drug-related ED visits increased 81% from 2004 (2.5 million) to 2009 (4.6 million). ED visits involving nonmedical use of pharmaceuticals increased 98.4% over the same period, from 627,291 visits to 1,244,679.

The largest pharmaceutical increases were observed for oxycodone products (242.2% increase), alprazolam (148.3% increase), and hydrocodone products (124.5%). Among ED visits involving illicit drugs, only those involving ecstasy increased more than 100% from 2004 to 2009 (123.2% increase).

For patients aged 20 or younger, ED visits resulting from nonmedical use of pharmaceuticals increased 45.4% between 2004 and 2009 (116,644 and 169,589 visits, respectively). Among patients aged 21 or older, there was an increase of 111.0%.

ED visits involving adverse reactions to pharmaceuticals increased 82.9% between 2005 and 2009, from 1,250,377 visits to 2,287,273. The majority of adverse reaction visits were made by patients 21 or older, particularly among patients 65 or older; the rate increased 89.2% from 2005 to 2009 among this age group.

Section 3.3

Increase in Emergency Room Visits Related to Ecstasy

"Emergency Department Visits Related to 'Ecstasy' Use Increased Nearly 75 Percent from 2004 to 2008," Substance Abuse and Mental Health Services Administration (www.samhsa.gov), March 24, 2011.

A new national study indicates that the number of hospital emergency visits involving the illicit drug ecstasy increased from 10,220 in 2004 to 17,865 visits in 2008—a 74.8% increase. According to this new study by SAMHSA most of these ecstasy-related visits (69.3%) involved patients aged 18 to 29, but notably 17.9% involved adolescents aged 12 to 17.

Ecstasy use can produce psychedelic and stimulant side effects such as anxiety attacks, tachycardia, hypertension, and hyperthermia. The variety and severity of adverse reactions associated with ecstasy use can increase when the drug is used in combination with other substances of abuse—a common occurrence among ecstasy users.

This SAMHSA study indicates that 77.8% of the emergency department visits involving ecstasy use also involve the use of at least one or more other substances of abuse. Among ecstasy-related emergency department cases involving patients aged 21 or older, 39.7% of the patients had used ecstasy with three or more other substances of abuse.

"The resurgence of ecstasy use is cause for alarm that demands immediate attention and action," said SAMHSA administrator Pamela S. Hyde, J.D. "The aggressive prevention efforts being put into place by SAMHSA will help reduce use in states and communities, resulting in less costly emergency department visits related to drug use."

This section is based on data from SAMHSA's 2004–2008 DAWN reports. A copy of the report is accessible at oas.samhsa.gov/2k11/dawn027/ecstasy.cfm.

Section 3.4

Deaths from Drug Overdoses

Excerpted from "Drug Poisoning Deaths in the United States, 1980–2008," National Center for Health Statistics, Centers for Disease Control and Prevention (www.cdc.gov/nchs), December 2011, and "Unintentional Drug Poisoning in the United States," Centers for Disease Control and Prevention (www.cdc.gov), July 2010.

Drug Poisoning Deaths in the United States, 1980–2008

In 2008, over 41,000 people died as a result of a poisoning. One of the Healthy People 2020 objectives is to reduce fatal poisonings in the United States. However, poisoning mortality increased during the Healthy People 2010 tracking period. Drugs—both legal and illegal—cause the vast majority of poisoning deaths. Misuse or abuse of prescription drugs, including opioid analgesic pain relievers, is responsible for much of the increase in drug poisoning deaths.

Poisoning is now the leading cause of death from injuries in the United States, and nearly 9 out of 10 poisoning deaths are caused by drugs. In 2008, the number of poisoning deaths exceeded the number of motor vehicle traffic deaths for the first time since at least 1980. In 2008, there were more than 41,000 poisoning deaths, compared with about 38,000 motor vehicle traffic deaths. In 2008, 89% of poisoning deaths were caused by drugs. During the past three decades, the poisoning death rate per 100,000 population nearly tripled from 4.8 in 1980 to 13.5 in 2008, while the motor vehicle traffic death rate decreased by almost one-half from 22.9 in 1980 to 12.5 in 2008. In the most recent decade, from 1999 to 2008, the poisoning death rate increased 90%, while the motor vehicle traffic death rate decreased 15%. From 1980 to 2008, the percentage of poisoning deaths caused by drugs increased from 56% to 89%. In 2008, about 77% of the drug poisoning deaths were unintentional, 13% were suicides, and 9% were of undetermined intent.

Poisoning is the leading cause of death from injury in 30 states. In 2008, age-adjusted poisoning death rates varied by state,

23

ranging from 7.6 to 30.8 per 100,000 population. In 20 states, the age-adjusted poisoning death rate was significantly higher than the U.S. rate of 13.4 deaths per 100,000 population. The five states with the highest poisoning death rates were New Mexico (30.8), West Virginia (27.6), Alaska (24.2), Nevada (21.0), and Utah (20.8). In 43 states over 80% of poisoning deaths were caused by drugs.

Opioid analgesics were involved in more than 40% of drug poisoning deaths in 2008. Of the 36,500 drug poisoning deaths in 2008, more than 40% (14,800) involved opioid analgesics. For about one-third (12,400) of the drug poisoning deaths, the type of drug(s) involved was specified on the death certificate but was not an opioid analgesic. The remaining 25% involved drugs, but the type of drugs involved was not specified on the death certificate (for example, "drug overdose" or "multiple drug intoxication" was written on the death certificate).

From 1999 to 2008, the number of drug poisoning deaths involving opioid analgesics increased from about 4,000 to 14,800, more rapidly than deaths involving only other types of drugs or only nonspecified drugs. From 1999 to 2008, the number of drug poisoning deaths involving only nonspecified drugs increased from about 3,600 to about 9,200. Some drug poisoning deaths for which the drug was not specified may involve opioid analgesics.

Natural and semi-synthetic opioid analgesics such as morphine, hydrocodone, and oxycodone were involved in over 9,100 drug poisoning deaths in 2008, up from about 2,700 in 1999. Of the 14,800 drug poisoning deaths involving opioid analgesics in 2008, the majority involved natural and semi-synthetic opioid analgesics such as morphine, hydrocodone, and oxycodone. The number of drug poisoning deaths involving natural and semi-synthetic opioid analgesics increased steadily each year from about 2,700 deaths in 1999 to over 9,100 deaths in 2008. The number of drug poisoning deaths involving methadone, which is a synthetic opioid analgesic used to treat opioid dependency as well as pain, increased sevenfold from about 800 deaths in 1999 to about 5,500 in 2007. Between 2007 and 2008, the number of deaths involving methadone decreased by nearly 600 deaths, the first decrease since 1999.

The number of drug poisoning deaths involving synthetic opioid analgesics other than methadone, such as fentanyl, tripled from about 700 in 1999 to 2,300 in 2008.

In 2008, the drug poisoning death rate was higher among those aged 45–54 years than among those in other age groups.

From 1999 to 2008, the drug poisoning death rate increased among all age groups. In 2004, the drug poisoning death rate among those aged 45–54 years surpassed the rate among those aged 35–44 years and became the age group with the highest drug poisoning death rate.

From 1999 to 2008, the age-adjusted drug poisoning death rate increased for males and females and for all race and ethnicity groups. In 2008, the rate was higher for males than for females, and higher for non-Hispanic American Indian or Alaska Native and non-Hispanic white persons than for those in other race and ethnicity groups.

Unintentional Drug Poisoning in the United States

Men and middle-aged people are more likely to die from drug overdose.

- In 2007, 18,029 drug overdose deaths occurred among males and 9,626 among females. Male rates exceeded female rates in almost every age group. Men have historically had higher rates of substance abuse than women.

- Male rates have doubled and female rates have tripled since 1999.

- For both sexes, the highest rates were in the 45–54 years old age group. Rates declined dramatically after the age of 54.

- After age 64, the male and female rates become comparable, probably as a result of the reduction in rates of substance abuse with age.

Among emergency department visits for the misuse or abuse of drugs, legal drugs have caught up with illegal drugs.

- The Drug Abuse Warning Network estimates ED visits caused by illicit drugs or the nonmedical use of legal drugs, which includes taking more than the prescribed amount, taking drugs prescribed for someone else, or substance abuse. Nonmedical use by this definition does not include use of drugs to harm oneself— e.g., suicide attempts or unintentional ingestions.

- In 2008, DAWN estimates show that prescription or over-the-counter drugs used nonmedically were involved in 1.0 million ED visits, and illicit drugs were involved in 1.0 million visits. Among the legal drugs, the most common drug categories involved were drugs acting on the central nervous system, especially opioid painkillers, and psychotherapeutic drugs, especially sedatives and antidepressants. Opioid painkillers were associated with approximately 306,000 visits and benzodiazepines (a type of sedative) with 272,000 visits.

- Among illicit drugs, cocaine was involved in 482,000 visits, and heroin was involved in 201,000 visits.

- People who abuse opioids have direct health care costs more than eight times those of nonabusers. A conservative estimate of the costs to society of prescription opioid abuse in the United States was $8.6 billion in 2001 ($9.5 billion in 2005 dollars).

Chapter 4

Understanding the Legal Use of Controlled Substances

Chapter Contents

Section 4.1

Schedule Classifications for Controlled Substances

"Drug Scheduling," Drug Enforcement Administration,
U.S. Department of Justice (www.justice.gov/dea), 2012.

Drugs, substances, and certain chemicals used to make drugs are classified into five distinct categories or schedules depending upon the drug's acceptable medical use and the drug's abuse or dependency potential. The abuse rate is a determinate factor in the scheduling of the drug; for example, schedule I drugs are considered the most dangerous class of drugs with a high potential for abuse and potentially severe psychological and/or physical dependence. As the drug schedule changes—schedule II, schedule III, etc.—so does the abuse potential; schedule V drugs represents the least potential for abuse. Listings of drugs and their schedule describe the basic or parent chemical and do not necessarily describe the salts, isomers and salts of isomers, esters, ethers, and derivatives that may also be classified as controlled substances.

Please note that a substance need not be listed as a controlled substance to be treated as a schedule I substance for criminal prosecution. A controlled substance analogue is a substance that is intended for human consumption and is structurally or pharmacologically substantially similar to or is represented as being similar to a schedule I or schedule II substance and is not an approved medication in the United States. (See 21 U.S.C. §802(32)(A) for the definition of a controlled substance analogue and 21 U.S.C. §813 for the schedule.)

Schedule I

Schedule I drugs, substances, or chemicals are defined as drugs with no currently accepted medical use and a high potential for abuse. Schedule I drugs are the most dangerous drugs of all the drug schedules with potentially severe psychological or physical dependence. Some examples of schedule I drugs are heroin, lysergic acid diethylamide (LSD), marijuana (cannabis), 3,4-methylenedioxymethamphetamine (ecstasy), methaqualone, and peyote.

Schedule II

Schedule II drugs, substances, or chemicals are defined as drugs with a high potential for abuse, less abuse potential than schedule I drugs, with use potentially leading to severe psychological or physical dependence. These drugs are also considered dangerous. Some examples of schedule II drugs are cocaine, methamphetamine, methadone, hydromorphone (Dilaudid), meperidine (Demerol), oxycodone (OxyContin), fentanyl, Dexedrine, Adderall, and Ritalin.

Schedule III

Schedule III drugs, substances, or chemicals are defined as drugs with a moderate to low potential for physical and psychological dependence. Schedule III drugs' abuse potential is less than schedule I and schedule II drugs but more than schedule IV. Some examples of schedule III drugs are combination products with less than 15 milligrams of hydrocodone per dosage unit (Vicodin), products containing less than 90 milligrams of codeine per dosage unit (Tylenol with codeine), ketamine, anabolic steroids, and testosterone.

Schedule IV

Schedule IV drugs, substances, or chemicals are defined as drugs with a low potential for abuse and low risk of dependence. Some examples of schedule IV drugs are Xanax, Soma, Darvon, Darvocet, Valium, Activan, Talwin, and Ambien.

Schedule V

Schedule V drugs, substances, or chemicals are defined as drugs with lower potential for abuse than schedule IV and consist of preparations containing limited quantities of certain narcotics. Schedule V drugs are generally used for antidiarrheal, antitussive, and analgesic purposes. Some examples of schedule V drugs are cough preparations with less than 200 milligrams of codeine or per 100 milliliters (Robitussin AC), Lomotil, Motofen, Lyrica, and Parepectolin.

Section 4.2

Prescriptions for Controlled Substances

"Questions & Answers: Prescriptions," Office of Diversion Control,
Drug Enforcement Administration, U.S. Department of Justice
(www.deadiversion.usdoj.gov), 2012.

What is a prescription?

A prescription is an order for medication that is dispensed to or for
an ultimate user. A prescription is not an order for medication that is
dispensed for immediate administration to the ultimate user (e.g., an
order to dispense a drug to an inpatient for immediate administration
in a hospital is not a prescription). To be valid, a prescription for a
controlled substance must be issued for a legitimate medical purpose
by a registered practitioner acting in the usual course of sound professional practice.

What information is required on a prescription for a controlled substance?

A prescription for a controlled substance must include the following information:

- Date of issue
- Patient's name and address
- Practitioner's name, address, and Drug Enforcement Administration (DEA) registration number
- Drug name
- Drug strength
- Dosage form
- Quantity prescribed
- Directions for use
- Number of refills (if any) authorized
- Manual signature of prescriber

A prescription must be written in ink or indelible pencil or typewritten and must be manually signed by the practitioner. An individual may be designated by the practitioner to prepare the prescriptions for his/her signature. The practitioner is responsible for making sure that the prescription conforms in all essential respects to the law and regulation.

Prescriptions for schedule II controlled substances must be written and be signed by the practitioner. In emergency situations, a prescription for a schedule II controlled substance may be telephoned to the pharmacy and the prescriber must follow up with a written prescription being sent to the pharmacy within seven days. Prescriptions for schedules III through V controlled substances may by written, oral, or transmitted by fax.

Can controlled substance prescriptions be refilled?

Prescriptions for schedule II controlled substances cannot be refilled. A new prescription must be issued. Prescriptions for schedules III and IV controlled substances may be refilled up to five times in six months. Prescriptions for schedule V controlled substances may be refilled as authorized by the practitioner.

Is it permissible to dispense a prescription for a quantity less than the face amount prescribed resulting in a greater number of dispensations than the number of refills indicated on the prescription?

Yes. Partial refills of schedules III and IV controlled substance prescriptions are permissible under federal regulations provided that each partial filling is dispensed and recorded in the same manner as a refilling (i.e., date refilled, amount dispensed, initials of dispensing pharmacist, etc.), the total quantity dispensed in all partial fillings does not exceed the total quantity prescribed, and no dispensing occurs after six months past the date of issue.

What changes may a pharmacist make to a prescription written for a controlled substance in schedule II?

On November 19, 2007, the DEA published in the Federal Register (FR) the Final Rule entitled *Issuance of Multiple Prescriptions for Schedule II Controlled Substances* (72 FR 64921). In the preamble to that Rule, DEA stated that "the essential elements of the [schedule II] prescription written by the practitioner (such as the name of the controlled substance, strength, dosage form, and quantity prescribed) ... may not be modified orally."

The instructions contained in the rule's preamble are in opposition to DEA's previous policy, which permitted the same changes a pharmacist may make to schedules III–V controlled substance prescriptions after oral consultation with the prescriber. DEA recognizes the resultant confusion regarding this conflict and plans to resolve this matter through a future rulemaking. Until that time, pharmacists are instructed to adhere to state regulations or policy regarding those changes that a pharmacist may make to a schedule II prescription after oral consultation with the prescriber.

Therefore, when information is missing from or needs to be changed on a schedule II controlled substance prescription, DEA expects pharmacists to use their professional judgment and knowledge of state and federal laws and policies to decide whether it is appropriate to make changes to that prescription.

What changes may a pharmacist make to a prescription written for a controlled substance in schedules III–V?

The pharmacist may add or change the patient's address upon verification. The pharmacist may add or change the dosage form, drug strength, drug quantity, directions for use, or issue date only after consultation with and agreement of the prescribing practitioner. Such consultations and corresponding changes should be noted by the pharmacist on the prescription. Pharmacists and practitioners must comply with any state/local laws, regulations, or policies prohibiting any of these changes to controlled substance prescriptions.

The pharmacist is never permitted to make changes to the patient's name, the controlled substance prescribed (except for generic substitution permitted by state law), or the prescriber's signature.

Can a practitioner prescribe methadone for the treatment of pain?

Federal law and regulations do not restrict the prescribing, dispensing, or administering of any schedule II, III, IV, or V narcotic medication, including methadone, for the treatment of pain, if such treatment is deemed medically necessary by a registered practitioner acting in the usual course of professional practice.

Confusion often arises due to regulatory restrictions concerning the use of methadone for the maintenance or detoxification of opioid-addicted individuals, in which case the practitioner is required to be registered with the DEA as a Narcotic Treatment Program (NTP).

Can an individual return his/her controlled substance prescription medication to a pharmacy?

No. An individual patient may not return his/her unused controlled substance prescription medication to the pharmacy. Federal laws and regulations make no provisions for an individual to return the controlled substance prescription medication to a pharmacy for further dispensing or for disposal. There are no provisions in the Controlled Substances Act or Code of Federal Regulations (CFR) for a DEA registrant (i.e., retail pharmacy) to acquire controlled substances from a nonregistrant (i.e., individual patient).

The CFR does have a provision for an individual to return his/her unused controlled substance medication to the pharmacy in the event of the controlled substance being recalled or a dispensing error having occurred.

An individual may dispose of his/her own controlled substance medication without approval from DEA. Medications should be disposed of in such a manner that does not allow for the controlled substances to be easily retrieved. In situations where an individual has expired, a caregiver or hospice staff member may assist the family with the proper disposal of any unused controlled substance medications.

Section 4.3

Purchasing Prescribed Controlled Substances over the Internet

Excerpted from: The National Center on Addiction and Substance Abuse at Columbia University (CASAColumbia™). (2008). *"You've got drugs!" V: Prescription drug pushers on the Internet.* New York: National Center on Addiction and Substance Abuse at Columbia University. © 2008. All rights reserved. Reviewed by David A. Cooke, MD, FACP, July 2013. Additional information from the U.S. Drug Enforcement Administration is cited separately within the section.

Prescription Drug Pushers on the Internet

In 2004, the National Center on Addiction and Substance Abuse (CASA) at Columbia University published its first report *You've Got Drugs! Prescription Drug Pushers on the Internet.* This report documented the widespread advertising and offers of sale for controlled prescription drugs—pain relievers like OxyContin and Percocet, depressants like Valium and Xanax, and stimulants like Ritalin and Adderall—online and without a prescription.

This report was inspired by early findings from CASA's study of the diversion and abuse of these drugs, published in 2005—*Under the Counter: The Diversion and Abuse of Controlled Prescription Drugs in the U.S.* Each year since 2004, CASA has replicated the analysis. Research for the 2004–2006 reports was contributed by Beau Dietl & Associates (BDA). This report is the fifth in the series.

Between 2004 and 2007, the number of Web sites identified that offer controlled prescription drugs for sale increased. This year, the number of such sites that CASA identified declined. It is possible that this decline is linked to growing efforts to reduce online access to controlled prescription drugs, but impossible to say with certainty. In spite of this decline, widespread availability continues and troubling facts remain in 2008:

- CASA identified a total of 365 Web sites either advertising or offering controlled prescription drugs for sale online; only two of those sites were registered Internet pharmacy practice sites.

- 85% of sites offering drugs for sale required no prescription from a patient's physician—the same as 2007 (84%).

- Of the 15% of sites offering drugs for sale that do indicate that a prescription is required, half simply ask that the prescription be faxed—increasing the risk of multiple use of one prescription or other fraud.

- There are no controls to block the sale of these drugs to children.

The Internet: A Pharmaceutical Candy Store

Today an estimated 200 million people in the U.S. are Internet users; 125 million access the World Wide Web at least weekly. While 63% of adults have access to the Internet, Internet users are disproportionately young, including nearly 100% of college students and 78% of 12- to 17-year-olds. The fact that children, teens, and college students are likelier to be online than adults makes online access to controlled prescription drugs even more troubling.

Not surprisingly, online trafficking of controlled prescription drugs grew rapidly since the first Internet pharmacies began in 1999. With cash, wire transfer, or access to a credit card and the click of a mouse, the Internet has offered a convenient and private means of purchasing controlled prescription drugs—completely lacking in scrutiny from parents and other family members, and frequently hidden from law enforcement.

Prescription Drug Abuse

CASA's landmark 2005 report, *Under the Counter: The Diversion and Abuse of Controlled Prescription Drugs in the U.S.*, documented the enormous increase in the manufacture and distribution of controlled prescription drugs. Between 1992 and 2002, while the U.S. population increased 13%, prescriptions filled for controlled drugs increased 154%. With increased availability has come increased abuse of these drugs.

The number of people who admit abusing controlled prescription drugs increased from 7.8 million in 1992 to 15.1 million in 2003—by 94%—seven times faster than the increase in the U.S. population. By 2006, 15.8 million people reported abusing controlled prescription drugs, more than the combined number who reported abusing cocaine (6.1 million), hallucinogens (4.0 million), inhalants (2.2 million), and heroin (0.5 million).

Children are especially at risk. In 2006, 2.2 million teens between the ages of 12 and 17 (8.5%) admitted abusing a prescription drug in the past year. A 2005 survey of teens found that nearly one in five (19% or 4.5

million) admit abusing prescription drugs in their lifetime. More teens have abused these drugs than many illegal drugs, including Ecstasy, cocaine, crack, and methamphetamine. More than half (56%) believe that prescription drugs are easier to obtain than illicit drugs and 52% believe that prescription pain relievers are "available everywhere."

The Regulatory Framework

Online pharmaceutical sales by state licensed, legitimate, and reputable Internet pharmacies can provide significant benefits to consumers. Legitimate online pharmacies operate much like traditional drugstores where drugs are dispensed only on receipt by the pharmacy of a valid prescription from the consumer or directly from the consumer's physician. But many pharmacies, so-called rogue pharmacies, do not obey the laws.

According to federal law outlined in the Controlled Substances Act (CSA), "it shall be unlawful for any person knowingly or intentionally to possess a controlled substance unless such substance was obtained directly, or pursuant to a valid prescription or order, from a practitioner, while acting in the course of his professional practice ..."

Federal regulation further states, "a prescription for a controlled substance to be effective must be issued for a legitimate medical purpose by an individual practitioner acting in the usual course of his professional practice." Under the law, the Drug Enforcement Administration (DEA) indicates that "for a doctor to be acting in the usual course of professional practice, there must be a bona fide doctor-patient relationship. For purposes of state law, many state authorities, with the endorsement of medical societies, consider the existence of the following four elements as an indication that a legitimate doctor-patient relationship has been established:

1. A patient has a medical complaint;

2. A medical history has been taken;

3. A physical examination has been performed; and,

4. Some logical connection exists between the medical complaint, the medical history, the physical examination and the drug prescribed."

Illegal Internet pharmacies have introduced a new avenue through which unscrupulous buyers and users can purchase controlled substances for unlawful purposes. These pharmacies—based both inside and outside the U.S.—sell a variety of prescription medications including controlled drugs.

Online Consultations

Many Internet pharmacies offer controlled drugs by advertising that no prescription is needed. Others dispense them after a patient completes an online questionnaire that may or may not be reviewed by a physician or a "script doctor" whose job is to write hundreds of prescriptions a day without ever seeing a patient. In any event, such sales do not constitute a legitimate doctor-patient relationship as described earlier.

The Federation of State Medical Boards of the United States, Inc., the American Medical Association, the National Association of Boards of Pharmacy, and the DEA all agree that online consultations cannot take the place of a face-to-face physical examination with a legitimate physician. For example, the Federation of State Medical Boards states that electronic technology "should supplement and enhance, but not replace, crucial interpersonal interactions that create the very basis of the physician-patient relationship."

In the case of online consultations, the consumer fills out an online questionnaire that is reportedly evaluated by a physician affiliated with the online pharmacy. Without ever meeting the patient face to face, allegedly a physician reviews the questionnaire and then authorizes the Internet pharmacy to send the drug to the patient.

Tens of thousands of "prescriptions" are written each year for controlled substances through such Internet pharmacies, which do not require medical records, examinations, lab tests, or follow-ups. The DEA reports that a maximum of about 11% of prescriptions filled by traditional (brick and mortar) pharmacies are for controlled substances. In contrast, 95% of prescriptions filled by Internet (cyber) pharmacies in 2006 were for controlled substances. One of the ways the DEA identifies rogue pharmacies is by their large percentage of prescriptions for controlled substances. The DEA reports that in response to detection and enforcement efforts, the percentage of prescriptions filled by cyber pharmacies for controlled substances dropped to 80% in 2007, and the number of such prescriptions fell significantly.

Some rogue Internet pharmacies provide online consultations free of charge; others refer customers to "script doctors" who are willing to write prescriptions for a fee. CASA's analysis identified fees ranging from $10 to $180. Some sites claim that a physician will contact the patient via telephone or e-mail. Others attempt to distance themselves from the consultation process by claiming that they merely are providing a referral service.

37

Verified Internet Pharmacy Practice Sites (VIPPS)

In an attempt to provide some assurance to consumers of legitimate online pharmacy practice sites, the National Association of Boards of Pharmacy established a process for certifying sites as legitimate. This process is known as becoming a Verified Internet Pharmacy Practice Site (VIPPS).

The VIPPS program "identifies to the public those online pharmacy practice sites that are appropriately licensed, are legitimately operating via the Internet, and that have completed successfully a rigorous criteria review and inspection." Certification is voluntary; fees range from $5,000 to $8,000 for initial certification and a minimum of $1,000 to $4,000 in yearly participation fees. There are currently 15 such sites.

Electronic Prescriptions and the Online Pharmacy Consumer Protection Act

The following excerpted from "Drugs of Abuse," U.S. Drug Enforcement Administration, U.S. Department of Justice (www.justice.gov/dea), 2011.

Electronic Prescriptions

On March 31, 2010, DEA published in the Federal Register the *Electronic Prescriptions for Controlled Substances* interim final rule which became effective June 1, 2010. The rule provides practitioners with the option of writing prescriptions for controlled substances electronically and also permits pharmacies to receive, dispense, and archive these electronic prescriptions.

Persons who wish to dispense controlled substances using electronic prescriptions must select software that meets the requirements of this rule. As of June 1, 2010, only those electronic applications that comply with all of DEA's requirements as set forth in 21 C.F.R. §1311 may be used to electronically create, transmit, receive/archive controlled substances prescriptions, and dispense controlled substances based on those prescriptions.

Ryan Haight Online Pharmacy Consumer Protection Act of 2008

On October 15, 2008, the president signed into law the Ryan Haight Online Pharmacy Consumer Protection Act of 2008, often referred to as the Ryan Haight Act. This law amends the CSA by adding a series of new regulatory requirements and criminal provisions designed to combat the proliferation of so-called "rogue Internet sites" that unlawfully dispense controlled substances by means of the Internet. The Ryan Haight Act applies to all controlled substances in all schedules. An online pharmacy is a person, entity, or Internet site, whether in the United States or abroad, that knowingly or intentionally delivers, distributes, or dispenses, or offers or attempts to deliver, distribute, or dispense, a controlled substance by means of the Internet.

This law became effective April 13, 2009. As of that date, it is illegal under federal law to deliver, distribute, or dispense a controlled substance by means of the Internet unless the online pharmacy holds a modification of DEA registration authorizing it to operate as an online pharmacy.

Section 4.4

Is Marijuana Medicine?

"DrugFacts: Is Marijuana Medicine?" National Institute on
Drug Abuse (www.drugabuse.gov), July 2012.

The use of marijuana to treat various medical conditions—or "medical marijuana"—is a controversial topic and has been for some time. Some people have argued that marijuana's reported beneficial effects on a variety of symptoms justify its legalization as a medicine for certain patients. Often the potential harm of marijuana use is not considered in these arguments, although risk is part of what the U.S. Food and Drug Administration (FDA) assesses when deciding whether to approve a medicine.

Under federal law, only FDA-approved medications are legal to prescribe—and marijuana is not one of those. Still, more than a dozen states have approved its use to alleviate a variety of symptoms.

What does marijuana do to the body?

Many of marijuana's effects (including its psychoactive or mind-altering properties) stem from an ingredient called delta-9-tetrahydrocannabinol (THC), which resembles a chemical that the body and brain make naturally. THC attaches to specialized proteins, called cannabinoid receptors (CBRs), to which the body's natural chemicals (e.g., anandamide) normally bind.

39

THC's chemical structure is similar to the brain chemical anandamide. Similarity in structure allows drugs to be recognized by the body and to alter normal brain communication. CBRs are part of a vast communication network known as the endocannabinoid system (ECS), which plays a role in normal brain development and function. They cluster in brain areas that influence pleasure, memory, thinking, concentration, movement, coordination, and sensory and time perception.

When someone smokes marijuana, THC stimulates the CBRs artificially, disrupting function of the natural cannabinoids. An overstimulation of these receptors in key brain areas produces the marijuana "high" as well as its other effects on mental processes.

Why isn't marijuana an FDA-approved medicine?

In fact, THC is an FDA-approved medication. It was shown in carefully controlled clinical trials to have therapeutic benefit for relieving nausea associated with cancer chemotherapy and stimulating appetite in patients with wasting syndrome (severe weight loss) that often accompanies AIDS.

However, the scientific evidence to date is not sufficient for the marijuana plant to gain FDA approval, and there are a number of reasons why:

First, there have not been enough clinical trials showing that marijuana's benefits outweigh its risks in patients with the symptoms it is meant to treat. The FDA requires carefully conducted studies in large numbers of patients (hundreds to thousands) to accurately assess the benefits and risks of a potential medication.

Second, to be considered a legitimate medicine, a substance must have well-defined and measureable ingredients that are consistent from one unit (such as a pill or injection) to the next. This consistency allows doctors to determine the dose and frequency.

Along with THC, the marijuana plant contains over 400 other chemical compounds, including other cannabinoids that may be biologically active and vary from plant to plant. This makes it difficult to consider its use as a medicine even though some of marijuana's specific ingredients may offer benefits.

Finally, marijuana has certain adverse health effects that also must be taken into account. Because it is usually smoked, marijuana can cause or worsen respiratory symptoms (e.g., bronchitis, chronic cough). It also impairs short-term memory and motor coordination; slows reaction time; alters mood, judgment, and decision making; and in some people can cause severe anxiety (paranoia) or psychosis (loss of touch with reality). And marijuana is addictive—about 4.5 million people in this country meet clinical criteria for marijuana abuse or dependence.

What's the difference between medical and "street" marijuana?

There is no difference between "medical-grade" marijuana and "street" marijuana. The marijuana sold in dispensaries as medicine is the same quality and carries the same health risks as marijuana sold on the street.

Section 4.5

Overview of the Medical Marijuana Debate

As efforts to make marijuana legal for medicinal use gain momentum, psychologists are studying the effects of the nation's most popular illicit drug—and several are sounding notes of caution.

As researchers, psychologists are exploring the risks of dependence, developing more effective interventions for marijuana users who want to quit, studying withdrawal, and evaluating medicinal uses of marijuana's main active chemical, delta-9-tetrahydrocannabinol (THC).

That research is more relevant than ever: 14 states have already legalized marijuana for medical purposes, with voters in 9 of those states approving medical marijuana by ballot initiative. A dozen more states are considering legislation this year [2010] to make marijuana available for medical use.

In California, the epicenter of what some describe as de facto legalization, voters will decide in November [2010] on whether marijuana's recreational use should be legalized, taxed, and regulated.

Meanwhile, public opinion polls continue to show growing acceptance for legalizing marijuana for personal use. An October Gallup poll found that 44% of adults favored legalizing marijuana, a group that's grown between 1% and 2% every year since 2000. In six Western states, most poll respondents favored outright legalization.

Support for medicinal uses for marijuana is even stronger: According to a January ABC News/Washington Post poll, 81% of Americans would allow physicians to prescribe marijuana for their patients, up from 69% in 1997.

But as the nation debates legalization, the public should know that about 10% of users go on to develop marijuana dependence, says Barbara Mason, PhD, co-director of the Pearson Center for Alcoholism and Addiction Research at the Scripps Research Institute in San Diego.

"90% of individuals will be able to use it in a way they find nonproblematic in terms of dependence but 10% will run the risk of developing dependence, and for that, effective treatments should be available," says Mason, the principal investigator for a National Institute on Drug Abuse [NIDA]–funded study of the neurobiological effects of marijuana use.

A secondary analysis of the 2005 National Survey on Drug Use and Health found that among people who had used heroin in the past year, 45.4% met the criteria for dependence. Among those who had smoked cigarettes in the past year, 35.3% were dependent on nicotine, and 20.4% of past-year cocaine users were dependent. The analysis, included in Chapter 22 of "Psychiatry Third Edition, Volume 1" (Wiley, 2008), found that 9.7% of people who used cannabis met criteria for dependence. Among past-year alcohol users, 4.9% met criteria for dependence.

While the percentage of American users who become dependent on marijuana wouldn't change after legalization, the absolute numbers probably would, says Columbia University neuroscience professor and marijuana researcher Margaret Haney, PhD. "Clearly, the more available something is, the more likely people will try it, and therefore a higher number will go on to develop problems with it," she says.

But some addiction researchers, including renowned researcher G. Alan Marlatt, PhD, aren't troubled by the trend toward legalization. In his view, many marijuana users who want to quit or cut back avoid treatment for fear of criminal repercussions.

"If it's decriminalized … that's going to open the door for more people to seek help," says Marlatt, who directs the University of Washington's Addictive Behaviors Research Center.

As society moves toward greater acceptance of marijuana, psychologists should make sure their research results are available to people who are considering using it, particularly adolescents and young adults, says Mason. They also need to develop more effective interventions for dependent users who want to stop.

"When an individual makes that decision that they want to quit, I want to meet them with the best possible strategy," she says.

Use and Abuse on the Rise

About 6% of Americans age 12 and older have used marijuana in the past month, according to the Substance Abuse and Mental Health Services Administration (SAMHSA)'s 2008 National Survey on Drug Use and Health—a trend that's held steady for the last seven years. However, the National Institute on Drug Abuse "Monitoring the Future" survey found that past-month marijuana use among high school seniors edged slightly upward over the past three years to 20.6% in 2009, reversing a decade-long downward trend. Although it's a concerning trend, it's a far cry from the peak of 37% in 1978. NIDA officials think use might continue to increase given the increasing percentage of high school seniors surveyed who don't view regular marijuana use as risky.

Marijuana use is, however, risky for some: About 4.2 million people are dependent on or abuse marijuana, almost twice the number of prescription drug abusers and three times the number of cocaine abusers, says Joseph Gfroerer, director of SAMHSA's Division of Population Surveys.

Complicating the picture is the fact that marijuana's main psychoactive component, THC, has FDA-approved medicinal uses in a nonsmoked form. People being treated for HIV smoke marijuana to deal with the nausea, anorexia, stomach upset, and anxiety associated with the disease and antiretroviral therapy. Cancer patients smoke it to relieve the side effects of chemotherapy. By relieving nausea and boosting appetite, marijuana can help patients in both groups avoid severe weight loss.

New research has found more potential uses for the drug. Five clinical trials funded by the University of California's Center for Medicinal Cannabis Research revealed that marijuana significantly decreases neuropathic pain—notoriously difficult-to-treat chronic discomfort, which can result from injuries, side effects of anti-HIV drugs, and diabetes, says Igor Grant, MD, executive vice chair of the department of psychiatry at the University of California, San Diego, School of Medicine.

One study funded by the center and published in the April 2008 *Journal of Pain* (Vol. 9, No. 6) found that both low-dose cannabis cigarettes (3.5% THC) and high-dose (7% THC) effectively reduced neuropathic pain from a variety of causes. According to NIDA, the average THC content of marijuana confiscated from the U.S. market was about 10% last year.

Two clinical trials examining the analgesic effects of THC on neuropathic pain will be completed by 2011, Grant says.

Overall, several of the studies showed that smoked marijuana reduced patient pain by more than 30%. That finding is important because in pain research, reducing pain by at least 30% is associated with "meaningful improvement in quality of life" for people dealing with chronic pain, according to a report Grant presented to the California Legislature in January.

Nationwide, 5% to 10% of Americans suffer some form of neuropathic pain, says Grant, so millions of people need more relief than they're currently receiving. "This pain doesn't respond as well to traditional pain medication, the opioid-type drugs, so what our studies showed is that cannabis has benefits with this kind of pain over and above the standard treatments patients were already receiving," says Grant.

Center-sponsored research also found that cannabis side effects were mild, not any worse than with other medications, and that they ceased once a participant stopped using marijuana. A separate, as-yet-unpublished study funded by the University of California center found that cannabis reduced muscle spasticity and pain intensity in people with multiple sclerosis beyond the relief available through conventional medication, Grant says.

Investigating Medical Benefits without Smoking

For all of the debate over the legalization of marijuana and the drug's possible medicinal uses, not enough is being done to study the possible benefits of the drug in its nonsmoked forms, says Haney.

In her research, Haney led a study comparing the relief offered by smoked marijuana with dronabinol, an oral form of THC, an FDA-approved treatment for nausea and disease-related weight loss.

In the study, a group of HIV patients who regularly smoked marijuana were given different concentrations of oral THC and smoked marijuana, or a placebo form of either drug. The researchers evaluated the effects THC had on diet, mood, cognitive performance, and sleep.

Her volunteers were all taking at least two antiretroviral medications, and a physician was managing their HIV.

When taken at doses eight times stronger than the current recommended dose, dronabinol achieved the same effects as smoked marijuana, Haney says. Participants ate more often, gained an average of almost one pound in four days, and experienced less anxiety on both forms of the drug as compared with a placebo, according to results published in the August 2007 *Journal of Acquired Immune Deficiency Syndrome* (Vol. 45, No. 5).

"What we found is that both oral THC and smoked marijuana work very nicely, they both increased appetite, and both were very well tolerated and had few side effects," she says. The results suggest that oral forms of THC, and a new form of delivery through a botanically derived oral spray called Sativex that combines cannabidiol and THC, may have many as-yet-unexplored medicinal uses, Haney says.

In her view, the state-by-state drive to legalize medical marijuana and promote its smoked form as the first choice for medical needs has diverted attention from finding better ways to use synthetic THC and nonsmoked marijuana—delivery methods that don't expose a patient to the harmful effects of smoking.

"From a scientist's perspective, it's been very frustrating that there hasn't been more science behind these [legalization] policies ... There's an awful lot of anecdote driving these policy changes," she says.

Living Dependent

For all of marijuana's possible medical benefits, it's an addictive drug for some people who try it, researchers say. Mason is looking at whether a nonaddictive, neuromodulating medication called gabapentin, prescribed for epilepsy and for some forms of neuropathic pain, can help people get through the initial withdrawal and avoid relapse. Results so far are promising, with less marijuana use and decreased withdrawal severity among a pilot study of 25 daily marijuana users, compared with 25 who received a placebo, she says. Both groups received behavioral therapy during treatment, but the users who took gabapentin had less severe withdrawal symptoms and were more successful at avoiding relapse longer. That's important because finding a way to ease withdrawal symptoms and decrease relapse, while starting behavioral therapy, could boost the percentage of people staying abstinent long-term, Mason says.

"There are a lot of individuals, perhaps leading lives of quiet desperation, who are really engaged in the marijuana culture and can't find their way out of it," Mason says.

A second study, with 150 participants given either gabapentin or a placebo, is now under way, she says.

Meanwhile, psychologists have also studied the life experiences of long-term, heavy marijuana users compared with people who briefly smoked marijuana—less than 50 times in adolescence and early adulthood. A case-control study of 108 long-term heavy cannabis users published in 2003 in *Psychological Medicine* (Vol. 33, No. 8) found that when compared with people who smoked marijuana briefly, matched by age and similar family backgrounds, heavy users reported lower income and lower educational achievement.

Heavy users—who reported smoking marijuana an average of 18,000 times in their lives—also rated their own quality of life much more negatively than study participants who used marijuana for only a short period of time and stopped. They had lower ratings across 10 measures, including quality of diet, overall satisfaction with self and life, and general happiness.

For users who become dependent, stopping brings a constellation of withdrawal symptoms that may lead to relapse, says Alan Budney, PhD, of the Center for Addiction Research at the University of Arkansas College of Medicine.

"In controlled outpatient studies, we observe increased irritability and anger," says Budney. "We observe sleep difficulties, and many [people] start to report strange or unusual dreaming. Restlessness, nervousness, and decreased appetite are also frequently reported."

Inpatient withdrawal research by Haney supports Budney's observations. Haney's team has regular users smoke marijuana under controlled conditions. When they're switched to marijuana free of THC, they experience irritability, restlessness, anxiety, sleep disturbances, and changes in appetite, with food intake dropping by as much as 1,000 calories a day.

Those effects were reversed when oral THC was administered or marijuana smoking was resumed, demonstrating the pharmacologic specificity of THC, according to a study published in 2004 in *Neuropsychopharmacology* (Vol. 29, No. 1).

"Once you do become dependent, it's difficult to stop," Haney says. "People who are seeking treatment relapse at rates as high as they are for cocaine, heroin, and alcohol."

Treating marijuana dependence is especially difficult when users don't believe they have a problem, says Gregory Brigham, PhD, a clinical psychologist at Maryhaven, a substance abuse and mental health treatment center in Columbus, Ohio.

Marijuana users often see it as fun and a key ingredient to an entire subculture, Brigham says. "With the relatively mild intoxication they experience, they're not alarmed by the consequences of being under the influence. It's difficult for them to make a connection between the problems in their life and the use of marijuana, and that's different from other drugs," he says.

Helping Users Quit

Despite these challenges, psychologists and other researchers have found that three types of interventions help people quit marijuana.

According to a 2007 study in *Addictive Behaviors* (Vol. 32, No. 6), when used together, these three interventions can result in an abstinence rate of about 27%, as measured at 14 months from treatment:

Motivational enhancement therapy: This approach uses motivational interviewing to get a person to consider the rewards and drawbacks of marijuana use. It focuses on helping clients acknowledge how marijuana use has affected their work, school, and family life. The goal is to help users see how marijuana use might conflict with their goals—such as completing college or applying for a job that requires drug testing. That realization helps many clients develop motivation to change.

Cognitive behavioral therapy: Following one to four sessions of motivational interviewing, if a client decides to quit, a therapist can help him or her develop skills to stay marijuana-free. For example, clients role-play situations where friends offer them marijuana. In a typical scenario, a friend invites them to get high. Combining a firm "no" with an explanation of "I'm not smoking pot anymore," the client proposes an alternative activity that doesn't involve smoking pot. The therapy includes relaxation techniques for falling asleep without using marijuana, as well as steps to alleviate depressed moods.

Contingency management: Adapted from techniques developed for people who abuse cocaine and other drugs, this intervention sets a client on a schedule of earning vouchers with a predetermined cash value that escalates in value, if urinalysis indicates abstinence, during a 14-week monitoring period. Contingency management provides a structure to abstain from marijuana through urine monitoring and, through the vouchers, an incentive to stay abstinent. One 2006 study found that combining an abstinence-based voucher program with cognitive behavioral therapy resulted in 37% abstinence at one year (*Journal of Consulting and Clinical Psychology*, Vol. 74, No. 2).

Looking to the future, even better interventions may come from boosting people's feelings of self-efficacy, says researcher Ronald Kadden, PhD, of the University of Connecticut Health Center. Previous research has found that marijuana users who reported significant improvements in feelings of self-efficacy while using coping skills learned to curtail cravings for marijuana stayed abstinent longer, says Kadden. To capitalize on this finding, Kadden is leading a NIDA-funded study to boost marijuana-dependent participants' self-efficacy using a more intense regimen of daily homework assignments.

"If we can enhance that in people, maybe we'll have better outcomes," he says.

Another area that needs further study is whether marijuana users whose cognitive abilities have been impaired by smoking large amounts daily can benefit from cognitive behavioral therapy delivered in shorter and more frequent sessions, says Karen Bolla, PhD, director of neuropsychology at Johns Hopkins Bayview Medical Center in Baltimore.

The Potential Costs of Legalization

Kadden's experiences working with people who are dependent on marijuana convinces him that legalization isn't a wise course to follow.

"We've got alcohol, and we're stuck with it. We do marijuana, and it's going to be another Pandora's box," he says.

A psychologist with very strong opinions on whether legalization is a wise course is A. Thomas McLellan, PhD, deputy director for the White House Office of National Drug Control Policy. As McLellan sees it, making marijuana more available will lead to more use, and more use will lead to greater dependence.

"Are you willing to say, 'Let's expand use, let's add another intoxicant into the public'? I don't like the odds," he says.

While noting that the cannabinoids found within marijuana show medicinal promise and will eventually be developed as a new class of pain reliever, smoked marijuana is not the best way to deliver those medical benefits, he says.

"Put it this way: We've got record unemployment, two wars, we have a bank collapse, a housing catastrophe. Oh, I know, let's add marijuana, let's add another intoxicant—that ought to fix things," McLellan says.

Editor's Note: As of spring 2013, medical marijuana is legal in 18 states and the District of Columbia. In addition, possession of marijuana for medical and nonmedical purposes is now legal in Colorado and Washington.

Chapter 5

Regulations Regarding Controlled Substances

Chapter Contents

Section 5.1

The Controlled Substances Act

Excerpted from "Drugs of Abuse," Drug Enforcement Administration, U.S. Department of Justice (www.justice.gov/dea), 2011.

Controlling Drugs or Other Substances through Formal Scheduling

The Controlled Substances Act (CSA) places all substances that were in some manner regulated under existing federal law into one of five schedules. This placement is based upon the substance's medical use, potential for abuse, and safety or dependence liability. The act also provides a mechanism for substances to be controlled (added to or transferred between schedules) or decontrolled (removed from control). The procedure for these actions is found in Section 201 of the act (21 U.S.C. § 811).

Proceedings to add, delete, or change the schedule of a drug or other substance may be initiated by the Drug Enforcement Administration (DEA), the Department of Health and Human Services (HHS), or by petition from any interested party, including the following:

- The manufacturer of a drug

- A medical society or association

- A pharmacy association

- A public interest group concerned with drug abuse

- A state or local government agency

- An individual citizen

When a petition is received by the DEA, the agency begins its own investigation of the drug. The DEA also may begin an investigation of a drug at any time based upon information received from law enforcement laboratories, state and local law enforcement and regulatory agencies, or other sources of information.

Once the DEA has collected the necessary data, the DEA administrator, by authority of the attorney general, requests from HHS a scientific and medical evaluation and recommendation as to whether the drug or other substance should be controlled or removed from control. This request is sent to the assistant secretary for health of HHS.

The assistant secretary, by authority of the secretary, compiles the information and transmits back to the DEA a medical and scientific evaluation regarding the drug or other substance, a recommendation as to whether the drug should be controlled, and in what schedule it should be placed.

The medical and scientific evaluations are binding on the DEA with respect to scientific and medical matters and form a part of the scheduling decision.

Once the DEA has received the scientific and medical evaluation from HHS, the administrator will evaluate all available data and make a final decision whether to propose that a drug or other substance should be removed or controlled and into which schedule it should be placed.

If a drug does not have a potential for abuse, it cannot be controlled. Although the term "potential for abuse" is not defined in the CSA, there is much discussion of the term in the legislative history of the act. The following items are indicators that a drug or other substance has a potential for abuse:

1. There is evidence that individuals are taking the drug or other substance in amounts sufficient to create a hazard to their health or to the safety of other individuals or to the community.

2. There is significant diversion of the drug or other substance from legitimate drug channels.

3. Individuals are taking the drug or other substance on their own initiative rather than on the basis of medical advice from a practitioner.

4. The drug is a new drug so related in its action to a drug or other substance already listed as having a potential for abuse to make it likely that the drug will have the same potential for abuse as such drugs, thus making it reasonable to assume that there may be significant diversions from legitimate channels, significant use contrary to or without medical advice, or a substantial capability of creating hazards to the health of the user or to the safety of the community. Of course, evidence of actual abuse of a substance is indicative that a drug has a potential for abuse.

In determining into which schedule a drug or other substance should be placed, or whether a substance should be decontrolled or rescheduled, certain factors are required to be considered. These factors are listed in Section 201(c), [21 U.S.C. § 811(c)] of the CSA as follows:

1. **The drug's actual or relative potential for abuse**

2. **Scientific evidence of the drug's pharmacological effect, if known:** The state of knowledge with respect to the effects of a specific drug is, of course, a major consideration. For example, it is vital to know whether or not a drug has a hallucinogenic effect if it is to be controlled due to that effect.

   The best available knowledge of the pharmacological properties of a drug should be considered.

3. **The state of current scientific knowledge regarding the substance:** Criteria 2 and 3 are closely related. However, 2 is primarily concerned with pharmacological effects and 3 deals with all scientific knowledge with respect to the substance.

4. **Its history and current pattern of abuse:** To determine whether or not a drug should be controlled, it is important to know the pattern of abuse of that substance.

5. **The scope, duration, and significance of abuse:** In evaluating existing abuse, the DEA administrator must know not only the pattern of abuse, but whether the abuse is widespread.

6. **What, if any, risk there is to the public health:** If a drug creates dangers to the public health, in addition to or because of its abuse potential, then these dangers must also be considered by the administrator.

7. **The drug's psychic or physiological dependence liability:** There must be an assessment of the extent to which a drug is physically addictive or psychologically habit forming.

8. **Whether the substance is an immediate precursor of a substance already controlled:** The CSA allows inclusion of immediate precursors on this basis alone into the appropriate schedule and thus safeguards against possibilities of clandestine manufacture.

After considering these listed factors, the administrator must make specific findings concerning the drug or other substance. This will determine into which schedule the drug or other substance will be placed. These schedules are established by the CSA.

When the DEA administrator has determined that a drug or other substance should be controlled, decontrolled, or rescheduled, a proposal to take action is published in the Federal Register. The proposal invites all interested persons to file comments with the DEA and may also request a hearing with the DEA. If no hearing is requested, the DEA will evaluate all comments received and publish a final order in the Federal Register, controlling the drug as proposed or with modifications based upon the written comments filed. This order will set the effective dates for imposing the various requirements of the CSA.

If a hearing is requested, the DEA will enter into discussions with the party or parties requesting a hearing in an attempt to narrow the issue for litigation. If necessary, a hearing will then be held before an administrative law judge. The judge will take evidence on factual issues and hear arguments on legal questions regarding the control of the drug. Depending on the scope and complexity of the issues, the hearing may be brief or quite extensive. The administrative law judge, at the close of the hearing, prepares findings of fact and conclusions of law and a recommended decision that is submitted to the DEA administrator. The DEA administrator will review these documents, as well as the underlying material, and prepare his/her own findings of fact and conclusions of law (which may or may not be the same as those drafted by the administrative law judge). The DEA administrator then publishes a final order in the Federal Register either scheduling the drug or other substance or declining to do so.

Once the final order is published in the *Federal Register*, interested parties have 30 days to appeal to a U.S. Court of Appeals to challenge the order. Findings of fact by the administrator are deemed conclusive if supported by "substantial evidence." The order imposing controls is not stayed during the appeal, however, unless so ordered by the court.

Emergency or Temporary Scheduling

The CSA was amended by the Comprehensive Crime Control Act of 1984. This act included a provision that allows the DEA administrator to place a substance, on a temporary basis, into schedule I, when necessary, to avoid an imminent hazard to the public safety. This emergency scheduling authority permits the scheduling of a substance that is not currently controlled, is being abused, and is a risk to the public health while the formal rulemaking procedures described in the CSA are being conducted. This emergency scheduling applies only to substances with no accepted medical use.

A temporary scheduling order may be issued for one year with a possible extension of up to six months if formal scheduling procedures have been initiated. The notice of intent and order are published in the Federal Register, as are the proposals and orders for formal scheduling [21 U.S.C. § 811(h)].

Controlled Substance Analogues

A new class of substances was created by the Anti-Drug Abuse Act of 1986. Controlled substance analogues are substances that are not controlled substances, but may be found in illicit trafficking. They are structurally or pharmacologically similar to schedule I or II controlled substances and have no legitimate medical use. A substance that meets the definition of a controlled substance analogue and is intended for human consumption is treated under the CSA as if it were a controlled substance in schedule I [21 U.S.C. § 802(32), 21 U.S.C. § 813].

International Treaty Obligations

United States treaty obligations may require that a drug or other substance be controlled under the CSA, or rescheduled if existing controls are less stringent than those required by a treaty. The procedures for these scheduling actions are found in Section 201(d) of the act [21 U.S.C. § 811(d)].

The United States is a party to the Single Convention on Narcotic Drugs of 1961, which was designed to establish effective control over international and domestic traffic in narcotics, coca leaf, cocaine, and cannabis. A second treaty, the Convention on Psychotropic Substances of 1971, which entered into force in 1976 and was ratified by Congress in 1980, is designed to establish comparable control over stimulants, depressants, and hallucinogens.

Section 5.2

Combat Methamphetamine Epidemic Act

Excerpted from "Combat Methamphetamine Epidemic Act of 2005: Questions & Answers," Office of Diversion Control, Drug Enforcement Administration, U.S. Department of Justice (www.deadiversion.usdoj.gov), 2007, accessed March 2013. Despite its older publication date, the material in this section is considered accurate and relevant.

What is the Combat Methamphetamine Epidemic Act of 2005?

The Combat Methamphetamine Epidemic Act of 2005 (CMEA) was signed into law on March 9, 2006, to regulate, among other things, retail over-the-counter sales of ephedrine, pseudoephedrine, and phenylpropanolamine products. Retail provisions of the CMEA include daily sales limits and monthly purchase limits, placement of product out of direct customer access, sales logbooks, customer ID, employee training, and self-certification of regulated sellers. The CMEA is found as Title VII of the USA PATRIOT Improvement and Reauthorization Act of 2005 (Public Law 109-177).

Why was the CMEA passed?

Ephedrine, pseudoephedrine, and phenylpropanolamine are precursor chemicals used in the illicit manufacture of methamphetamine or amphetamine. They are also common ingredients used to make cough, cold, and allergy products. Methamphetamine laboratories have been found in homes, cars, hotel rooms, storage facilities—these are generally referred to as "small toxic labs." Passage of the CMEA was accomplished to curtail the illicit production of methamphetamine and amphetamine. States that have enacted similar or more restrictive retail regulations have seen a dramatic drop in small toxic labs.

What is methamphetamine?

Methamphetamine is a powerfully addictive drug that severely affects users' minds and bodies, ruins lives, and endangers communities and the environment. Chronic use can lead to extremely violent behavior, the neglect of a user's children, and an inability to cope with the ordinary demands of life. Unfortunately, methamphetamine is unique in that making it is easy but dangerous, posing the risk of explosion, exposing families, children, and neighborhoods to toxic chemicals.

Is methamphetamine production and abuse a nationwide problem?

Methamphetamine, or "meth," has become a tremendous challenge for the entire nation. A clandestine methamphetamine laboratory has been found in every state over the past five years. A July 18, 2006, National Association of Counties Survey found that meth is the leading drug-related local law enforcement problem in the country. The survey of 500 county law enforcement officials in 44 states found that meth continues to be the number one drug problem—more counties (48%) report that meth is the primary drug problem—more than cocaine (22%), marijuana (22%), and heroin (3%) combined. In addition, according to the survey, crimes related to meth continue to grow—55% of law enforcement officials report an increase in robberies or burglaries in the last year and 48% report an increase in domestic violence.

Does methamphetamine production have an impact on the environment?

Clandestine methamphetamine laboratories pose a significant danger in the community, as they contain highly flammable and explosive materials. Additionally, for each pound of methamphetamine produced, five to seven pounds of toxic waste remain, which is often introduced into the environment via streams, septic systems, and surface water run-off.

Do the Combat Meth Act and the implementing regulations preempt state laws?

State laws vary considerably. Some parts of a state law may be less stringent than the CMEA requirements; other parts may be more stringent. The CMEA does not preempt those requirements under state laws/regulations that are more stringent than the act's requirements. Simply put, all persons subject to the CMEA must comply with the act and the laws in the state(s) in which they sell scheduled listed chemical products at retail. Where the CMEA is less stringent than a state law (e.g., the state limits sales to licensed pharmacists or pharmacy technicians where the act does not), the state requirements continue to be in force. If there are state requirements that are less stringent than the CMEA provisions (e.g., exemptions of some products), the act supersedes the provisions.

Chapter 6

Substance Abuse Treatment Statistics

Chapter Contents

Section 6.1

Treatment Received for Substance Abuse

"DrugFacts: Treatment Statistics," National Institute on Drug Abuse (www.drugabuse.gov), March 2011, and excerpts from "Results from the 2011 National Survey on Drug Use and Health: Summary of National Findings," Substance Abuse and Mental Health Services Administration (www.samhsa.gov), September 2012.

Treatment Statistics

According to the Substance Abuse and Mental Health Services Administration (SAMHSA)'s National Survey on Drug Use and Health, 23.5 million persons aged 12 or older needed treatment for an illicit drug or alcohol abuse problem in 2009 (9.3% of persons aged 12 or older). Of these, only 2.6 million—11.2% of those who needed treatment—received it at a specialty facility.

SAMHSA also reports characteristics of admissions and discharges from substance abuse treatment facilities in its Treatment Episode Data Set (TEDS). According to TEDS, there were 1.8 million admissions in 2008 for treatment of alcohol and drug abuse to facilities that report to state administrative data systems. Most treatment admissions (41.4%) involved alcohol abuse. Heroin and other opiates accounted for the largest percentage of drug-related admissions (20.0%), followed by marijuana (17.0%).

Admissions to publicly funded substance abuse treatment programs are as follows:

- **Alcohol only:** 23.1%

- **Alcohol + another drug:** 18.3%

- **Marijuana:** 17.0%

- **Heroin:** 14.1%

- **Smoked cocaine (crack):** 8.1%

- **Stimulants:** 6.5% (Methamphetamine accounted for 6.1% of admissions, and the remaining 0.4% were categorized as "Other Amphetamine.")

- **Opiates (not heroin):** 5.9% (These drugs include codeine, hydrocodone, hydromorphone, meperidine, morphine, opium, oxycodone, pentazocine, propoxyphene, tramadol, and any other drug with morphine-like effects. Nonprescription use of methadone is not included.)

- **Nonsmoked cocaine (e.g., cocaine powder):** 3.2%

- **Tranquilizers:** 0.6%

- **PCP (phencyclidine):** 0.2%

- **Sedatives:** 0.2%

- **Hallucinogens:** 0.1%

- **Inhalants:** 0.1%

- **Other drugs:** 0.4%

- **None reported:** 2.2%

About 60% of admissions were white, 21% were African American, and 14% were Hispanic or Latino. Another 2.3% were American Indian or Alaska Native, and 1% were Asian/Pacific Islander.

The age range with the highest proportion of treatment admissions was the 25–29 group at 14.8%, followed by those 20–24 at 14.4% and those 40–44 at 12.6%.

Admissions to publicly funded substance abuse treatment programs are as follows:

- **14.8%:** 25–29

- **14.4%:** 20–24

- **12.6%:** 40–44

- **11.7%:** 35–39

- **11.5%:** 45–49

- **11.3%:** 30–34

- **10.4%:** 50–59

- **7.5%:** 12–17

- **4.1%:** 18–19

- **1.2%:** 60–64

- **0.6%:** 65 or older

Results from the 2011 National Survey on Drug Use and Health

Past-Year Treatment for a Substance Use Problem

Estimates described in this section refer to treatment received for illicit drug or alcohol use, or for medical problems associated with the use of illicit drugs or alcohol. This includes treatment received in the past year at any location, such as a hospital (inpatient), rehabilitation facility (outpatient or inpatient), mental health center, emergency room, private doctor's office, prison or jail, or a self-help group, such as Alcoholics Anonymous or Narcotics Anonymous.

Persons could report receiving treatment at more than one location. Note that the definition of treatment in this section is different from the definition of specialty treatment, which includes treatment only at a hospital (inpatient), a rehabilitation facility (inpatient or outpatient), or a mental health center.

Individuals who reported receiving substance use treatment but were missing information on whether the treatment was specifically for alcohol use or illicit drug use were not counted in estimates of either illicit drug use treatment or alcohol use treatment; however, they were counted in estimates for "drug or alcohol use" treatment.

- In 2011, 3.8 million persons aged 12 or older (1.5% of the population) received treatment for a problem related to the use of alcohol or illicit drugs. Of these, 1.2 million received treatment for the use of both alcohol and illicit drugs, 0.8 million received treatment for the use of illicit drugs but not alcohol, and 1.4 million received treatment for the use of alcohol but not illicit drugs. (Note that estimates by substance do not sum to the total number of persons receiving treatment because the total includes persons who reported receiving treatment but did not report for which substance the treatment was received.)

- The rate and the number of persons in the population aged 12 or older receiving substance use treatment within the past year was stable between 2010 (1.6% and 4.2 million) and 2011 (1.5% and 3.8 million) and between 2002 (1.5% and 3.5 million) and 2011.

- In 2011, among the 3.8 million persons aged 12 or older who received treatment for alcohol or illicit drug use in the past year, 2.1 million persons received treatment at a self-help group, and 1.5 million received treatment at a rehabilitation facility as an outpatient. There were 1.0 million persons who received treatment at a mental health center as an outpatient, 1.0 million persons who received treatment at a rehabilitation facility as an inpatient, 871,000 at a hospital as an inpatient, 700,000 at a private doctor's office, 574,000 at an emergency room, and 435,000 at a prison or jail. None of these estimates changed significantly between 2010 and 2011. Except for persons who received treatment at a prison or jail, these estimates also did not change between 2002 and 2011; the number of persons who received treatment at a prison or jail increased from 259,000 in 2002 to 435,000 in 2011.

- In 2011, during their most recent treatment in the past year, 2.4 million persons aged 12 or older reported receiving treatment for alcohol use, and 872,000 persons reported receiving treatment for marijuana use. Estimates for receiving treatment for the use of other drugs were 726,000 persons for pain relievers, 511,000 for cocaine, 430,000 for heroin, 318,000 for tranquilizers, 309,000 for stimulants, and 293,000 for hallucinogens. None of these estimates changed significantly between 2010 and 2011.

- The numbers of persons aged 12 or older who received treatment for the use of pain relievers and tranquilizers increased between 2002 and 2011. Numbers who received treatment for pain relievers in 2009 to 2011 ranged from 726,000 to 761,000 persons and were greater than the numbers in 2002 to 2005.

- The numbers of persons aged 12 or older who received treatment for marijuana, hallucinogens, and stimulants were stable between 2002 and 2011. (Note that respondents could indicate that they received treatment for more than one substance during their most recent treatment.)

Illicit Drug Use Treatment and Treatment Need

- In 2011, the number of persons aged 12 or older needing treatment for an illicit drug use problem was 7.2 million (2.8% of the total population). Both the rate and the number declined between 2010 (3.1% and 7.9 million) and 2011. Although the percentage of persons needing treatment for an illicit drug use problem declined between 2002 (3.3%) and 2011, the corresponding number of persons did not differ between 2002 (7.7 million) and 2011.

- Of the 7.2 million persons aged 12 or older who needed treatment for an illicit drug use problem in 2011, 1.4 million (0.5%

of the total population and 18.8% of persons who needed treatment) received treatment at a specialty facility for an illicit drug use problem in the past year. The rate and the number were similar between 2010 and 2011 and between 2002 and 2011.

• There were 5.8 million persons (2.3% of the total population) who needed but did not receive treatment at a specialty facility for an illicit drug use problem in 2011, which declined between 2010 (6.4 million and 2.5%) and 2011. The rate declined between 2002 (2.7%) and 2011, but the numbers in 2002 (6.3 million) and 2011 were similar.

• Of the 5.8 million people aged 12 or older who needed but did not receive specialty treatment for illicit drug use in 2011, 488,000 (8.4%) reported that they perceived a need for treatment for their illicit drug use problem, and 5.3 million did not perceive a need for treatment. The number of persons who needed treatment for an illicit drug use problem but did not perceive the need declined between 2010 (6.0 million) and 2011 (5.3 million).

• Of the 488,000 persons who felt a need for treatment in 2011, 187,000 reported that they made an effort to get treatment, and 301,000 reported making no effort to get treatment. These estimates were similar to the estimates in 2010.

• Among youths aged 12 to 17, there were 1.2 million persons (4.7%) who needed treatment for an illicit drug use problem in 2011. Of this group, only 125,000 received treatment at a specialty facility (10.5% of youths aged 12 to 17 who needed treatment), leaving 1.1 million youths who needed treatment but did not receive it at a specialty facility.

• Among people aged 12 or older who needed but did not receive illicit drug use treatment and felt they needed treatment (based on 2008–2011 combined data), the most often reported reasons for not receiving treatment were (a) no health coverage and could not afford cost (43.6%), (b) not ready to stop using (29.0%), (c) concern that receiving treatment might cause neighbors/community to have negative opinion (14.6%), (d) possible negative effect on job (14.1%), (e) not knowing where to go for treatment (14.0%), and (f) having health coverage that did not cover treatment (10.6%).

Section 6.2

Increase in Treatment Admissions for Prescription Pain Medicine Abuse

"New Report Shows Treatment Admissions for Abuse of Prescription Pain Relievers Have Risen 430 Percent from 1999–2009," Substance Abuse and Mental Health Services Administration (www.samhsa.gov), December 8, 2011.

A new report shows that while the overall rate of substance abuse treatment admissions among those aged 12 and older in the U.S. has remained nearly the same from 1999 to 2009, there has been a dramatic rise (430%) in the rate of treatment admissions for the abuse of prescription pain relievers during this period. The report by SAMHSA shows that the rate of treatment admissions primarily linked to these drugs rose from 10 per 100,000 in the population in 1999 to 53 per 100,000 population in 2009.

The rise in treatment admissions related to the abuse of prescription drug pain relievers occurred in every region of the country but was highest in the states of Maine, Vermont, Delaware, Kentucky, Maryland, Arkansas, Rhode Island, and West Virginia.

The report finds that while the overall rate of substance abuse treatment admissions has remained virtually the same for the U.S during this period (759 per 100,000 population in 1999 versus 753 per 100,000 population in 2009) there have also been significant changes in the rates involving specific substances of abuse and various regions of the country.

For example, the rate for admissions primarily related to marijuana disorders has climbed 33%—from 102 per 100,000 population in 1999 to 136 per 100,000 population in 2009. Nearly all areas of the nation experienced this sharp rise except for the Mountain region, particularly the states of Idaho, Montana, Colorado, Nevada, and Utah.

On the other hand, the admissions rate for the treatment of primary cocaine abuse dropped by 34% during this same period—from 107 per 100,000 population in 1999 to 71 per 100,000 population in 2009. This drop was experienced throughout every region of the country.

"While some aspects of substance abuse treatment admissions have changed—meeting the overall need remains an essential public health priority," said SAMHSA administrator Pamela S. Hyde. "The increasing numbers of people entering treatment for prescription drug abuse is the latest indicator of the severity of the problem. Concerned family members or friends who think a substance abuse problem may exist should seek help. Treatment is effective and people recover."

SAMHSA offers an online treatment locator service that can be accessed at www.samhsa.gov/treatment or by calling 800-662-HELP (4357).

In April 2011, the administration released a comprehensive action plan designed to address the national prescription drug abuse epidemic while protecting the delivery of effective pain-management. Titled "Epidemic: Responding to America's Prescription Drug Abuse Crisis," the plan includes support for the expansion of state-based prescription drug monitoring programs, more convenient and environmentally responsible disposal methods to remove unused medications from the home, education for patients and health care providers, and support for law enforcement efforts that reduce the prevalence of "pill mills" and doctor shopping.

The other major findings from the SAMHSA report include the following:

- The admission rate for the treatment of primary alcohol abuse was 14% lower in 2009 than it was in 1999—314 per 100,000 population versus 364 per 100,000 population.

- The admission rate for treatment of primary alcohol abuse was higher than the admission rate for treatment of illicit drug abuse in 46 out of the 50 reporting states and jurisdictions.

- Admissions for the treatment of methamphetamine/amphetamine soared between 1999 and 2005, from 32 per 100,000 population to 69 per 100,000 population, and then dropped every year through 2009—down to a rate of 44 per 100,000.

The report, "Treatment Episode Data Set (TEDS) 1999 to 2009, State Admissions to Substance Abuse Treatment Services," is based on the report of thousands of substance abuse treatment facilities throughout the nation and Puerto Rico. TEDS is an administrative data system providing descriptive information about the national flow of admissions to specialty providers of substance abuse treatment. Copies of this report and all its detailed findings are available at wwwdasis.samhsa.gov/teds09/teds2009stweb.pdf.

Section 6.3

Predictors of Substance Abuse Treatment Completion

Excerpted from "The TEDS Report—Predictors of Substance Abuse Treatment Completion or Transfer to Further Treatment, by Service Type," Substance Abuse and Mental Health Services Administration (www.samhsa.gov), February 26, 2009.

- In 2005, clients discharged from short-term residential treatment were more likely to complete treatment than clients discharged from long-term residential, outpatient, or intensive outpatient treatment settings.

- Significant predictors of treatment completion or transfer among clients who were discharged from outpatient, intensive outpatient, long-term residential, or short-term residential treatment included: alcohol as the primary substance of abuse, less than daily use at admission, being over age 40, having 12 or more years of education, being white, referral to treatment by the criminal justice system, and being employed.

- Among clients who were discharged from intensive outpatient treatment, men were more likely than women to complete treatment or transfer to another program or facility; however, among clients who were discharged from outpatient or long-term residential treatment, women were more likely than men to complete treatment or transfer to another facility.

Among adults who seek treatment for an alcohol or drug abuse problem, many do not complete an entire course of treatment. This finding is a concern given the research showing that length of stay in treatment is one of the strongest predictors of positive treatment outcomes. Identifying factors that predict treatment completion is an important step toward understanding what leads to successful treatment.

The Treatment Episode Data Set is an annual compilation of data on the demographic characteristics and substance abuse problems of those admitted to and discharged from substance abuse treatment.

TEDS also collects information on reasons for leaving substance abuse treatment. These include treatment completion, transfer to another substance abuse program or facility within a single episode of treatment, left against professional advice (i.e., dropped out), terminated by the facility (i.e., discharge was not because the client dropped out, was incarcerated, or any other client reason), and other reasons, such as death. Clients' treatment may be terminated by a facility for a variety of reasons, such as not following facility rules or exhibiting violent behavior.

This section focuses on the 973,000 clients who were discharged from outpatient, intensive outpatient, long-term residential (more than 30 days), and short-term residential (30 days or fewer) treatment in 2005. Specifically, it examines the proportion of clients discharged who completed treatment or transferred to further treatment and the demographic and substance use characteristics that predict treatment completion and transfer. Because treatment completion and transfer to further treatment represent positive conclusions to a treatment episode, understanding the characteristics of clients who are completing treatment or transferring to further treatment may assist providers to tailor programs that will yield more successful outcomes for their clients.

Treatment Completion and Transfer to Further Treatment, by Treatment Type

In 2005, clients discharged from short-term residential treatment were more likely to complete treatment than clients discharged from long-term residential, outpatient, or intensive outpatient treatment settings (57% vs. 38% or less). Clients discharged from intensive outpatient and short-term residential treatment were more likely to transfer to another program or facility than clients discharged from long-term residential and outpatient treatment settings (19% and 17% vs. 13% and 12%).

Demographic and Substance Use Characteristics That Predict Treatment Completion or Transfer to Further Treatment

To examine the client characteristics associated with treatment completion or transfer to further treatment, a statistical analysis was conducted. This analysis identifies the likelihood of one group completing treatment or transferring to further treatment compared with another group.

Across the four treatment types (outpatient, intensive outpatient, short-term residential, and long-term residential), the strongest predictors of treatment completion or transfer to further treatment were use of alcohol as the primary substance, being referred to treatment from the criminal justice system, and being employed. However, the strength of each predictor varied across service types. For example, clients referred from the criminal justice system (versus any other referral source) were 58% more likely to complete outpatient treatment or be transferred to further treatment, 37% more likely to complete short-term residential treatment or be transferred to further treatment, 34% more likely to complete intensive outpatient treatment or be transferred to further treatment, and 28% more likely to complete long-term residential treatment or be transferred to further treatment.

The results show that the client characteristics that most strongly predicted treatment completion varied depending on the type of treatment (outpatient, intensive outpatient, short-term residential, or long-term residential). The findings underscore the strong positive influence of being employed on the likelihood of completing treatment or transferring to further treatment. These findings provide important insights to treatment providers and policy makers as they work to ensure that treatment is successful for all clients in all service settings.

Part Two

Drug Abuse and Specific Populations

Chapter 7

Initiation of Drug Abuse

Chapter Contents

Section 7.1

Estimates of Drug Use Initiation

Excerpted from "Results from the 2011 National Survey on Drug Use and Health: Summary of National Findings," Substance Abuse and Mental Health Services Administration (www.samhsa.gov), September 2012.

Initiation of Substance Use (Incidence, or First-Time Use) within the Past 12 Months

• In 2011, an estimated 3.1 million persons aged 12 or older used an illicit drug for the first time within the past 12 months. This averages to about 8,400 initiates per day and was similar to the estimate for 2010 (3.0 million). A majority of these past-year illicit drug initiates reported that their first drug was marijuana (67.5%). More than one in five initiated with psychotherapeutics (22.0%, including 14.0% with pain relievers, 4.2% with tranquilizers, 2.6% with stimulants, and 1.2% with sedatives). In 2011, 7.5% of initiates reported inhalants as their first illicit drug, and 2.8% used hallucinogens as their first drug.

• In 2011, the illicit drug categories with the largest number of past-year initiates among persons aged 12 or older were marijuana use (2.6 million) and nonmedical use of pain relievers (1.9 million). These estimates were not significantly different from the numbers in 2010. However, the number of marijuana initiates increased between 2008 (2.2 million) and 2011 (2.6 million).

• In 2011, the average age of marijuana initiates among persons aged 12 to 49 was 17.5 years, which was higher than the average age of marijuana initiates in 2002 (17.0 years).

• The number of past-year initiates of methamphetamine among persons aged 12 or older was 133,000 in 2011. This estimate was lower than the estimates in 2002 to 2006, which ranged from 192,000 to 318,000.

- The number of past-year initiates of ecstasy aged 12 or older was similar in 2011 (922,000) and 2010 (949,000), but the number in 2011 increased from 2005 (615,000).

- In 2011, there were 1.1 million persons aged 12 or older who had used hallucinogens for the first time within the past 12 months.

- The number of past-year cocaine initiates aged 12 or older declined from 1.0 million in 2002 to 670,000 in 2011. The number of initiates of crack cocaine declined during this period from 337,000 to 76,000.

- In 2011, there were 178,000 persons aged 12 or older who used heroin for the first time within the past year, not significantly different from the estimates from 2009 and 2010. However, this was an increase from the annual numbers of initiates during 2005 to 2007 (between 90,000 and 108,000).

- In 2011, there were 719,000 persons aged 12 or older who had used inhalants for the first time within the past 12 months, which was lower than the numbers in prior years from 2002 to 2005 (ranging from 849,000 to 877,000). An estimated 67.1% of past-year initiates of inhalants in 2011 were under age 18 when they first used.

- Psychotherapeutics include the nonmedical use of any prescription-type pain relievers, tranquilizers, stimulants, or sedatives. Over-the-counter substances are not included. In 2011, there were 2.3 million persons aged 12 or older who used psychotherapeutics nonmedically for the first time within the past year, which averages to around 6,400 initiates per day.

- Over half of initiates (55.5%) were younger than age 18 when they first used, and 55.8% of new users were female. The 2011 average age at initiation among persons aged 12 to 49 was 18.1 years, which was similar to the 2010 estimate (19.1 years).

Initiation of Substance Use Discussion

Information on substance use initiation, also known as incidence or first-time use, is important for policy makers and researchers. Measures of initiation are often leading indicators of emerging patterns of substance use. They provide valuable information that can be used to assess the effectiveness of current prevention programs and to focus prevention efforts. With its large sample size and over-sampling of youths aged 12 to 17 and young adults aged 18 to 25, the

National Survey on Drug Use and Health (NSDUH) provides estimates of recent or past-year initiation of use of illicit drugs, tobacco, and alcohol based on reported age and on year and month at first use. Recent or past-year initiates are defined as those who reported use of a particular substance for the first time within 12 months preceding the date of interview.

There is a caveat to the past-year initiation measure worth mentioning. Because the survey interviews persons aged 12 or older, the past-year initiation estimates reflect only a portion of the initiation that occurred at age 11 and none of the initiation that occurred at age 10 or younger. This underestimation primarily affects estimates of initiation for cigarettes, alcohol, and inhalants because they tend to be initiated at a younger age than other substances.

Regarding the age at first use estimates, means, as measures of central tendency, are heavily influenced by the presence of extreme values in the data for persons aged 12 or older. To reduce the effect of extreme values, the mean age at initiation was calculated for persons aged 12 to 49, leaving out those few respondents who were past-year initiates at age 50 or older. Including data from initiates aged 26 to 49 in this broad age group also can cause instability of estimates of the mean age at initiation among persons aged 12 to 49, but this effect is less than that of including data from initiates aged 50 or older. Nevertheless, caution is needed in interpreting these trends for persons aged 12 to 49.

Other estimates in this section, including the numbers and percentages of past-year initiates, are not affected by extreme ages at initiation and therefore are reported for all persons aged 12 or older.

Another important consideration in examining incidence estimates across different drug categories is that substance users typically initiate use of different substances at different times in their lives. Thus, the estimates for past-year initiation of each specific illicit drug cannot be added to obtain the total number of overall illicit drug initiates because some of the initiates previously had used other drugs. The initiation estimate for any illicit drug represents the past-year initiation of use of a specific drug that was not preceded by use of other illicit drugs. For example, a respondent who reported initiating marijuana use in the past 12 months is counted as a marijuana initiate. The same respondent also can be counted as an illicit drug initiate with marijuana as the first drug only if his or her marijuana use initiation was not preceded by use of any other drug (cocaine, heroin, hallucinogens, inhalants, pain relievers, tranquilizers, stimulants, or sedatives).

Section 7.2

Dependence Following Drug Use Initiation

Excerpted from "Substance Use and Dependence Following Initiation of Alcohol or Illicit Drug Use," Substance Abuse and Mental Health Services Administration (www.samhsa.gov), March 27, 2008. Reviewed by David A. Cooke, MD, FACP, July 2013.

- Among persons who initiated alcohol use 13 to 24 months prior to the survey interview ("year-before-last initiates"), 3.2% were dependent on alcohol in the past 12 months ("past year").

- Among year-before-last marijuana initiates, 5.8% were dependent on marijuana in the past year.

- More than one-tenth (13.4%) of year-before-last heroin initiates were dependent on heroin in the past year, and 9.2% of year-before-last crack initiates were dependent on any type of cocaine in the past year.

A series of recent research reports has examined the characteristics associated with the development of dependence soon after the initiation of alcohol, marijuana, cocaine, and hallucinogen use. These studies suggest that each drug class has a different trajectory from first use to cessation of use, continuation of use without dependence, or dependence upon the drug.

The National Survey on Drug Use and Health asks persons aged 12 or older to report on their use of alcohol and illicit drugs during their lifetime and in the past year. Respondents who reported use of a given substance were asked when they first used it.

NSDUH also asks questions to assess symptoms of substance dependence during the past year. NSDUH defines substance dependence using criteria specified by the 4th edition of the *Diagnostic and Statistical Manual of Mental Disorders* (DSM-IV). It includes such symptoms as withdrawal, tolerance, unsuccessful attempts to cut down on use, and continued use despite health and emotional problems caused by the substance.

This section examines the development of dependence upon a substance in the two years following substance use initiation (i.e., 1 to 24 months after initiation). Persons who initiated use of a substance 13 to 24 months prior to the interview are referred to as "year-before-last initiates." Year-before-last initiates were assigned to three mutually exclusive categories reflecting their substance use trajectories following initiation: those who had not used the substance in the past 12 months ("past year"), those who had used the substance during the past year but were not dependent on the substance during the past year, and those who had used the substance and were dependent on the substance during the past year.

Comparisons are made across substance classes in terms of the percentages of these year-before-last initiates classified in each of these three past year categories. All findings presented in this report are annual averages based on combined 2004, 2005, and 2006 NSDUH data.

Noncontinuation of substance use following initiation: Among year-before-last initiates of specific substances, over two-thirds of crack cocaine, inhalant, and heroin initiates did not use the drug in the past year. Alcohol and marijuana were the only substances for which the majority of year-before-last initiates used the substance in the past year.

Risk for developing alcohol dependence following initiation: Among year-before-last initiates of alcohol, one-fourth (25.7%) had not used alcohol during the past year, 71.1% had used alcohol in the past year but were not dependent on alcohol, and 3.2% were both using and dependent on alcohol during the past year.

Risk for developing marijuana dependence following initiation: Among year-before-last initiates of marijuana, 42.4% had not used marijuana during the past year, 51.8% had used marijuana in the past year but were not dependent on marijuana, and 5.8% were both using and dependent on marijuana in the past year.

Risk for developing cocaine dependence following initiation: Year-before-last initiates of cocaine were examined in two subgroups: initiates of crack and initiates of cocaine other than crack. Approximately 9.2% of year-before-last crack initiates were dependent on any type of cocaine in the past year, whereas 3.7% of initiates of cocaine other than crack were dependent on any type of cocaine in the past year.

Risk for developing other drug dependence following initiation: More than one-tenth (13.4%) of year-before-last initiates of heroin were dependent on heroin in the past year, while less than 1% (0.9%)

of year-before-last inhalant initiates were dependent on inhalants in the past year and less than 2% (1.9%) of year-before-last hallucinogen initiates were dependent on hallucinogens in the past year. About 5% (4.7%) of year-before-last initiates of nonmedical use of stimulants were dependent on stimulants in the past year, whereas in the past year, 3.1% of year-before-last initiates of nonmedical pain reliever use were dependent on pain relievers, 2.4% of initiates of nonmedical sedative use were dependent on sedatives, and 1.2% of initiates of nonmedical tranquilizer use were dependent on tranquilizers.

Chapter 8

The Effect of Adult Substance Abuse on Children

Chapter Contents

Section 8.1

Concerns about Drug Abuse during Pregnancy

Nearly 4% of pregnant women in the United States use illicit drugs such as marijuana, cocaine, Ecstasy and other amphetamines, and heroin. These and other illicit drugs may pose various risks for pregnant women and their babies. Some of these drugs can cause a baby to be born too small or too soon, or to have withdrawal symptoms, birth defects, or learning and behavioral problems.

Because many pregnant women who use illicit drugs also use alcohol and tobacco, which also pose risks to unborn babies, it often is difficult to determine which health problems are caused by a specific illicit drug. Additionally, illicit drugs may be prepared with impurities that may be harmful to a pregnancy.

Finally, pregnant women who use illicit drugs may engage in other unhealthy behaviors that place their pregnancy at risk, such as having extremely poor nutrition or developing sexually transmitted infections. All of these factors make it difficult to know exactly what the effects of illicit drugs are on pregnancy.

What are the risks with use of marijuana during pregnancy?

Marijuana is the most frequently used illicit drug among women of childbearing age in the United States. Some studies suggest that use of marijuana during pregnancy may slow fetal growth and slightly decrease the length of pregnancy (possibly increasing the risk of premature birth). These effects are seen mainly in women who use marijuana regularly (six or more times a week).

After delivery, some babies who were regularly exposed to marijuana before birth appear to undergo withdrawal-like symptoms, including excessive crying and trembling. These babies have difficulty with state regulation (the ability to easily adjust to touch and changes in their environment), are more sensitive to stimulation, and have poor sleep patterns.

Couples who are planning pregnancy should keep in mind that marijuana can reduce fertility in both men and women, making it more difficult to conceive.

What is the long-term outlook for babies exposed to marijuana before birth?

There have been a limited number of studies following marijuana-exposed babies through childhood. Some did not find any increased risk of learning or behavioral problems. However, others found that children who were exposed to marijuana before birth are more likely to have subtle problems that affect their ability to pay attention. Exposed children do not appear to have a decrease in IQ.

What are the risks with use of Ecstasy, methamphetamine, and other amphetamines during pregnancy?

The use of Ecstasy, methamphetamine, and other amphetamines has increased dramatically in recent years. There have been few studies on how Ecstasy may affect pregnancy. One small study did find a possible increase in congenital heart defects and, in females only, of a skeletal defect called clubfoot. Babies exposed to Ecstasy before birth also may face some of the same risks as babies exposed to other types of amphetamines.

Another commonly abused amphetamine is methamphetamine, also known as speed, ice, crank, and crystal meth. A 2006 study found that babies of women who used this drug were more than three times as likely than unexposed babies to grow poorly before birth. Even when born at term, affected babies tend to be born with low birthweight (less than 5 1/2 pounds) and have a smaller-than-normal head circumference.

Use of methamphetamine during pregnancy also increases the risk of pregnancy complications, such as premature birth and placental problems. There also have been cases of birth defects, including heart defects and cleft lip/palate, in exposed babies, but researchers do not yet know whether the drug contributed to these defects.

After delivery, some babies who were exposed to amphetamines before birth appear to undergo withdrawal-like symptoms, including jitteriness, drowsiness, and breathing problems.

What is the long-term outlook for babies exposed to Ecstasy, methamphetamine, and other amphetamines before birth?

The long-term outlook for these children is not known. Children who are born with low birthweight are at increased risk of learning and other problems. Children with reduced head circumference are more likely to have learning problems than those with low birthweight and normal head size. One study reported increased rates of anxious/depressed symptoms at three to five years of age, and higher rates of ADHD at five years of age, among children whose mothers used methamphetamine during pregnancy. More studies are needed to determine the long-term outlook for children exposed to amphetamines before birth.

What are the risks with use of heroin during pregnancy?

Women who use heroin during pregnancy greatly increase their risk of serious pregnancy complications. These risks include poor fetal growth, premature rupture of the membranes (the bag of waters that holds the fetus breaks too soon), premature birth, and stillbirth.

As many as half of all babies of heroin users are born with low birthweight. Many of these babies are premature and often suffer from serious health problems during the newborn period, including breathing problems. They also are at increased risk of lifelong disabilities.

Use of heroin in pregnancy may increase the risk of a variety of birth defects. What is not entirely clear is whether these effects are caused by the drug itself or related to the poor health behaviors that women who take heroin often have. The substances that the heroin often is mixed with when it is made also may play a role.

Most babies of heroin users show withdrawal symptoms during the three days after birth, including fever, sneezing, trembling, irritability, diarrhea, vomiting, continual crying, and seizures. These symptoms usually subside by one week of age. The severity of a baby's symptoms is related to how long the mother has been using heroin or other narcotics and how high a dose she has taken. The longer the baby's exposure in the womb and the greater the dose, the more severe the withdrawal. Babies exposed to heroin before birth also face an increased risk of sudden infant death syndrome (SIDS).

While heroin can be sniffed, snorted, or smoked, most users inject the drug into a muscle or vein. Pregnant women who share needles are at risk of contracting HIV (the virus that causes AIDS) and the hepatitis C virus. These infections can be passed on to the infant during pregnancy or at birth. Intravenous drug use carries a high risk of serious complications, regardless of which drug is being used.

A pregnant woman who uses heroin should not attempt to suddenly stop taking the drug. This can put her baby at increased risk of death. She should consult a health care provider or drug-treatment center about treatment one of two drugs, methadone or buprenorphine. Both help addicted women to stay away from heroin and are much safer than heroin during pregnancy.

Infants born to mothers taking methadone have withdrawal symptoms that can be safely treated. Methadone-exposed babies have higher birthweights than babies born to women who continue to use heroin. It is important for families to be aware that infants who are withdrawing from narcotics, including methadone, may continue to have symptoms of withdrawal for weeks after discharge from the nursery. There are effective ways to reduce the baby's discomfort using pacifiers, swaddling, and cuddling. Parents and caregivers benefit from support from family and friends and should seek out assistance if they are feeling stressed or overwhelmed.

What is the long-term outlook for babies exposed to heroin before birth?

The outlook for these children depends on a number of factors, including whether they suffered serious prematurity-related or other complications. Some studies suggest that children exposed to heroin before birth are at increased risk of learning and behavioral problems.

What are the risks of use of "T's and Blues" and opioid painkillers during pregnancy?

This is the street name for a mixture of a prescription opioid (related to morphine) painkiller called pentazocine and an over-the-counter allergy medicine. Individuals who abuse the mixture inject it into a vein. Babies of women who use T's and Blues during pregnancy are at increased risk of slow growth and may suffer withdrawal symptoms.

Babies of women who abuse prescription oral (taken by mouth) opioid painkillers, such as oxycodone (OxyContin), also may undergo withdrawal. Treatment with methadone or buprenorphine are also safer options for pregnant women who are addicted to prescription opioids.

What are the risks with use of cocaine during pregnancy?

Cocaine use during pregnancy can affect a pregnant woman and her baby in many ways. During the early months of pregnancy, cocaine may increase the risk of miscarriage. Later in pregnancy, it may trigger preterm labor (labor that occurs before 37 completed weeks of pregnancy) or cause the baby to grow poorly. As a result, cocaine-exposed babies are more likely than unexposed babies to be born prematurely and with low birthweight. Premature and low-birthweight babies are at increased risk of health problems during the newborn period, lasting disabilities such as intellectual disabilities and cerebral palsy, and even death. Cocaine-exposed babies also tend to have smaller heads, which generally reflect smaller brains and an increased risk of learning problems.

Some studies suggest that cocaine-exposed babies are at increased risk of birth defects involving the urinary tract and, possibly, other birth defects. Cocaine may cause an unborn baby to have a stroke, which can result in irreversible brain damage and sometimes death.

Cocaine use during pregnancy can cause placental problems, including placental abruption. In this condition, the placenta pulls away from the wall of the uterus before labor begins. This can lead to heavy bleeding that can be life threatening for both mother and baby. The baby may be deprived of oxygen and adequate blood flow when an abruption occurs. Prompt cesarean delivery, however, can prevent most deaths but may not prevent serious complications for the baby caused by lack of oxygen.

After birth, some babies who were regularly exposed to cocaine before birth may have mild behavioral disturbances. As newborns, some are jittery and irritable, and they may startle and cry at the gentlest touch or sound. These babies may be difficult to comfort and may be withdrawn or unresponsive. Other cocaine-exposed babies "turn off" surrounding stimuli by going into a deep sleep for most of the day. Generally, these behavioral disturbances are temporary and resolve over the first few months of life.

Cocaine-exposed babies may be more likely than unexposed babies to die of SIDS. However, studies suggest that poor health practices that often accompany maternal cocaine use (such as use of other drugs and smoking) may play a major role in these deaths.

What is the long-term outlook for babies who were exposed to cocaine before birth?

Most children who were exposed to cocaine before birth have normal intelligence. This is encouraging, in light of earlier predictions that many of these children would be severely brain damaged. A 2004 study at Case Western Reserve University found that four-year-old children who were exposed to cocaine before birth scored just as well on intelligence tests as unexposed children.

However, the Case Western and other studies suggest that cocaine may sometimes contribute to subtle learning and behavioral problems, including language delays and attention problems. A good home environment appears to help reduce these effects. A recent study also suggests that cocaine-exposed children grow at a slower rate through age 10 than unexposed children, suggesting some lasting effect on development.

What are the risks of "club drugs," such as PCP (angel dust), ketamine (Special K), and LSD (acid)?

There are few studies on the risks of these drugs during pregnancy. Babies of mothers who used PCP in pregnancy may have withdrawal symptoms. Babies exposed before birth to PCP or ketamine may be at increased risk of learning and behavioral problems. There have been occasional reports of birth defects in babies of women who used LSD during pregnancy, but it is not known whether or not the drug contributed to the defects.

What are the risks of inhaling glues and solvents during pregnancy?

Individuals, pregnant or not, who inhale these substances risk liver, kidney, and brain damage and even death. Abusing these substances during pregnancy can contribute to miscarriage, slow fetal growth, preterm birth, and birth defects. They also may cause withdrawal symptoms in the newborn.

How can a woman protect her baby from the dangers of illicit drugs?

Birth defects and other problems caused by illicit drugs are completely preventable. The March of Dimes advises women who use illicit drugs to stop before they become pregnant or to delay pregnancy until they believe they can avoid the drug completely throughout pregnancy. The March of Dimes also encourages pregnant women who use illicit drugs (with the exception of heroin) to stop using the drug immediately, because of the harm continued drug use may cause. Women who use heroin should consult their health care provider or a drug treatment center about methadone treatment.

Section 8.2

Negative Consequences of Prenatal Exposure to Drugs

Excerpted from "Protecting Children in Families Affected by Substance Use Disorders. Chapter 3, How Parental Substance Use Disorders Affect Children," Child Welfare Information Gateway, U.S. Department of Health and Human Services (www.childwelfare.gov), 2009, and "Prenatal Methamphetamine Exposure Linked with Problems," National Institute on Drug Abuse (www.drugabuse.gov), December 21, 2012.

Protecting Children in Families Affected by Substance Use Disorders: The Impact on Prenatal Development

In 2006 and 2007, an average of 5.2% of pregnant women aged 15 to 44 years used an illicit drug during the month prior to being surveyed, and 11.6% had consumed alcohol. Nationwide, between 550,000 and 750,000 children are born each year after prenatal exposure to drugs or alcohol. These children often are medically fragile or born with a low birth weight. Some are born prematurely and require intensive care.

Identifying the effects of drugs and alcohol on fetuses has posed challenges for researchers. While there has been some success researching the effects of alcohol on fetal development, securing accurate information regarding the use of illicit drugs from pregnant women or women who have given birth has proven to be very difficult. In addition, women who abuse substances often have other risk factors in their lives (e.g., a lack of prenatal care, poor nutrition, stress, violence, poor social support) that can contribute significantly to problematic pregnancies and births.

Pregnancy and Substance Use Disorders (SUDs)

Women who use alcohol or illicit drugs may find it difficult or seemingly impossible to stop, even when they are pregnant. Moreover, pregnancy can be stressful and uncomfortable. For someone who commonly uses drugs and alcohol to minimize pain or stress, this practice may not only continue, but also become worse. Pregnant women can face significant stigma and prejudice when their SUDs are discovered. For these reasons, some women avoid seeking treatment or adequate prenatal care. Other pregnant women, however, do seek treatment. According to the Substance Abuse and Mental Health Services Administration, 3.9% of the women admitted to state-licensed or certified SUD treatment programs were pregnant at the time of admission. In another study, pregnant women aged 15 to 44 years were more likely than nonpregnant women of the same age group to enter treatment for cocaine abuse.

Screening Newborns at Birth

Opinions differ about how best to respond to prenatal substance exposure. Some hospitals are reconsidering whether they should test newborns for drugs, and some courts are treating prenatal substance exposure as a public health matter, turning to Child Protective Services (CPS) only if they determine the child was harmed. Decisions regarding whether and when to screen newborns for prenatal substance exposure are beyond the purview of CPS.

Child welfare legislation has provided some guidance regarding how such cases should be handled. The Keeping Children and Families Safe Act of 2003 requires that health care providers notify CPS, as appropriate, to address the needs of infants born exposed to drugs, and requires the development of a plan of safe care for any affected infants. In 2006, statutes in 15 states and the District of Columbia specified reporting procedures when there is evidence at birth that an infant was exposed prenatally to drugs, alcohol, or other controlled substances. Additionally, 13 states and the District of Columbia included prenatal substance exposure in their definitions of child abuse or neglect.

The Effects of Prenatal Exposure to Alcohol

Drinking alcohol during pregnancy can have serious effects on fetal development. Alcohol consumed by a pregnant woman is absorbed by the placenta and directly affects the fetus. A variety of birth defects to the major organs and the central nervous system, which are permanent, can occur due to alcohol use during pregnancy, though the risk of harm decreases if the pregnant woman stops drinking completely. Collectively, these defects are called fetal alcohol syndrome (FAS). FAS is one of the most commonly known birth defects related to prenatal drug exposure. Children with FAS may exhibit these symptoms:

- Growth deficiencies, both prenatally and after birth

- Problems with central nervous system functioning

- IQs in the mild to severely retarded range
- Small eye openings and poor development of the optic nerve
- A small head and brain
- Joint, limb, ear, and heart malformations

Alcohol-related neurodevelopmental disorder (ARND) and alcohol-related birth defects (ARBD) are similar to FAS. ARND and ARBD encompass the functional and physiological problems associated with prenatal alcohol exposure but are less severe than FAS. Children with ARND can experience functional or mental impairments as a result of prenatal alcohol exposure, and children with ARBD can have malformations in the skeletal and major organ systems. Not all children who are exposed prenatally to alcohol develop FAS, ARND, or ARBD, but for those who do, these effects continue throughout their lives and at all the stages of development, although they are likely to present themselves differently at each developmental stage. Table 8.1 compares typical childhood behavior at each developmental stage with behaviors and characteristics associated with FAS, ARND, and ARBD.

More information on FAS is available from the National Organization on Fetal Alcohol Syndrome (www.nofas.org) and the National Center on Birth Defects and Developmental Disabilities (www.cdc.gov/ncbddd/fas).

The Effects of Prenatal Exposure to Drugs

Similar to alcohol use, use of other substances can have significant effects on the developing fetus. For example, cocaine or marijuana use during pregnancy may result in premature birth, low birth weight, decreased head circumference, or miscarriage. Prenatal exposure to marijuana has been associated with difficulties in functioning of the brain. Even if there are no noticeable effects in the children at birth, the impact of prenatal substance use often can become evident later in their lives. As they get older, children who were exposed to cocaine prenatally can have difficulty focusing their attention, be more irritable, and have more behavioral problems. Difficulties surface in sorting out relevant versus irrelevant stimuli, making school participation and achievement more challenging.

Pregnancy as a Motivation for Treatment

Given the dangers associated with substance use during pregnancy, women who abuse substances during pregnancy should receive treatment as early as possible. Research has found that women often are more amenable to entering treatment when they are pregnant.

Once their babies are born, significant changes can occur in the lives of women who abused alcohol or drugs during pregnancy. In the case of babies who test positive for substances at birth, the mothers may experience remorse and sadness over the actual or potential consequences of their substance use, which also can be a motivating factor to seek treatment. Mothers may admit to enough drug use to explain a positive drug test, but not to an addiction, due to the fear of losing custody of their children. They may comply with treatment requirements in order to compensate for the problems their SUD may have caused their children. Nevertheless, new difficulties may begin when CPS closes the case and the pressure is off the mothers to stay clean. For instance, they may be tempted to use drugs and alcohol again.

Table 8.1. Childhood Behavior and Characteristics Associated with FAS, ARND, and ARBD

Developmental Stage	Typical Behaviors or Characteristics	FAS/ARND/ARBD Behaviors or Characteristics
Infants	Develop mental and physical skills; bond with caretakers	Problems with spatial and depth perception, muscle coordination and development, facility with speech, and processing information; attention deficit disorder; inability to focus; possible attachment disorders
Toddlers	Develop sense of self; assert independence by saying no	Difficulty exercising self-control, which leads to self doubt and feelings of inadequacy
5- to 7-year-olds	Try new things; meet or exceed academic standards; learn new social skills	Overwhelmed with new situations and interactions with other children; inability to pick up social skills by observation; problems meeting academic standards
8- to 12-year-olds	Increased influence of peers; games become important method of bonding and developing interpersonal skills	Difficulty remembering rules of games; lack of remorse in breaking rules; become depressed and exhibit other behavior problems
Teenagers	Continued detachment from parents; development of individual identity; learn to identify with larger community	May lack skills to become good community members; become socially isolated; may find their way to peer groups that engage in high risk behaviors; may withdraw altogether from groups

Prenatal Methamphetamine Exposure Linked with Problems

In the latest findings from an ongoing study of the effects of prenatal methamphetamine exposure on child development, primary caregivers reported more signs of increased emotionality, anxiety, and depression in exposed than nonexposed children at ages three and five years. The caregivers also reported that at age five, methamphetamine-exposed children were less able to sustain attention and more prone to act out aggressively or destructively than were nonexposed children.

The National Institute on Drug Abuse (NIDA)-supported Infant Development, Environment, and Lifestyle (IDEAL) study has followed more than 200 children exposed to methamphetamine prenatally, along with matched controls, since birth. Previous IDEAL reports linked prenatal methamphetamine exposure to reduced neonatal size and alertness as well as deficits in fine motor skills through age three years.

The new findings reflect primary caregivers' responses to the Child Behavior Checklist when the children were three and five years old. In both assessments, the caregivers rated the exposed children higher on emotional reactivity and anxiety/depression. In the assessment at age five, the caregivers also scored the exposed children higher on externalizing behaviors (e.g., defiance, aggression) and attention-deficit/hyperactivity disorder (ADHD). Although the average scores of exposed and nonexposed children were within normal limits, more exposed five-year olds were in the range indicating a clinically significant externalizing problem.

The IDEAL investigators also reported that 26 children whose mothers used methamphetamine at least three days a week throughout their pregnancy scored lower on a test of inhibitory control at age 5.5 than did nonexposed children. The ability to resist an initial impulse or to stay focused despite distractions provides a foundation for academic and psychosocial success during later childhood and adolescence.

These data suggest that methamphetamine use during pregnancy could disrupt the normal development of the frontal cortex, says Dr. Linda LaGasse at the Warren Alpert Medical School of Brown University and Women and Infants Hospital in Providence, Rhode Island. Disrupted frontal cortex circuitry may impair inhibitory control, which, in turn, may lead to attention deficits and behavioral problems. The researchers note that studies have pointed to such a sequence of effects following prenatal exposure to cocaine, a stimulant similar to methamphetamine.

Identifying such problems at an early age is critical to prevent a child's emotional and behavioral difficulties from escalating, says Dr. LaGasse. "It is imperative that these children continue to be followed in order to understand the long-term implications of these findings. As we map out the developmental trajectories of these children, we will be able to identify key touchpoints for the development of preventive interventions," says Dr. Barry Lester, principal investigator of the IDEAL study.

Section 8.3

Drug Endangered Children

Excerpted from "Protecting Children in Families Affected by Substance Use Disorders. Chapter 3, How Parental Substance Use Disorders Affect Children," Child Welfare Information Gateway, U.S. Department of Health and Human Services (www.childwelfare.gov), 2009, and excerpts from "Drug Endangered Children," White House Office of National Drug Control Policy (www.whitehouse.gov/ondcp), 2010.

Protecting Children in Families Affected by Substance Use Disorders: The Impact on Childhood Development

Exposure to parental SUDs during childhood also can have dire consequences for children. Compared to children of parents who do not abuse alcohol or drugs, children of parents who do, and who also are in the child welfare system, are more likely to experience physical, intellectual, social, and emotional problems. Among the difficulties in providing services to these children is that problems affected or compounded by their parents' SUDs might not emerge until later in their lives.

This section summarizes some of the consequences of SUDs on childhood development, including a disruption of the bonding process; emotional, academic, and developmental problems; lack of supervision; parentification; social stigma; and adolescent substance use and delinquency.

Disruption of the Bonding Process

When mothers or fathers abuse substances after delivery, their ability to bond with their child—so important during the early stages of life—may be weakened. In order for an attachment to form, it is necessary that caregivers pay attention to and notice their children's attempts to communicate. Parents who use marijuana, for example, may have difficulty picking up their babies' cues because marijuana dulls response time and alters perceptions. When parents repeatedly miss their babies' cues, the babies eventually stop providing them. The result is disengaged parents with disengaged babies. These parents and babies then have difficulty forming a healthy, appropriate relationship.

Neglected children who are unable to form secure attachments with their primary caregivers may show these characteristics:

- May become more mistrustful of others and may be less willing to learn from adults

- May have difficulty understanding the emotions of others, regulating their own emotions, or forming and maintaining relationships with others

- May have a limited ability to feel remorse or empathy, which may mean that they could hurt others without feeling their actions were wrong

- May demonstrate a lack of confidence or social skills that could hinder them from being successful in school, work, and relationships

- May demonstrate impaired social cognition, which is awareness of oneself in relation to others as well as of others' emotions. Impaired social cognition can lead a person to view many social interactions as stressful

Emotional, Academic, and Developmental Problems

Children who experience either prenatal or postnatal drug exposure are at risk for a range of emotional, academic, and developmental problems. For example, they are more likely to show these characteristics:

- Experience symptoms of depression and anxiety

- Suffer from psychiatric disorders

- Exhibit behavior problems

- Score lower on school achievement tests

- Demonstrate other difficulties in school

These children may behave in ways that are challenging for biological or foster parents to manage, which can lead to inconsistent caregiving and multiple alternative care placements.

Positive social and emotional child development generally has been linked to nurturing family settings in which caregivers are predictable, daily routines are respected, and everyone recognizes clear boundaries for acceptable behaviors. Such circumstances often are missing in the homes of parents with SUDs. As a result, extra supports and interventions are needed to help children draw upon their strengths and maximize their natural potential despite their home environments. Protective factors, such as the involvement of other supportive adults (e.g., extended family members, mentors, clergy, teachers, neighbors), may help mitigate the impact of parental SUDs.

Lack of Supervision

The search for drugs or alcohol, the use of scarce resources to pay for them, the time spent in illegal activities to raise money for them, or the time spent recovering from hangovers or withdrawal symptoms can leave parents with little time or energy to care properly for their children. These children frequently do not have their basic needs met and often do not receive appropriate supervision. In addition, rules about curfews and potentially dangerous activities may not be enforced or are enforced haphazardly. As a result, SUDs are often a factor in neglect cases.

Parentification

As children grow older, they may become increasingly aware that their parents cannot care for them. To compensate, the children become the caregivers of the family, often extending their caregiving behavior to their parents as well as younger siblings. This process is labeled "parentification."

Parentified children carry a great deal of anxiety and sometimes go to great lengths to control or to eliminate their parents' use of drugs or alcohol. They feel responsible for running the family. These feelings are reinforced by messages from the parents that the children cause the parents' SUDs or are at fault in some way if the family comes to the attention of authorities. Sometimes these children must contact medical personnel in the case of a parent's overdose, or they may be left supervising and caring for younger children when their parents are absent while obtaining or abusing substances.

Social Stigma

Adults with SUDS may engage in behaviors that embarrass their children and may appear disinterested in their children's activities or school performance. Children may separate themselves from their parents by not wanting to go home after school, by not bringing friends to the house, or by not asking for help with homework. These children may feel a social stigma attached to certain aspects of their parents' lives, such as unemployment, homelessness, an involvement with the criminal justice system, or SUD treatment.

Adolescent Substance Use and Delinquency

Adolescents whose parents have SUDs are more likely to develop SUDs themselves. Some adolescents mimic behaviors they see in their families, including ineffective coping behaviors such as using drugs and alcohol. Many of these children also witness or are victims of violence. It is hypothesized that substance abuse is a coping mechanism for such traumatic events. Moreover, adolescents who use substances are more likely to have poor academic performance and to be involved in criminal activities. The longer children are exposed to parental SUD, the more serious the negative consequences may be for their overall development and well-being.

Child Abuse as a Precursor to Substance Use Disorders

Many people view SUDs as a phenomenon that leads to or exacerbates the abuse or neglect of children. Research also suggests, however, that being victimized by child abuse, particularly sexual abuse, is a common precursor of SUDs. Sometimes, victims of abuse or neglect "self-medicate" (i.e., drink or use drugs to escape the unresolved trauma of the maltreatment). One study found that women with a history of childhood physical or sexual abuse were nearly five times more likely to use street drugs and more than twice as likely to abuse alcohol as women who were not maltreated. In another study, childhood abuse predicted a wide range of problems, including lower self-esteem, more victimization, more depression, and chronic homelessness, and indirectly predicted drug and alcohol problems.

Drug Endangered Children

A drug endangered child is a person, under the age of 18, who lives in or is exposed to an environment where drugs, including pharmaceuticals, are illegally used, possessed, trafficked, diverted, and/or manufactured and, as a result of that environment: the child experiences, or is at risk of experiencing, physical, sexual, or emotional abuse; the child experiences, or is at risk of experiencing, medical, educational, emotional, or physical harm, including harm resulting or possibly resulting from neglect; or the child is forced to participate in illegal or sexual activity in exchange for drugs or in exchange for money likely to be used to purchase drugs.

—Federal Interagency Task Force for Drug
Endangered Children (2010)

Background and History

Stemming in part from the methamphetamine crisis, the Drug Endangered Children (DEC) movement began in the last decade to respond to the growing phenomenon of finding children living among the squalor of meth labs located in homes and other areas where children were living or playing. The children found in these situations were often severely harmed or neglected, and in many instances tested positive for drugs. To rescue these children, local DEC programs were created all over the country and a national DEC program was created in 2003.

Since that time, the movement to identify and aid drug endangered children has expanded in scope and impact to include partners on the federal, state, tribal, and local levels. Through this collaboration, the definition of drug endangered children expanded beyond only those children confronted by meth, and it broadened to include children that faced dangerous exposure to any type of drug. The DEC movement also sought to assist parents/guardians with substance use disorders and help address family issues surrounding the problem.

Around the country, the DEC movement has rescued thousands of children and led to the development of numerous programs that have coordinated the efforts of law enforcement, medical services, and child welfare services to ensure that drug endangered children receive appropriate attention and care. Up to this point, however, a cohesive and coordinated federal response had been lacking. For this reason, an Interagency Task Force on Drug Endangered Children was formed.

The Federal Interagency Task Force on Drug Endangered Children is focused on gathering and producing educational resources (model protocols, programming, and promising practices) that can aid law enforcement, child welfare workers, health and education professionals, and children's advocates nationwide in protecting children and responding to their needs and the needs of their caregivers. By working together with its federal, state and local partners, the task force aims to end this vicious cycle.

Research and Statistics

- Between 2002 and 2007, an estimated 2.1 million children in the U.S. (3.0%) lived with at least one parent who abused or was dependent on illicit drugs.

- Studies of children in foster care find that 40% to 80% of families involved with child welfare having substance abuse problems.

- A 2003 study analyzing administrative data regarding persons treated for substance abuse in California found that 60% of persons treated for substance abuse in California's publicly funded treatment system were parents of minor children. Of those treated, 295,000 parents (or 27%) had one or more children removed from their custody by child welfare services.

Chapter 9

Adolescent Drug Abuse

Chapter Contents

Section 9.1

Trends in Adolescent Drug Abuse

Excerpted from "DrugFacts: High School and Youth Trends,"
National Institute on Drug Abuse (www.drugabuse.gov), December 2012.

Every year, the Monitoring the Future (MTF) survey measures drug, alcohol, and tobacco use and related attitudes among 8th, 10th, and 12th graders. Following are facts and statistics about youth substance use from the 2012 MTF report.

Illicit drug use among teenagers has continued at high rates, largely due to the popularity of marijuana. Marijuana use by adolescents declined from the late 1990s until the mid-to-late 2000s but has been on the increase since then. In 2012, 6.5% of 8th graders, 17.0% of 10th graders, and 22.9% of 12th graders used marijuana in the past month—an increase among 10th and 12th graders from 14.2% and 18.8% in 2007. Daily use has also increased; 6.5% of 12th graders now use marijuana every day, compared to 5.1% in 2007.

Rising marijuana use reflects changing perceptions and attitudes. Historically, as perception of risks goes down, use goes up (and vice versa). Young people are showing decreased perception that marijuana is dangerous. The growing perception of marijuana as a safe drug may reflect recent public discussions over medical marijuana and marijuana legalization.

Synthetic marijuana is a new and major concern. Also known as Spice or K2, synthetic marijuana refers to herbal mixtures laced with synthetic cannabinoids, chemicals that act in the brain similarly to THC, the main active ingredient in marijuana. These mixtures could be obtained legally until recently and are still wrongly perceived as a safe alternative to marijuana. Synthetic marijuana was added to the MTF survey in 2011. In that year, 11.4% of 12th graders—one in nine—reported using it in the past year. This year 4.4% of 8th graders, 8.8% of 10th graders, and 11.3% of 12th graders reported past-year use.

Nonmedical use of prescription and over-the-counter medicines remains a significant part of the teen drug problem. In 2012, 14.8% of high-school seniors used a prescription drug nonmedically in the past year. Data for specific drugs show that the most commonly abused prescription drugs by teens are the stimulant Adderall and the pain reliever Vicodin.

Past year illicit use among 12th graders is as follows:

- **Marijuana:** 36.4%

- **Synthetic marijuana:** 11.3%

- **Adderall:** 7.6%

- **Vicodin:** 7.5%

- **Cough medicine:** 5.6%

- **Tranquilizers:** 5.3%

- **Hallucinogens:** 4.8%

- **Sedatives:** 4.5%

- **Salvia:** 4.4%

- **OxyContin:** 4.3%

- **Ecstasy (MDMA):** 3.8%

- **Inhalants:** 2.9%

- **Cocaine:** 2.7%

- **Ritalin:** 2.6%

Positive trends in the past several years include reduced use of inhalants and less use of cocaine. Inhalant use is at its lowest levels in the history of the survey. Past-year inhalant use by younger teens dropped significantly between 2007 and 2012, from 8.3% of 8th graders and 6.6% of 10th graders to 6.2% and 4.1%, respectively. Past-year use of cocaine by 12th graders dropped from 5.2% to 2.7% from 2007 to 2012. Other drugs, such as heroin, methamphetamine, and hallucinogens, are holding fairly steady.

Ecstasy is seeing a significant drop among teens. Past-year use of ecstasy by 12th graders decreased from 5.3% in 2011 to 3.8% in 2012. Among 10th and 8th graders it dropped from 4.5% to 3.0% and from 1.7% to 1.1%, respectively.

Learn More

Complete MTF survey results are available at www.monitoringthefuture .org. For more information on the survey and its findings, also visit www .drugabuse.gov/related-topics/trends-statistics/monitoring-future.

Other sources of information on drug use trends among youth are available:

The annual National Survey of Drug Use and Health (NSDUH), conducted by the Substance Abuse and Mental Health Services Administration, gathers detailed data on drug, alcohol, and tobacco use by all age groups. It is a comprehensive source of information on substance use and dependence among Americans aged 12 and older. Data and reports can be found at www.oas.samhsa.gov/NSDUHLatest.htm.

The Youth Risk Behavior Survey is a school-based survey conducted every other year by the Centers for Disease Control and Prevention. It gathers data on a wide variety of health-related risk behaviors, including drug abuse, from students in grades 9–12. More information is available at www.cdc.gov/nccdphp/dash/yrbs/index.htm.

Section 9.2

Reasons Adolescents Try Drugs and Alcohol and Understanding Risk Factors

Know Your Child's Risk Level for Developing a Substance Abuse Problem

Several decades of research shows that some teens are more at risk for developing a substance abuse problem than other teens. Why is that? Well, there is no single factor. However, the more risk factors a teen has, the more likely he or she will abuse drugs or alcohol. Conversely, the fewer the number of risk factors, the less likely he or she will develop a drug or alcohol problem. Also, it's important to recognize that even children raised in the same home may have varying levels of risk.

It is important to keep in mind that risk factors do not determine a child's destiny. Instead, they provide a general gauge as to the likelihood of drug or alcohol abuse.

But it is safe to say that addressing risk factors early and paying careful attention to children at higher risk can reduce that child's likelihood of a future problem with drugs or alcohol. Understanding risk factors is also very important when a child with more risk has already experimented with substances or has a problem. In that case, you will have a clearer picture of why things might have happened and know how to get the right kind of treatment. (Example: Treating a mental health problem.)

Here are four common risk factors associated with teen drug and alcohol abuse

- **Family history:** Family history of drug or alcohol problems, especially when a parent has a drug or alcohol problem, can place a child at increased risk for developing a problem him- or herself. Children can inherit genes that increase their risk of alcoholism, so having a parent or grandparent with alcohol problems may indicate increased risk for the child, although inheriting the gene does not mean the child will automatically become dependent on alcohol. If there is a history of a drug or alcohol problem in your family, you should let your child know since he or she is at a higher risk for developing a drug or alcohol problem. These conversations should take place when you feel your child is able to understand the information.

- **Mental or behavioral disorder:** If your child has a psychiatric condition like depression, anxiety, or Attention Deficit Hyperactivity Disorder (ADHD), he or she is at more risk for a drug or alcohol problem. Although not all teenagers with these disorders will develop a substance abuse problem, the chances are higher when they have difficulty regulating their thoughts and emotions. Therefore parents with children with psychiatric conditions should be vigilant about the possibility of their teen using drugs or alcohol.

  It is also a good idea to talk with your health care providers about the connection between psychiatric conditions and substance use. Managing and treating underlying psychiatric conditions, or understanding how emotional and behavioral problems can trigger or escalate a substance use problem, is important for preventing or reducing risk.

- **Trauma:** Children who have had a history of traumatic events (such as witnessing or experiencing a car accident or natural disaster; being a victim of physical or sexual abuse) have been shown to be more at risk for substance use problems later in life. Therefore, it is important for parents to recognize and address the possible impact of trauma on their child and get help for their child.

- **Impulse control problems:** Children who frequently take risks or have difficulty controlling impulses are more at risk for substance use problems. While most teens understand the dangers of taking risks, some have particular difficulty resisting impulses to engage in risky behavior.

Remember: Think about your child's risk factors and review them at least annually (Example: On your child's birthday). If your child's risk factors are high or increase over time, watch more carefully for behavioral, psychological, and social problems. Take action to address risk factors and don't hesitate to seek professional help if you cannot manage the problems yourself.

Don't: Ignore risk factors and assume your child will be okay or just ignore a problem because you think it is a stage of development. If something is apparent, seek help.

The Best Prevention

There is one thing all parents can do to help protect their kids against teenage drinking: build strong family bonds. "Teenagers who say they can go to at least one parent to confide in or seek advice when they're dealing with a personal issue are much less likely to use," says [Ken] Winters [Ph.D., Director of the Center for Adolescent Substance Abuse Research and Senior Scientist at the Treatment Rsearch Institute].

A Parent's Guide to the Teen Brain

From mood swings to risk taking, "normal teenage behavior" can appear to be anything-but-normal to parents! Do you ever find yourself asking, "Who is this kid?" Then check out *A Parent's Guide to the Teen Brain* [at teenbrain.drugfree.org].

Top Eight Reasons Why Teens Try Alcohol and Drugs

There is no single reason for teenage drug use and alcohol use. In *How to Keep Your Teenager Out of Trouble and What to Do if You Can't,*

Dr. Neil I. Bernstein details some of the core issues and influences behind teenage drug and alcohol use. It's important that you, as a parent, understand these reasons and talk to your kids about the dangers of drinking and using drugs.

- **Other people:** Teenagers see lots of people using various substances. They see their parents and other adults drinking alcohol, smoking, and, sometimes, abusing other substances. Also, the teen social scene often revolves around drinking and smoking pot. Sometimes friends urge one another to try a drink or smoke something, but it's just as common for teens to start using a substance because it's readily available and they see all their friends enjoying it. In their minds, they see drug use as a part of the normal teenage experience.

- **Popular media:** 47% of teens agreed that movies and TV shows make drugs seem like an OK thing to do, according to a 2011 study. Not surprisingly, 12- to 17-year-olds who viewed three or more "R" rated movies per month were seven times more likely to smoke cigarettes, six times more likely to use marijuana, and five times more likely to drink alcohol, compared to those who hadn't watched "R" rated films.

- **Escape and self-medication:** When teens are unhappy and can't find a healthy outlet for their frustration or a trusted confidant, they may turn to chemicals for solace. Depending on what substance they're using, they may feel blissfully oblivious, wonderfully happy, or energized and confident. The often rough teenage years can take an emotional toll on children, sometimes even causing depression, so when teens are given a chance to take something to make them feel better, many can't resist.

- **Boredom:** Teens who can't tolerate being alone, have trouble keeping themselves occupied, or crave excitement are prime candidates for substance abuse. Not only do alcohol and marijuana give them something to do, but those substances help fill the internal void they feel. Further, they provide a common ground for interacting with like-minded teens, a way to instantly bond with a group of kids.

- **Rebellion:** Different rebellious teens choose different substances to use based on their personalities. Alcohol is the drug of choice for the angry teenager because it frees him to behave aggressively. Methamphetamine, or meth, also encourage aggressive, violent behavior, and can be far more dangerous and potent than alcohol. Marijuana, on the other hand, often seems to reduce aggression and is more of an avoidance drug. LSD [lysergic acid diethylamide] and hallucinogens are also escape drugs, often used by young people who feel misunderstood and may long to escape to a more idealistic, kind world. Smoking cigarettes can be a form of rebellion to flaunt their independence and make their parents angry. The reasons for teenage drug use are as complex as teenagers themselves.

- **Instant gratification:** Drugs and alcohol work quickly. The initial effects feel really good. Teenagers turn to drug use because they see it as a short-term shortcut to happiness.

- **Lack of confidence:** Many shy teenagers who lack confidence report that they'll do things under the influence of alcohol or drugs that they might not otherwise. This is part of the appeal of drugs and alcohol even for relatively self-confident teens; you have the courage to dance if you're a bad dancer, or sing at the top of your lungs even if you have a terrible voice, or kiss the girl you're attracted to. And alcohol and other drugs tend not only to loosen your inhibitions but to alleviate social anxiety. Not only do you have something in common with the other people around you, but there's the mentality that if you do anything or say anything stupid, everyone will just think you had too many drinks or smoked too much weed.

- **Misinformation:** Perhaps the most avoidable cause of substance abuse is inaccurate information about drugs and alcohol. Nearly every teenager has friends who claim to be experts on various recreational substances, and they're happy to assure her that the risks are minimal. Educate your teenager about drug use, so they get the real facts about the dangers of drug use.

Please note that information from the book has been edited for length.

Section 9.3

Adolescents and Prescription Drug Abuse

"Teens and Prescription Drugs," © 2007 New York State Office of Alcoholism and Substance Abuse Services (www.oasas.ny.gov). Reprinted with permission. Reviewed by David A. Cooke, MD, FACP, July 2013. Other information from National Institute on Drug Abuse is cited separately within the section.

The availability of over-the-counter and prescription medications in the family medicine cabinet provides easy access for teens. Teens often mistakenly believe that these medications are safe because they are approved by the FDA [U.S. Food and Drug Administration] and are prescribed by a physician. A National Center for Addiction and Substance Abuse (CASA) at Columbia University report (2005) found a 154% increase in the total number of prescriptions for controlled substances written by physicians between 1992 and 2002. Increased prescriptions allow for increased access and increased potential for diversion of medications at all points along the distribution chain. Internet sites also provide ready access to teens. CASA, in cooperation with Beau Dietl and Associates, surveyed a sample of Internet pharmacies and found that only 6% required a prescription, 41% reported that no prescription was needed, and 49% provided the medication after an "online consultation."

Why Might Teens Use Drugs?

- To enhance pleasure
- To have fun
- To vary their conscious experience
- To self-medicate
- As a way to cope with trauma
- To relieve anxiety, depression, insomnia
- To relieve pain
- To promote and enhance social interaction

- To stimulate artistic creativity and performance

- To rebel

- To improve physical/mental performance

- To fend off withdrawal

- To lose weight

"Pharming" is the new lexicon for grabbing a handful of prescription drugs and ingesting some or all of them. Teens bring prescription drugs from their home medicine cabinets and mix them all together in a grab bag. This can be an activity at adolescent parties and the medications can be mixed with alcohol, compounding the dangers.

Cold medicines such as Robitussin, Nyquil, Vicks Formula 44, and Coricidin HBP Cough and Cold tablets contain a chemical called dextromethorphan (DXM), which is found in more than 120 nonprescription cough and cold medications. DXM is a synthetic drug and has been added to cough syrups and some cold medications since the 1970s. Authorities say that DXM overdoses typically occur in clusters, as word of mouth about DXM use spreads through community middle schools and high schools.

- Teenagers have various nicknames for DXM including: Robo, Skittles, Triple C's, Dex, Vitamin D, and Tussin.

- Cough and cold tablets contain much more potent doses of DXM than cough syrups, so the kids don't need to drink a whole bottle of nasty-tasting cough syrup. They can easily and conveniently take a few pills containing DXM to get high.

- DXM costs just a few dollars as compared to other much more expensive illicit drugs. Unfortunately, there is quite a bit of information on the Internet regarding how much DXM it takes kids to get high, and teens can easily log on to get the information they need.

- The Drug Enforcement Administration classifies DXM as a "drug of concern" because if misused it can be very dangerous. However, there are no legal restrictions on purchasing the drug.

- Growing concerns about DXM have led to some store chains and drugstores restricting access to products containing DXM, and to limiting the amount that can be purchased at any one time.

DXM is not the only over-the-counter drug that teenagers are abusing. The list also includes diet pills, sleep aids, and motion sickness medication. Some teenagers use excessive amounts of diet pills in an attempt to lose weight quickly, others take them to get high. Diet pills are not meant for teens as they contain potentially dangerous ingredients. Even herbal diet pills can be dangerous as they are not well regulated by the FDA.

- Motion sickness pills such as Dramamine are being used by teens; taken in large doses (one entire package or more), Dramamine can cause hallucinations.

- Sleep aids such as Tylenol PM, Excedrin PM, and Sominex can cause extreme drowsiness when abused.

Another risk is that many medications (prescription and over the counter) contain Tylenol (acetaminophen) and if greater than 4,000 mg [milligrams] are ingested over a short period of time, severe liver damage can occur.

A new mixture, Cheese Heroin is made with Mexican black tar heroin and Tylenol PM, an over-the-counter drug found in many in medicine cabinets right now. Also known as cheeze, chees, cheez, chez, chz, queso, keso, and ksoh, this mix of drugs can cause:

- brief but intense euphoria;

- alternate states of restlessness and lethargy disorientation;

- constricted pupils;

- slowed breathing;

- irregular heartbeat;

- changes in appetite.

Behavioral Warning Signs for the Adolescent Abusing Prescription and Over-the-Counter Medications

- Loss of enthusiasm and signs of depression

- Withdrawal from normal activities

- Truancy and unexplained drop in grades

- Irritability and overreaction to criticism

- Unusual requests for money

- Decreased interest in appearance

- Unexplained changes in friends

• Frequent nasal or sinus infections

Note: There are many other reasons for these behaviors and parents need to talk to their children about the signs and symptoms that they are seeing.

Adolescents and Young Adults

"Prescription Drugs: Abuse and Addiction: Adolescents and Young Adults," National Institute on Drug Abuse (www.drugabuse.gov), October 2011.

Abuse of prescription drugs is highest among young adults aged 18 to 25, with 5.9% reporting nonmedical use in the past month (NS-DUH, 2010). Among youth aged 12 to 17, 3.0% reported past-month nonmedical use of prescription medications.

According to the 2010 MTF, prescription and over-the-counter (OTC) drugs are among the most commonly abused drugs by 12th graders, after alcohol, marijuana, and tobacco. While past-year nonmedical use of sedatives and tranquilizers decreased among 12th graders over the last five years, this is not the case for the nonmedical use of amphetamines or opioid pain relievers.

When asked how prescription opioids were obtained for nonmedical use, more than half of the 12th graders surveyed said they were given the drugs or bought them from a friend or relative. Interestingly, the number of students who purchased opioids over the Internet was negligible.

Youth who abuse prescription medications are also more likely to report use of other drugs. Multiple studies have revealed associations between prescription drug abuse and higher rates of cigarette smoking; heavy episodic drinking; and marijuana, cocaine, and other illicit drug use among adolescents, young adults, and college students in the United States.

Section 9.4

Adolescent Marijuana Use Increases over Alcohol and Tobacco

"Adolescent Smoking and Drinking at Historic Lows," July 20, 2012, and "Teen Marijuana Use Increases, Especially among Eighth-Graders," December 14, 2010, National Institute on Drug Abuse (www.drugabuse.gov).

Adolescent Smoking and Drinking at Historic Lows

Rates of adolescent cigarette smoking and alcohol drinking stood at historic lows in 2011, but marijuana use trended upward, according to the 2011 Monitoring the Future survey. The findings reflect the responses of 46,773 8th, 10th, and 12th graders in 400 public and private secondary schools nationwide.

In all three grades, rates of smoking and alcohol consumption were the lowest that they have been in the survey's 37-year history. Binge drinking was also reported at record lows.

Illicit drug use by adolescents, however, has risen gradually from 2008 through 2011, driven by the increase in marijuana use over the four-year period. One in four students surveyed reported past-year marijuana use in 2011, an increase of nearly 17% since 2007.

NIDA officials point to two worrisome findings. Daily use of marijuana rose in all three grades and, among 12th graders, stood at its highest rate (6.6%) in 30 years. In addition, the perception of harm associated with marijuana use declined in all three grades—an indication that use is likely to continue to rise.

Questions on synthetic marijuana, also known as K2 and spice, were added to the survey in 2011, allowing researchers to quantify the growing popularity of products called herbal mixtures—plant materials sprayed with synthetic chemicals that mimic the effects of marijuana. In the survey, 11.4% of high school seniors said they had used synthetic marijuana in the past year.

This rate is "very high and unexpected" given that synthetic marijuana is a new drug, says NIDA director Dr. Nora D. Volkow. "The students' willingness to experiment at such a high level with a drug for which there is not much experience underlies the urgency of addressing this problem so that we can prevent further escalation," she adds.

Poison control centers across the nation received 5,741 calls pertaining to synthetic marijuana in the first 10 months of 2011, nearly twice the number of calls received in all of 2010.

In 2011, the Drug Enforcement Administration added five of the chemicals used in synthetic marijuana to its list of controlled substances, making it illegal to possess or sell them. The U.S. House of Representatives approved legislation to ban the sale of synthetic marijuana in 2011; a similar bill is pending in the U.S. Senate. At least 18 states have banned the sale of synthetic marijuana.

"Next year's survey results should tell us a lot more about how successful these new control efforts are," says Dr. Lloyd Johnston of the University of Michigan, lead investigator of the survey.

Further details on the survey are available at www.monitoringthe future.org.

Teen Marijuana Use Increases

Fueled by increases in marijuana use, the rate of 8th graders saying they have used an illicit drug in the past year jumped to 16%, up from last year's 14.5%, with daily marijuana use up in all grades surveyed, according to the 2010 Monitoring the Future Survey.

For 12th graders, declines in cigarette use accompanied by recent increases in marijuana use have put marijuana ahead of cigarette smoking by some measures. In 2010, 21.4% of high school seniors used marijuana in the past 30 days, while 19.2% smoked cigarettes.

The survey also shows significant increases in use of ecstasy. In addition, nonmedical use of prescription drugs remains high.

Most measures of marijuana use increased among 8th graders, and daily marijuana use increased significantly among all three grades. The 2010 use rates were 6.1% of high school seniors, 3.3% of 10th graders, and 1.2% of 8th graders compared to 2009 rates of 5.2%, 2.8%, and 1.0%, respectively.

"These high rates of marijuana use during the teen and pre-teen years, when the brain continues to develop, places our young people at particular risk," said NIDA director Nora D. Volkow, M.D. "Not only does marijuana affect learning, judgment, and motor skills, but research tells us that about one in six people who start using it as adolescents become addicted."

"The increases in youth drug use reflected in the Monitoring the Future Study are disappointing," said Gil Kerlikowske, director of the White House Office of National Drug Control Policy. "Mixed messages about drug legalization, particularly marijuana, may be to blame. Such messages certainly don't help parents who are trying to prevent kids from using drugs. The Obama administration is aggressively addressing the threat of drug use and its consequences through a balanced and comprehensive drug control strategy, but we need parents and other adults who influence children as full partners in teaching young people about the risks and harms associated with drug use, including marijuana."

The MTF survey also showed a significant increase in the reported use of MDMA, or ecstasy, with 2.4% of 8th graders citing past-year use, compared to 1.3% in 2009. Similarly, past-year MDMA use among 10th graders increased from 3.7% to 4.7% in 2010.

Also of concern is that the downward trend in cigarette smoking has stalled in all three grades after several years of marked improvement on most measures. Greater marketing of other forms of tobacco prompted the 2010 survey to add measures for 12th graders' use of small cigars (23.1%) and of tobacco with a smoking pipe known as a hookah (17.1%).

Prescription drug abuse remains a major problem. Although Vicodin abuse decreased in 12th graders this year to 8%, down from around 9.7% the past four years, other indicators confirm that nonmedical use of prescription drugs remains high. For example, the use of OxyContin, another prescription opiate, stayed about the same for 12th graders at 5.1% in 2010. And 6 of the top 10 illicit drugs abused by 12th graders in the year prior to the survey were prescribed or purchased over the counter. The survey again found that teens generally get these prescription drugs from friends and family, whether given, bought, or stolen.

However, the survey says binge drinking continued its downward trend. Among high school seniors, 23.2% report having five or more drinks in a row during the past two weeks, down from 25.2% in 2009 and from the peak of 31.5% in 1998. In addition, 2010 findings showed a drop in high school seniors' past-year consumption of flavored alcoholic beverages, to 47.9% in 2010 from 53.4% in 2009. Past-year use of flavored alcohol by 8th graders was at 21.9%, down from 27.9% in 2005.

The MTF survey also measures teen attitudes about drugs, including perceived harmfulness, perceived availability, and disapproval, all of which can predict future abuse. Related to its increased use, the perception that regular marijuana smoking is harmful decreased for 10th graders (down from 59.5% in 2009 to 57.2% in 2010) and 12th graders (from 52.4% in 2009 to 46.8% in 2010). Moreover, disapproval of smoking marijuana decreased significantly among 8th graders.

"We should examine the extent to which the debate over medical marijuana and marijuana legalization for adults is affecting teens' perceptions of risk," said Dr. Volkow. "We must also find better ways to communicate to teens that marijuana use can harm their short-term performance as well as their long-term potential."

Additional information on the MTF Survey, as well as comments from Dr. Volkow, can be found at www.drugabuse.gov/drugpages/MTF.html.

Section 9.5

Social Networking Increases Risk of Teen Drug Abuse

Excerpted from: The National Center on Addiction and Substance Abuse at Columbia University (CASAColumbia™). (2011). *National Survey of American Attitudes on Substance Abuse XVI: Teens and Parents.* New York: National Center on Addiction and Substance Abuse at Columbia University. © 2011. All rights reserved.

American teens ages 12–17 who in a typical day spend any time on social networking sites are at increased risk of smoking, drinking, and drug use, according to the *National Survey of American Attitudes on Substance Abuse XVI: Teens and Parents,* the 16th annual back-to-school survey conducted by The National Center on Addiction and Substance Abuse at Columbia University (CASA Columbia).

For the first time this year, the survey asked 12- to 17-year-olds whether they spend time on Facebook, MySpace, or other social networking sites in a typical day. Seventy percent of teens report spending time on social networking sites in a typical day compared to 30% of teens who say they do not. This means that 17 million 12- to 17-year-olds are social networking in a typical day.

Social Networking Teens at Increased Substance Abuse Risk

Compared to teens that spend no time on social networking sites in a typical day, teens that do are:

112

- five times likelier to use tobacco;
- three times likelier to use alcohol; and
- twice as likely to use marijuana.

Teen Substance Abuse Photos Rampant on Social Networking Sites

The CASA Columbia survey found that 40% of all teens surveyed have seen pictures on Facebook, Myspace, or other social networking sites of kids getting drunk, passed out, or using drugs. Half of teens who have seen pictures of kids drunk, passed out, or using drugs on Facebook and other social networking sites first saw such pictures when they were 13 years of age or younger; more than 90% first saw such pictures when they were 15 or younger.

Compared to teens that have never seen pictures of kids getting drunk, passed out, or using drugs on social networking sites, teens that have seen these images are:

- three times likelier to use alcohol;
- four times likelier to use marijuana;
- four times likelier to be able to get marijuana, almost three times likelier to be able to get controlled prescription drugs without a prescription, and more than twice as likely to be able to get alcohol in a day or less; and
- much likelier to have friends and classmates who abuse illegal and prescription drugs.

Teens Viewing Suggestive Teen Programming at Increased Substance Abuse Risk

This year's survey explored teen TV viewing habits in relation to teen substance abuse. One-third of teens (32%) watch teen reality shows like *Jersey Shore*, *Teen Mom*, or *16 and Pregnant* or teen dramas like *Skins* or *Gossip Girl* in a typical week.

Compared to teens who do not watch suggestive teen programming, teens who typically watch one or more such programs per week are:

- twice as likely to use tobacco;
- almost twice as likely to use alcohol;
- more than one-and-a-half times likelier to use marijuana;

113

- twice as likely to be able to get marijuana within a day or less; and

- more than one-and-a-half times likelier to be able to get prescription drugs without a prescription within a day or less.

"The relationship of social networking site images of kids drunk, passed out, or using drugs and of suggestive teen programming to increased teen risk of substance abuse offers grotesque confirmation of the adage that a picture is worth a thousand words," said Joseph A. Califano, Jr., CASA Columbia's founder and chairman and former U.S. secretary of health, education, and welfare. "The time has come for those who operate and profit from social networking sites like Facebook to deploy their technological expertise to curb such images and to deny use of their sites to children and teens who post pictures of themselves and their friends drunk, passed out, or using drugs. Continuing to provide the electronic vehicle for transmitting such images constitutes electronic child abuse."

Parental Perceptions Out of Touch with Reality

Eighty-seven percent of parents said they think spending time on social networking sites does not make it more likely their child will drink alcohol; 89% of parents felt it would not make their child more likely to use drugs.

Cyber Bullying and Substance Abuse

The CASA Columbia survey also found that 19% of teens ages 12–17 (more than 4.5 million teens) report being cyber bullied (having someone post mean or embarrassing things about them on a social networking site). Compared to teens who are not cyber bullied, teens who have been cyber bullied are more than twice as likely to use tobacco, alcohol, and marijuana.

"The anything goes, free-for-all world of Internet expression and suggestive television programming that teens are exposed to on a daily basis puts them at increased risk of substance abuse," said Califano. "The findings in this year's survey should strike Facebook fear into the hearts of parents of young children and drive home the need for parents to give their children the will and skill to keep their heads above the water of the corrupting cultural currents their children must navigate."

Other Key Findings Related to Teen Substance Abuse

Teens whose parents don't agree completely with each other on what to say to their teen about drug use are more than three times likelier to use marijuana, and three-and-a-half times likelier to expect to try drugs in the future, than teens whose parents agree completely on what to say about drug use.

Teens whose parents do not agree completely with each other on what to say to their teen about drinking alcohol are twice as likely to use alcohol than teens whose parents agree completely on what to say about drinking.

Teens who agreed with any of the following statements—"If a friend of mine uses illegal drugs, it's none of my business," "I should be able to do what I want with my own body," or "It's not a big deal to have sex with someone you don't care that much about"—are three times likelier to use marijuana, twice as likely to drink alcohol, and much more likely to smoke cigarettes, compared to teens who disagreed with the statements.

For the fifth straight year, more than 60% of high school students say they attend schools where drugs are used, kept, or sold on school grounds.

Forty-two percent of 12- to 17-year-olds report knowing at least one friend or classmate who uses illegal drugs, like acid, ecstasy, methamphetamine, cocaine, or heroin, a 24% increase since 2007.

CASA Columbia's back-to-school survey was conducted using two concurrent surveys. CASA Columbia used Knowledge Networks to do an Internet-based survey administered to a nationally representative sample of 1,037 teens (546 boys, 491 girls), and 528 of their parents, from March 27 to April 27, 2011. Sampling error is +/- 3.1 for teens and +/- 4.4 for parents. As in the past, CASA Columbia used QEV Analytics to do a survey of trend questions at home by telephone which was administered to a nationally representative sample of 1,006 teens (478 boys, 528 girls) from March 29 to May 9, 2011. Sampling error is +/- 3.1.

Chapter 10

Drug Use among College Students

The Size and Shape of the Problem

From 1993 to 2005, there has been no significant reduction in the levels of drinking and binge drinking among college students. In 2005, 67.9% of students (approximately 5.3 million students) reported drinking in the past month and 40.1% (approximately 3.1 million students) reported binge drinking. However, from 1993 to 2001 rates of riskier drinking—frequent binge drinking, being intoxicated, drinking to get drunk—have increased.

The proportion of students reporting frequent binge drinking increased 15.7% (from 19.7% to 22.8%). Other indicators of increased risky drinking showed even greater increases over that period: a 24.9% increase in drinking on 10 or more occasions in the past month (18.1% to 22.6%); a 25.6% increase in being intoxicated three or more times in the past month (23.4% to 29.4%); and a 20.8% increase in drinking for the purpose of getting drunk in the past month (39.9% to 48.2%).

Between 1993 and 2005, there has been a 342.9% increase in the proportion of students abusing prescription opioids like Percocet, Vicodin, and OxyContin in the past month (0.7% to 3.1%, approximately 240,000 students); a 93.3% increase in those abusing prescription

Excerpted from: The National Center on Addiction and Substance Abuse at Columbia University (CASAColumbia™). (2007). *Wasting the best and the brightest: Substance abuse at America's colleges and universities.* New York: National Center on Addiction and Substance Abuse at Columbia University. © 2007. All rights reserved. Reviewed by David A. Cooke, MD, FACP, July 2013.

stimulants like Ritalin and Adderall (1.5% to 2.9%, approximately 225,000 students); a 450% increase in those abusing prescription tranquilizers like Xanax and Valium (0.4% to 2.2%, approximately 170,000 students); and a 225% increase in those abusing prescription sedatives like Nembutal and Seconal (0.4% to 1.3%, approximately 101,000 students).

Between 1993 and 2005, the proportion of students using illicit drugs other than marijuana in the past month increased 51.9% from 5.4% to 8.2% (approximately 636,000 students). The proportion of students who are daily marijuana users increased 110.5%, from 1.9% to 4.0% (approximately 310,000 students).

During the 1993 to 2005 period, smoking among college students rose and then leveled off at about the same rates as they were a decade ago. More than 1.8 million full-time college students still are current smokers. One positive note is that reported rates of daily smoking (15.2% in 1993, 12.4% in 2005, approximately 960,000 students) and daily heavy smoking (8.9% in 1993, 6.7% in 2005, approximately 520,000 students) showed declines.

In 2005, 69.0% or 5.4 million full-time college students reported drinking, abusing controlled prescription drugs, using illicit drugs, or smoking in the past month; 49.4% or 3.8 million reported binge drinking, abusing controlled prescription drugs, or using illicit drugs in the past month. Almost one-half (45% or 2.3 million) of those who drink engage in two or more other forms of substance use (binge drinking, illicit drug use, prescription drug abuse, or smoking).

Gender

When definitions of binge drinking are adjusted for differences in female physiology, virtually the same proportion of male and female students binge drink on a typical drinking occasion. The relative increase between 1993 and 2001 in frequent binge drinking, being drunk three or more times, and drinking on 10 or more occasions in the past 30 days was greater for college women than it was for college men. Rates of controlled prescription drug abuse and illicit drug use increased more sharply for college men than for college women between 1993 and 2005. College women are somewhat likelier than college men to be daily smokers and daily heavy smokers.

Race and Ethnicity

White students are likelier to use and abuse all forms of drugs than are minority students. Students attending historically black colleges and universities (HBCUs)—regardless of their race/ethnicity—use all forms of substances at much lower rates than other students.

The Consequences

The harmful consequences linked to college student substance abuse are on the rise. There is no one data source for these consequences so CASA [National Center on Addiction and Substance Abuse] has assembled the best and most up-to-date information available from a variety of sources.

Between 1993 and 2001, there has been a 37.6% increase in the proportion of college students hurt or injured as a result of their alcohol use (9.3% vs. 12.8%). In 2001, 1,717 college students died from unintentional alcohol-related injuries—up 6% from 1998.

Compared to 22 other countries, college students in the U.S. who drive have the highest rate of drinking and driving (50% of male drinkers and 35% of female drinkers). In 1993, 26.6% of college students drove under the influence of alcohol; in 2001 29% did so.

The average number of alcohol-related arrests per campus increased 21% between 2001 and 2005. In 2005, alcohol-related arrests constituted 83% of campus arrests.

When drunk or high, college students are more likely to be sexually active and to have sex with someone they just met. More than three-fourths (78%) of college students who have used illicit drugs have had sexual intercourse compared to 44% of those who never used drugs. In 1993, 19.2% of college students who used alcohol in the past year reported engaging in alcohol-related unplanned sexual activity; in 2001, 21.3% of student drinkers did so.

The most common secondary effects of college student drinking are property damage and vandalism, fights, rape and other sexual violence, and disruption to other students' quality of life. Financial costs include damage to campus property, increase in security staff and counselors, lost tuition from dropouts, and legal costs of suits against the college for liability. Residents living within a mile of college campuses report more incidents of public drunkenness, drug use, crime, vandalism, and loitering than those living more than a mile away.

Young people who report current alcohol use give significantly lower ratings of their own health than do alcohol abstainers or past users. Depression, anxiety, and personality disturbances in young adulthood are associated with marijuana and other illicit drug use during the teen years. In recent years, there has been a sharp increase in the number of students in need of mental health services. Young smokers are three times more likely than nonsmokers to have consulted a doctor or mental health professional because of emotional or psychological problems and almost twice as likely to develop symptoms of depression.

College students who report seriously having considered attempting suicide in the past 12 months are likelier than other students to engage in current binge drinking (41.9% vs. 39.6%), marijuana use (23.2% vs. 16.1%), other illicit drug use (6.7% vs. 2.8%), and smoking (31.9% vs. 19.9%), even after taking into consideration age, gender, and race.

Student drinking and drug use are linked to lower grade point averages (GPA). Drinking impairs learning, memory, abstract thinking, problem solving, and perceptual motor skills (such as eye-hand coordination). More than 5% of binge-drinking students report having been suspended; 50.6% have gotten behind in their schoolwork and 68.1% report missing classes. Alcohol and drug law violations by students also can mar their academic and legal records, compromising their career options.

Almost one in four (22.9% or 1.8 million) full-time college students already meet the DSM-IV diagnostic criteria for alcohol and/or drug abuse (12.3% for alcohol abuse; 2.5% for drug abuse) or alcohol and/or drug dependence (7.7% for alcohol dependence, 4.7% for drug dependence) in the past year. This is compared to less than one in 10 (8.5%) in the general population who meet the DSM-IV diagnostic criteria for alcohol and/or drug abuse or dependence.

Nonsmokers exposed to secondhand smoke are at a 25% to 30% increased risk of developing heart disease and at a 20% to 30% increased risk of developing lung cancer.

Chapter 11

Substance Abuse Issues of Concern to Women

Chapter Contents

Section 11.1

Women's and Girls' Use of Illicit Drugs

"Women, Girls, Families, and Substance Abuse" and excerpts from
"Women and Treatment," White House Office of National Drug Control
Policy (www.whitehouse.gov/ondcp), accessed March 19, 2013.

Women, Girls, Families, and Substance Abuse

Certain risk factors may make the female population vulnerable
to substance abuse. A three-year study on women and young girls
(aged 8–22) revealed that girls and young women use substances for
different reasons than boys and young men. The study found that risk
factors such as low self-esteem, peer pressure, and depression make
girls and young women more vulnerable to substance use as well as
addiction, in that females become dependent faster and suffer the
consequences sooner, compared to males (National Center on Addiction
and Substance Abuse at Columbia University, *The Formative Years:
Pathways to Substance Abuse Among Girls and Young Women Ages
8–22*, February 2003).

Substance use is a growing problem among females. The 2009 National Survey on Drug Use and Health (NSDUH) reported that approximately 6.6% of women aged 12 and older reported past-month
use of an illicit drug (Substance Abuse and Mental Health Services Administration, *2009 National Survey on Drug Use and Health (NSDUH)*,
September 2010).

Women in the criminal justice system display an even higher rate of
substance use. According to data from the Bureau of Justice Statistics,
approximately 59.3% of state and 47.6% of federal female prisoners
surveyed in 2004 indicated that they had used drugs in the month prior
to their offense. Additionally, approximately 60.2% of state and 42.8%
of federal female prisoners surveyed in 2004 met drug dependence or
abuse criteria.

Women and Treatment

With the rising prevalence of female substance abuse, more women
are in need of treatment. In 2007, 32.3% of the approximately 1.8

million admissions to drug/alcohol treatment in the U.S. were female admissions. Because women are more likely to be victims of physical or sexual abuse, which contribute to drug and alcohol abuse, depression, and criminal activity, there is a growing need for more gender-specific substance use treatment services for women. Effective substance abuse prevention and treatment for girls and women requires crafting programs to address the specific risks and consequences of substance use that are more frequently associated with females.

The *2011 National Drug Control Strategy* acknowledges the high substance abuse rate of females and works to reverse this trend. The *Strategy* specifically stresses the need to create more treatment centers that address female-specific challenges. Seeking treatment for drug addiction poses hurdles specific to women because many treatment programs are designed for and used mostly by men, and many women must weigh competing family concerns against the need for substance abuse treatment.

As many traditional treatment programs do not allow for the inclusion of children, a woman may be torn between the need to care for her dependent children and the need for treatment. Involvement with the child welfare system also complicates a woman's decision to seek care, because admitting to a substance abuse problem may lead to involvement with the criminal justice system and/or the loss of custody of children. This must change; women should not feel torn between seeking treatment and caring for their families. There are many model family-based treatment programs around the country that prove families do not need to be separated in order for them to achieve success in treatment and recovery.

The Office of National Drug Control Policy (ONDCP) is also committed to working with our interagency partners, both through the Interagency Working Groups established by our office and through external partnerships, to address the needs of dependent women and their children. ONDCP supports interventions that are gender responsive and trauma informed, including sentencing alternatives to incarceration, expansion of family-based treatment, improved conditions of maternal incarceration, and increased support for programming focused on parent-child relationships during a mother's sentence.

Prevention for Teens—National Media Campaign

ONDCP's National Youth Anti-Drug Media Campaign utilizes a blend of paid advertising and public communications in its brand, Above the Influence, which empowers all teens to reject drugs and any other negative influence in their lives. By embracing challenges that more frequently affect teen girls, the Media Campaign facilitates healthy decisions to reject drugs. The Above the Influence messaging highlights short-term and long-term social and health consequences, has national reach, involves multiple channels, and engages teen girls in print, television, radio, and online messaging.

Section 11.2

What Women Need to Know about Date Rape Drugs

"Date Rape Drugs Fact Sheet," U.S. Department of Health and Human Services Office on Women's Health (www.womenshealth.gov), December 5, 2008. Reviewed by David A. Cooke, MD, FACP, July 2013.

What are date rape drugs?

These are drugs that are sometimes used to assist a sexual assault. Sexual assault is any type of sexual activity that a person does not agree to. It can include touching that is not okay, putting something into the vagina, sexual intercourse, rape, and attempted rape. These drugs are powerful and dangerous. They can be slipped into your drink when you are not looking. The drugs often have no color, smell, or taste, so you can't tell if you are being drugged. The drugs can make you become weak and confused—or even pass out—so that you are unable to refuse sex or defend yourself. If you are drugged, you might not remember what happened while you were drugged. Date rape drugs are used on both females and males.

The three most common date rape drugs are the following:

- **Rohypnol:** The trade name for flunitrazepam (abuse of two similar drugs appears to have replaced Rohypnol abuse in some parts of the United States; these are clonazepam—marketed as Klonopin in the U.S. and Rivotril in Mexico—and alprazolam— marketed as Xanax)

- **GHB:** Short for gamma hydroxybutyric acid

• **Ketamine**

These drugs also are known as "club drugs" because they tend to be used at dance clubs, concerts, and "raves."

The term "date rape" is widely used. But most experts prefer the term "drug-facilitated sexual assault." These drugs also are used to help people commit other crimes, like robbery and physical assault. They are used on both men and women. The term "date rape" also can be misleading because the person who commits the crime might not be dating the victim. Rather, it could be an acquaintance or stranger.

What do the drugs look like?

Rohypnol comes as a pill that dissolves in liquids. Some are small, round, and white. Newer pills are oval and green-gray in color. When slipped into a drink, a dye in these new pills makes clear liquids turn bright blue and dark drinks turn cloudy. But this color change might be hard to see in a dark drink, like cola or dark beer, or in a dark room. Also, the pills with no dye are still available. The pills may be ground up into a powder.

GHB has a few forms: a liquid with no odor or color, white powder, and pill. It might give your drink a slightly salty taste. Mixing it with a sweet drink, such as fruit juice, can mask the salty taste.

Ketamine comes as a liquid and a white powder.

What effects do these drugs have on the body?

These drugs are very powerful. They can affect you very quickly and without your knowing. The length of time that the effects last varies. It depends on how much of the drug is taken and if the drug is mixed with other drugs or alcohol. Alcohol makes the drugs even stronger and can cause serious health problems—even death.

Rohypnol: The effects of Rohypnol can be felt within 30 minutes of being drugged and can last for several hours. If you are drugged, you might look and act like someone who is drunk. You might have trouble standing. Your speech might be slurred. Or you might pass out. Rohypnol can cause these problems:

• Muscle relaxation or loss of muscle control

• Difficulty with motor movements

• Drunk feeling

• Problems talking

- Nausea
- Can't remember what happened while drugged
- Loss of consciousness (black out)
- Confusion
- Problems seeing
- Dizziness
- Sleepiness
- Lower blood pressure
- Stomach problems
- Death

GHB: GHB takes effect in about 15 minutes and can last three to four hours. It is very potent: a very small amount can have a big effect. So it's easy to overdose on GHB. Most GHB is made by people in home or street "labs." So, you don't know what's in it or how it will affect you. GHB can cause these problems:

- Relaxation
- Drowsiness
- Dizziness
- Nausea
- Problems seeing
- Loss of consciousness (black out)
- Seizures
- Can't remember what happened while drugged
- Problems breathing
- Tremors
- Sweating
- Vomiting
- Slow heart rate
- Dream-like feeling
- Coma
- Death

Ketamine: Ketamine is very fast-acting. You might be aware of what is happening to you, but unable to move. It also causes memory problems. Later, you might not be able to remember what happened while you were drugged. Ketamine can cause these problems:

- Distorted perceptions of sight and sound

- Lost sense of time and identity

- Out of body experiences

- Dream-like feeling

- Feeling out of control

- Impaired motor function

- Problems breathing

- Convulsions

- Vomiting

- Memory problems

- Numbness

- Loss of coordination

- Aggressive or violent behavior

- Depression

- High blood pressure

- Slurred speech

Are these drugs legal in the United States?

Some of these drugs are legal when lawfully used for medical purposes. But that doesn't mean they are safe. These drugs are powerful and can hurt you. They should only be used under a doctor's care and order.

- Rohypnol is not legal in the United States. It is legal in Europe and Mexico, where it is prescribed for sleep problems and to assist anesthesia before surgery. It is brought into the United States illegally.

- Ketamine is legal in the United States for use as an anesthetic for humans and animals. It is mostly used on animals. Veterinary clinics are robbed for their ketamine supplies.

- GHB was recently made legal in the United States to treat problems from narcolepsy (a sleep disorder). Distribution of GHB for this purpose is tightly restricted.

Is alcohol a date rape drug? What about other drugs?

Any drug that can affect judgment and behavior can put a person at risk for unwanted or risky sexual activity. Alcohol is one such drug. In fact, alcohol is the drug most commonly used to help commit sexual assault.

The club drug "ecstasy" (MDMA) has been used to commit sexual assault. It can be slipped into someone's drink without the person's knowledge. Also, a person who willingly takes ecstasy is at greater risk of sexual assault. Ecstasy can make a person feel "lovey-dovey" toward others. It also can lower a person's ability to give reasoned consent. Once under the drug's influence, a person is less able to sense danger or to resist a sexual assault.

Even if a victim of sexual assault drank alcohol or willingly took drugs, the victim is not at fault for being assaulted. You cannot "ask for it" or cause it to happen.

How can I protect myself from being a victim?

- Don't accept drinks from other people.

- Open containers yourself.

- Keep your drink with you at all times, even when you go to the bathroom.

- Don't share drinks.

- Don't drink from punch bowls or other common, open containers. They may already have drugs in them.

- If someone offers to get you a drink from a bar or at a party, go with the person to order your drink. Watch the drink being poured and carry it yourself.

- Don't drink anything that tastes or smells strange. Sometimes, GHB tastes salty.

- Have a nondrinking friend with you to make sure nothing happens.

- If you realize you left your drink unattended, pour it out.

- If you feel drunk and haven't drunk any alcohol—or, if you feel like the effects of drinking alcohol are stronger than usual—get help right away.

Are there ways to tell if I might have been drugged and raped?

It is often hard to tell. Most victims don't remember being drugged or assaulted. The victim might not be aware of the attack until 8 or 12 hours after it occurred. These drugs also leave the body very quickly. Once a victim gets help, there might be no proof that drugs were involved in the attack. But there are some signs that you might have been drugged:

- You feel drunk and haven't drunk any alcohol—or, you feel like the effects of drinking alcohol are stronger than usual.

- You wake up feeling very hung over and disoriented or having no memory of a period of time.

- You remember having a drink, but cannot recall anything after that.

- You find that your clothes are torn or not on right.

- You feel like you had sex, but you cannot remember it.

What should I do if I think I've been drugged and raped?

- Get medical care right away. Call 911 or have a trusted friend take you to a hospital emergency room. Don't urinate, douche, bathe, brush your teeth, wash your hands, change clothes, or eat or drink before you go. These things may give evidence of the rape. The hospital will use a "rape kit" to collect evidence.

- Call the police from the hospital. Tell the police exactly what you remember. Be honest about all your activities. Remember, nothing you did—including drinking alcohol or doing drugs—can justify rape.

- Ask the hospital to take a urine (pee) sample that can be used to test for date rape drugs. The drugs leave your system quickly. Rohypnol stays in the body for several hours and can be detected in the urine up to 72 hours after taking it. GHB leaves the body in 12 hours. Don't urinate before going to the hospital.

- Don't pick up or clean up where you think the assault might have occurred. There could be evidence left behind—such as on a drinking glass or bed sheets.

- Get counseling and treatment. Feelings of shame, guilt, fear, and shock are normal. A counselor can help you work through these emotions and begin the healing process. Calling a crisis center or a hotline is a good place to start. One national hotline is the National Sexual Assault Hotline at 800-656-HOPE.

Chapter 12

Drug Use and Socioeconomic Status

Chapter Contents

Section 12.1

Substance Use and Treatment among People Living in Poverty

Excerpted from "The NSDUH Report: Substance Use Treatment Need and Receipt among People Living in Poverty," Substance Abuse and Mental Health Services Administration (www.samhsa.gov), January 14, 2010.

- Combined 2006 to 2008 data indicate that 3.7 million persons aged 12 or older living in poverty were in need of substance use treatment in the past year; of these, 17.9% received treatment at a specialty facility during this time period.

- Males living in poverty were nearly twice as likely as their female counterparts to have been in need of substance use treatment in the past year (17.1% vs. 8.9%), but males who needed treatment were as likely as their female counterparts to have received treatment.

- Among persons living in poverty, those aged 18 to 25 had the highest rate of past-year treatment need; however, this age group had the lowest rate of treatment receipt.

Substance use disorders affect people in all economic circumstances, and all face challenges in trying to overcome these disorders. The difficulties faced by persons living in poverty, however, may be even more formidable as they may lack health insurance coverage. Considering that the number of people living in poverty has increased for three consecutive years—reaching a near record high of 39.8 million in 2008—understanding the gap between service needs and service receipt may help policy makers and program managers ensure that the gap does not widen in the future.

Characteristics of Persons in Poverty

An annual average of 12.2% of persons aged 12 or older—an estimated 30.0 million persons—were living in poverty. Females comprised 58.4% of the persons living in poverty compared with 51.5% of the total household population. In addition, persons living in poverty tended to be younger than those in the total population; persons aged 12 to 34 accounted for 55.0% of persons in poverty compared with 37.4% of the overall household population.

About two-fifths (42.3%) of those living in poverty were white, 26.7% were Hispanic, and 23.8% were black. By comparison, 68.1% of the total U.S. household population were white, 13.8% were Hispanic, and 11.8% were black. Nearly one in three (30.6%) persons living in poverty were without health insurance coverage compared with about one in seven (14.5%) of the total household population.

Treatment Need

Among individuals aged 12 or older living in poverty, 12.3% (3.7 million persons) were classified as being in need of substance use treatment in the past year. The need for substance use treatment varied by demographic characteristics. Males living in poverty were nearly twice as likely as their female counterparts to have been in need of treatment (17.1% vs. 8.9%). Among persons living in poverty, those aged 18 to 25 had a higher rate of treatment need than those in any of the other age groups. Need for treatment also varied by race/ethnicity among those living in poverty, ranging from 21.6% among American Indians or Alaska Natives to 6.3% among Asians.

Among persons living in poverty, those with no health insurance coverage were more likely than those with coverage to have been in need of substance use treatment in the past year (14.9% vs. 11.2%). An estimated 1.4 million persons living in poverty and with no health insurance coverage were in need of treatment.

Treatment Receipt

Of the persons living in poverty who were in need of substance use treatment in the past year, 17.9% (an estimated 663,000 persons) received treatment at a specialty facility during this time period. Nearly one-third (30.8%) of persons aged 35 to 49 living in poverty and in need of treatment received it compared with one-quarter of their counterparts aged 26 to 34 (23.1%) and less than one-tenth of young adults aged 18 to 25 and adolescents aged 12 to 17 (8.7% and 9.3%, respectively). There were no statistically significant differences in receipt of treatment by gender or health insurance coverage.

Discussion

Thirty million Americans aged 12 or older are living in poverty, and for some, their financial challenges are made even more difficult because of substance use problems. The data in this report indicate that there is a substantial unmet need for substance use treatment among individuals living in poverty, particularly among young adults and adolescents. Addressing the substance use treatment needs of individuals living in poverty may result in increases in economic sufficiency and employment, while decreasing health care costs and other adverse factors associated with substance use disorders (e.g., unintentional injuries, incarceration, and physical and mental health problems). Similarly, assessing needs for ancillary services, from basic subsistence needs to job hunting and placement, must be considered as essential components of the pathway to achieving recovery and sustaining resilience.

Section 12.2

High Socioeconomic Status Also a Risk Factor for Substance Abuse

Humensky, J. Are adolescents with high socioeconomic status more likely to engage in alcohol and illicit drug use in early adulthood? *Substance Abuse Treatment, Prevention, and Policy.* 2010 5:19. © 2010 Humensky; licensee BioMed Central Ltd. This is an Open Access article distributed under the terms of the Creative Commons Attribution License (http://creativecommons.org/licenses/by/3.0).

Background

Previous literature has shown a divergence by age in the relationship between socioeconomic status (SES) and substance use: adolescents with low SES are more likely to engage in substance use, as are adults with high SES. However, there is growing evidence that adolescents with high SES are also at high risk for substance abuse. The objective of this study is to examine this relationship longitudinally, that is, whether wealthier adolescents are more likely than those with lower SES to engage in substance use in early adulthood. The study analyzed data from the National Longitudinal Survey of Adolescent Health (AddHealth), a longitudinal, nationally representative survey of secondary school students in the United States.

Discussion

The results from this study indicate that higher SES in adolescence, as measured by parental education and household income in adolescence, is associated with higher rates of substance use, particularly binge drinking, marijuana use, and cocaine use, in early adulthood. No statistically significant results were found for crystal methamphetamine or other drug use. Results were consistent when controlling for college attendance by young adulthood as a sensitivity analysis.

Previous literature has shown that the relationships between SES and substance use vary by age. The results in this study are somewhat contrary to previous literature in youth which has shown that lower SES is associated with higher rates of substance use problems. However, the results of this study are consistent with previous research in adults, which found that demand for illicit substances is price sensitive, and thus predicts that substance use will increase as income is higher. This therefore indicates that the behavior of young adults more closely reflects that of adults rather than that of youth. The results are also consistent with Bellis and colleagues ["Predictors of Risky Alcohol Consumption in Schoolchildren and Their Implications for Preventing Alcohol-Related Harm," *Substance Abuse Treatment, Prevention and Policy*, 2007], who found that adolescents with more spending money reported greater substance use and with Martin and colleagues ["The Role of Monthly Spending Money in College Student Drinking Behaviors and their Consequences," *Journal of American College Health*, 2009], who found that college students with more spending money engaged in greater alcohol use. This study provides additional evidence for these earlier findings in a longitudinal, nationally representative sample of adolescents in the United States, and in illicit substances in addition to alcohol use. In addition, it is possible that parental education may have a distinct influence on subsequent college attendance by the adolescent, distinct from general socioeconomic status. Parents with higher education may have a greater influence on their adolescent's choice to attend college, as the intergenerational transfer of education has been well-established in previous literature. It is possible that this college attendance could in turn provide greater opportunities for substance use. However, the relationships observed in this study were found for both measures of SES, parental education and household income, indicating that these relationships were consistent across measures and not limited to parental education.

Several limitations to this study must be noted. AddHealth is an observational study, not a randomized control trial, thus causality is difficult to establish with certainty. However, the longitudinal nature of this analysis helps somewhat to address this issue. Sample loss due to attrition and item non-response is also problematic. Additionally, the outcome variables measure self-reported substance use, rather than clinically diagnosed substance abuse or dependence. It should be noted that AddHealth is a nationally representative sample of U.S. secondary school students at the time of data collection and thus does not capture adolescents who are not enrolled in school. It also does not offer extensive data on early childhood, as data collection begins when participants are in grades 7–12.

Despite its limitations, the AddHealth data allows for a longitudinal analysis of the relationship between SES in adolescence and subsequent substance use in early adulthood. The richness of the AddHealth data allows for the consideration of a number of facets of SES and use of a wide range of substances. It also includes a large set of individual, family, school, and community characteristics assessed at baseline, including substance use and mental health at baseline.

Conclusions

This study examines the relationship between adolescent SES and subsequent substance use in early adulthood. The association varies somewhat by the type of substance used. Higher adolescent SES, as measured by parental education and household income in adolescence, is associated with higher rates of binge drinking, marijuana, and cocaine use in early adulthood. No statistically significant results were found for crystal methamphetamine or other drug use.

Previous research has shown that substance use can lead to numerous problems for young adults, including difficulties in school, in the labor market, and in the criminal justice system. As much of the previous scientific literature often focuses on substance abuse in lower SES populations, it is possible that teachers and school administrators in wealthier schools may be less likely to recognize the need for substance abuse treatment programs, if the current policy focus is on lower SES populations. Likewise, administrators of drug abuse prevention programs may be less likely to focus their efforts in higher-income areas. This study offers evidence that wealthier students may be at risk for substance use problems in the future, particularly for binge drinking, marijuana, and cocaine use. As previous evidence shows that students with more spending money might be more likely to engage in substance use into adulthood, access to allowances and other forms of spending money may be issues that parents can address if they are concerned with the possibility of substance abuse among their children. School administrators seeking to identify substance use education policies in their schools can find a listing of programs shown to be effective on the website for the National Institute on Drug Abuse (NIDA) [at www .nida.nih.gov/prevention/examples.html]. Examining the substance abuse problems facing students with higher SES can help teachers, school administrators, and parents recognize the needs that may be present in their schools and communities, and the need for programs to effectively address substance use.

Chapter 13

Substance
Abuse in the Workplace

The majority of people with substance use and mental disorders are employed. In fact, of the 20.8 million adults aged 18 or older classified with substance use dependence or abuse, 70% were employed full or part time. In addition, depression—the most common mental health problem in the workplace—affects about 1 in 10 employees. These problems are medical conditions that if left untreated or undertreated can affect individual employees as well as entire businesses. By increasing access to treatment and recovery support services, employers will reap the following benefits:

- Improve employee health

- Lower health care costs

- Reduce absenteeism

- Reduce the risk of injury

- Improve job performance and productivity

Education, Awareness, and Support in the Workplace

Employee education, awareness, and support campaigns are effective in preventing problems both in and out of the workplace. Prevention, treatment, and wellness programs incorporate several

Excerpted from "2012 Toolkit: Addressing Substance Use and Mental Disorders in the Workplace," Substance Abuse and Mental Health Services Administration, National Recovery Month (www.recoverymonth.gov), 2012.

components, including substance use and mental health awareness, assessment of risk, brief screenings, drug testing, intervention, treatment, recovery support, and assistance back into the workforce for employees, families, and their communities. Through its Public Awareness and Recovery Support Strategic Initiatives, the Substance Abuse and Mental Health Services Administration (SAMHSA) increases the understanding of substance use and mental health prevention and treatment services and attempts to educate all individuals that recovery is much more than just abstinence from substance use or a reduction in symptoms of a mental health problem. True recovery means that individuals can live a quality, self-directed, satisfying life in the community, which includes good health, a home, and a purpose.

Prevention, treatment, and wellness programs can be provided in or out of the workplace. They are designed to inform employees about the importance of addressing mental health problems at work and at home and educating them about risks associated with substance misuse and the impact of alcohol and/or drug use on their family and co-workers. Through these programs, employers can promote healthy lifestyles and reinforce the following positive messages to their employees:

- Drug-free workplace policies protect the health and safety of all employees, customers, and the public. They also safeguard employer assets from theft and destruction and maintain product quality and company integrity and reputation.

- By effectively addressing substance use and mental disorders, employers can see benefits such as improved employee morale, quality of work, employee satisfaction, and decision making, as well as reduced absenteeism and tardiness.

- Implementing exercise programs and other health-oriented activities can help improve physical and emotional health issues among employees, such as weight problems, high blood pressure, diabetes, depression, or gastric problems, and can help reduce stress.

- In short, prevention works, treatment is effective, and people do recover from substance use and mental disorders while contributing to their jobs.

Prevalence of Substance Use and Mental Disorders in the Workplace

Use of substances may occur both on and off the job, equally affecting one's overall health, well-being, and work performance. According to a national survey, in the course of a year, more than 2 million people used illicit drugs during work hours, and approximately 3 million workers used an illicit drug within two hours of reporting to work. Additionally, 7% of Americans used alcohol during the workday, and 9% of Americans claimed they had worked "hungover," experiencing the physical effects following the heavy use of alcohol, ultimately affecting their work performance. The following occupations have the highest rate of reported substance use:

- Construction workers

- Sales personnel

- Restaurant workers

- Transportation and material movers

High-paying occupations and positions, including company directors, military personnel, lawyers, police officers, and doctors, also have high alcohol and drug consumption rates.

Mental health problems, such as depression or anxiety, also have a significant impact on the workplace. For example, depression, the most common mental health problem in the workplace, affects nearly 1 in 10 employees. It's estimated that 72% of people in the workforce who have depression are not properly diagnosed, causing over $63 billion lost annually due to decreased productivity. When left untreated, these health conditions can affect performance, resulting in a loss of productivity and absenteeism.

In addition, mental health problems contribute to more work impairment and absences than other chronic health conditions such as diabetes, asthma, arthritis, back pain, hypertension, and heart disease. Prevention, awareness, and support campaigns in and out of the workplace are essential to combat these treatable, yet common, public health problems. Outpatient programs that treat mental health problems can produce savings for employers; research has shown that after three weeks of treatment, work impairment was cut nearly in half, from 31% to 18% for employees with mental health problems.

Contributing Factors to Substance Use and Mental Disorders in the Workplace

Occupational, personal, and social factors play a role in increased substance use and mental disorders in and outside the workplace.

- Job responsibilities that are high stress or have low satisfaction, long or irregular shifts, repetitive duties, or inconsistent supervision are common elements that may contribute to increased substance use and mental disorders.

- Personal stressors such as illness, death in the family, marital strain, financial problems, internal conflicts, emotional or physical abuse, and trauma are common troubles that can contribute to increased alcohol and/or drug use and can affect one's everyday work.

- Economic worries, including increased unemployment, foreclosures, loss of investments, and other financial distress can cause mental health problems such as depression, anxiety, and compulsive behaviors, as well as substance misuse.

The following signs may be present in employees who are dealing with these personal or work issues, which can contribute to substance use and mental disorders:

- Lack of attention to job tasks

- Increased work absences and on-the-job accidents

- Inconsistent work quality or work not up to its usual standards

- Disregarded work safety procedures

- Extended lunch breaks, late arrivals, or early departures

One-fourth of employees view their jobs as the number one stressor in their lives. While nearly one-half of large companies in the United States provide some type of stress management training, all employers should work with their employees to reduce and manage any stress and establish EAPs (employee assistance programs) so that employees become familiar with prevention and referral programs available to them. Employers should encourage employees and company leaders to brainstorm and apply positive ways to help prevent problems of substance use and mental disorders within the workplace.

Chapter 14

Drug Abuse in Other Populations

Chapter Contents

Section 14.1

Veterans and Drug Abuse

"DrugFacts: Substance Abuse in the Military," National Institute on Drug Abuse (www.drugabuse.gov), March 2013, and excerpts from "Address Mental and/or Substance Use Disorders among Active Military, Veterans, and Their Families," Substance Abuse and Mental Health Services Administration, Recovery Month (www.recoverymonth.gov), September 2012.

Substance Abuse in the Military

Members of the armed forces are not immune to the substance use problems that affect the rest of society. Although illicit drug use is lower among U.S. military personnel than among civilians, heavy alcohol and tobacco use, and especially prescription drug abuse, are much more prevalent and are on the rise.

The stresses of deployment during wartime and the unique culture of the military account for some of these differences. Zero-tolerance policies and stigma pose difficulties in identifying and treating substance use problems in military personnel, as does lack of confidentiality that deters many who need treatment from seeking it.

Those with multiple deployments and combat exposure are at greatest risk of developing substance use problems. They are more apt to engage in new-onset heavy weekly drinking and binge drinking, to suffer alcohol- and other drug-related problems, and to have greater prescribed use of behavioral health medications. They are also more likely to start smoking or relapse to smoking.

Illicit and Prescription Drugs

According to the 2008 Department of Defense (DoD) Survey of Health Related Behaviors among Active Duty Military Personnel, just 2.3% of military personnel were past-month users of an illicit drug, compared with 12% of civilians. Among those age 18–25 (who are most likely to use drugs), the rate among military personnel was 3.9%, compared with 17.2% among civilians.

A policy of zero tolerance for drug use among DoD personnel is likely one reason why illicit drug use has remained at a low level in the military for two decades. The policy was instituted in 1982 and is currently enforced by frequent random drug testing; service members face dishonorable discharge and even criminal prosecution for a positive drug test.

However, in spite of the low level of illicit drug use, abuse of prescription drugs is higher among service members than among civilians and is on the increase. In 2008, 11% of service members reported misusing prescription drugs, up from 2% in 2002 and 4% in 2005. Most of the prescription drugs misused by service members are opioid pain medications.

Mental Health Problems in Returning Veterans

Service members may carry the psychological and physical wounds of their military experience with them into subsequent civilian life. In one study, one in four veterans returning from Iraq and Afghanistan reported symptoms of a mental or cognitive disorder; one in six reported symptoms of posttraumatic stress disorder (PTSD). These disorders are strongly associated with substance abuse and dependence, as are other problems experienced by returning military personnel, including sleep disturbances, traumatic brain injury, and violence in relationships.

Young adult veterans are particularly likely to have substance use or other mental health problems. According to a report of veterans in 2004–2006, a quarter of 18- to 25-year-old veterans met criteria for a past-year substance use disorder, which is more than double the rate of veterans aged 26–54 and five times the rate of veterans 55 or older.

The greater availability of these medications and increases in prescriptions for them may contribute to their growing misuse by service members. Pain reliever prescriptions written by military physicians quadrupled between 2001 and 2009—to almost 3.8 million. Combat-related injuries and the strains from carrying heavy equipment during multiple deployments likely play a role in this trend.

Drinking and Smoking

Alcohol use is also higher among men and women in military service than among civilians. Almost half of active duty service members (47%) reported binge drinking in 2008—up from 35% in 1998. In 2008, 20% of military personnel reported binge drinking every week in the past month; the rate was considerably higher—27%—among those with high combat exposure.

In 2008, 30% of all service members were current cigarette smokers—comparable to the rate for civilians (29%). However, as with alcohol use, smoking rates are significantly higher among personnel who have been exposed to combat.

Suicides and Substance Use

Suicide rates in the military were traditionally lower than among civilians in the same age range, but in 2004 the suicide rate in the U.S. Army began to climb, surpassing the civilian rate in 2008. Substance use is involved in many of these suicides. The 2010 report of the Army Suicide Prevention Task Force found that 29% of active duty Army suicides from fiscal year (FY) 2005 to FY 2009 involved alcohol or drug use; and in 2009, prescription drugs were involved in almost one-third of them.

Addressing the Problem

A 2012 report prepared for the DoD by the Institute of Medicine (IOM Report) recommended ways of addressing the problem of substance use in the military, including increasing the use of evidence-based prevention and treatment interventions and expanding access to care. The report recommends broadening insurance coverage to include effective outpatient treatments and better equipping health care providers to recognize and screen for substance use problems so they can refer patients to appropriate, evidence-based treatment when needed. It also recommends measures like limiting access to alcohol on bases.

The IOM Report also notes that addressing substance use in the military will require increasing confidentiality and shifting a cultural climate in which drug problems are stigmatized and evoke fear in people suffering from them.

Branches of the military have already taken steps to curb prescription drug abuse. The Army, for example, has implemented changes that include limiting the duration of prescriptions for opioid pain relievers to six months and having a pharmacist monitor a soldier's medications when multiple prescriptions are being used.

NIDA and other government agencies are currently funding research to better understand the causes of drug abuse and other mental health problems among military personnel, veterans, and their families and how best to prevent and treat them.

Address Mental and/or Substance Use Disorders among Active Military, Veterans, and Their Families

It's important to monitor for signs and symptoms of substance use disorders and to prevent the misuse of alcohol and/or drugs. Individuals, families, and members of the military community should be aware of the following signs and consequences associated with substance use:

- Failure to fulfill major personal and professional obligations

- Recurrent use of substances in situations in which they are physically hazardous

- Recurrent alcohol or substance-related legal problems

- Persistent or recurrent social or interpersonal problems caused or exacerbated by the effects of alcohol or substance use, while this use often continues without stopping

- Mood and behavior problems

- Work-related/financial difficulties

- Hurt social relationships

The Extended Impact on Families

In the United States, there are approximately 700,000 military spouses, and more than 700,000 children have experienced the deployment of a parent. Military families play an active role in the recovery of a relative's disorder, while at the same time they may also experience difficulties dealing with situations that can arise due to a family member's deployment, injury, or death.

Families of military personnel can directly experience both the emotional and physical effects of behavioral health conditions, particularly during their loved one's long absence(s). Studies show that parental deployment has a cumulative effect on children, while prolonged deployment is associated with more mental health diagnosis among U.S. Army wives. The effects of deployment are significant, as evidenced by the following findings:

- Children of deployed military personnel have more school, family, and peer-related emotional difficulties, compared with the civilian public.

- Women whose husbands have been deployed for 1 to 11 months are diagnosed with more depressive disorders, sleep disorders,

147

anxiety, and acute stress reaction and adjustment disorders than those whose husbands are not deployed.

- For children who were between ages 3 and 8 when a parent was deployed, 19% showed an increase in behavioral issues while their parent was gone.

- In one year, 34% of caregivers in military families reported that their children experienced moderate to high levels of emotional and behavioral problems, compared with 19% of all youth nationally.

To prevent the onset of these issues, families need to identify the signs of mental and/or substance use disorders among loved ones—and monitor for symptoms even after a parent or spouse returns home. Reintegration challenges exist for children, including increased attachment behavior when parents return, compared with children whose parents have not recently been deployed. Like recovery, reintegration for both the military personnel and the family members is a journey that takes time and effort.

Section 14.2

Inmate Populations and Substance Abuse

Excerpted from: The National Center on Addiction and Substance Abuse at Columbia University (CASAColumbia™). (2010). *Behind Bars II: Substance Abuse and America's Prison Population*. New York: National Center on Addiction and Substance Abuse at Columbia University. © 2010. All rights reserved.

Substance-Involved Inmates on the Rise

Between 1996 and 2006, the U.S. population grew by 12.5%. While the percentage of adults incarcerated in federal, state, and local correctional facilities grew by 32.8% during that period, the percentage of substance-involved offenders behind bars in America rose even more rapidly, by 43.2%.

Substance misuse and addiction are key factors in the continuous growth of the U.S. inmate population. By 2006, a total of 2.3 million people—one in every 133 adult Americans—were behind bars; 84.8% of all inmates (1.9 million) were substance involved; 86.2% of federal inmates (0.2 million), 84.6% of state inmates (1.1 million), and 84.7% of local jail inmates (0.6 million).

Alcohol and Other Drug Use Is Implicated in All Types of Crime

Substance misuse and addiction are overwhelming factors in all types of crime, not just alcohol and drug law violations. Thirty-seven percent of federal, state, and local prison and jail inmates in 2006 were serving time for committing a violent crime as their controlling offense; of these inmates, 77.5% were substance involved. Those serving time for property crimes comprise 19.2% of the inmate population; 83.4% were substance involved. Those whose controlling offense was a supervision violation, public order offense, immigration offense, or weapon offense comprise 13.3% of the inmate population; 76.9% were substance involved.

149

Alcohol Plays a Dominant Role; Few Incarcerated for Marijuana Possession Only

Alcohol is implicated in the incarceration of over half (56.6%) of all inmates in America. In addition to the inmates who were convicted of an alcohol law violation, 51.6% of drug law violators, 55.9% of those who committed a property crime, 57.7% of inmates who committed a violent crime, and 52.0% of those who committed other crimes were either under the influence of alcohol at the time of the crime, had a history of alcohol treatment, or had an alcohol use disorder.

While illicit drugs are implicated in three-quarters of incarcerations (75.9%), few inmates are incarcerated for marijuana possession as their controlling or only offense. Inmates incarcerated in federal and state prisons and local jails for marijuana possession as the controlling offense accounted for 1.1% (25,235) of all inmates and 4.4% of those incarcerated for drug law violations. Those incarcerated for marijuana possession as their only offense accounted for 0.9% (20,291) of all inmates and 2.9% of those incarcerated for drug law violations.

Tobacco Use High among Inmates

In 2005, 37.8% of state inmates and 38.6% of federal inmates smoked in the month of their arrest. In contrast, approximately 24.9% of the population was a current smoker. State and federal inmates who met clinical criteria for alcohol or other drug use disorders had even higher rates of use; 66.5% of state inmates and 51.5% of federal inmates with a substance use disorder smoked in the month of their arrest.

Arrests, Convictions, Sentencing, and Recidivism

While arrest rates have declined overall between 1998 and 2004, arrests for drug law violations have increased. The number of arrestees convicted of a crime is up overall including federal convictions for drug law violations, but the number of state convictions for these offenses has declined. The number of convicted offenders sentenced to prison or jail also has risen overall, as have the number of federal and state drug law violators sentenced to prison or jail. Although re-incarceration rates have declined slightly, they remain high, particularly among substance-involved offenders. In 2006, 48.4% of all inmates had a previous incarceration, down from 50.3% in 1996.

Substance-involved inmates are likelier to begin their criminal careers at an early age and to have more contacts with the criminal justice system than inmates who are not substance involved. Among substance-involved inmates, those who have committed a crime to get money to buy drugs have the highest average number of past arrests (6.6), followed by inmates who had a history of alcohol treatment (6.3) or were under the influence of alcohol or other drugs at the time of their crime (5.9).

Substance Use and Mental Health Disorders

Substance use disorders among inmates are at epidemic proportions. Almost two-thirds (64.5%) of the inmate population in the U.S. (1.5 million) meet medical criteria for an alcohol or other drug use disorder. Prison and jail inmates are seven times likelier than are individuals in the general population to have a substance use disorder. One-third (32.9%) of the 2.3 million prison and jail inmates has a diagnosis of a mental illness. A quarter (24.4%) of prison and jail inmates has both a substance use disorder and a co-occurring mental health problem.

Female inmates make up 8.4% of the total inmate population—up from 7.7% in 1996. Women inmates are somewhat likelier to have a substance use disorder than are male inmates (66.1% vs. 64.3%) and significantly more likely to have co-occurring substance use and mental health disorders (40.5% vs. 22.9%). These co-occurring conditions are linked to the fact that female inmates are more than seven times likelier to have been sexually abused and almost four times likelier to have been physically abused before incarceration than male inmates.

Income, Education, Age, and Family History

Compared with inmates who are not substance involved, substance-involved inmates are:

- four times likelier to receive income through illegal activity (24.6% vs. 6.0%);

- almost twice as likely to have had at least one parent abuse alcohol or other drugs (34.5% vs. 18.4%);

- 40.6% likelier to have some family criminal history (42.6% vs. 30.3%);

- 29.2% less likely to have completed at least high school (30.4% vs. 39.3%); and

- 20.0% likelier to be unemployed a month before incarceration (32.1% vs. 26.8%).

Inmates who are substance involved also are likelier than those who are not substance involved: to be younger (average age 33.9 vs. 36.2); to have lived only with their mother during childhood (39.6% vs. 32.5%); and to have ever spent time in foster care (12.2% vs.7.3%).

The Treatment Gap

Of the 1.5 million prison and jail inmates who met clinical diagnostic criteria for a substance use disorder in 2006, only 11.2% had received any type of professional treatment since admission. Only 16.6% of facilities offer treatment in specialized settings which can produce better outcomes for offenders as measured by drug use and arrests post-release. Few inmates actually receive evidence-based services, including access to pharmacological treatments, and the availability of highly trained staff is limited. Simply offering treatment, even in specialized settings, does not mean that the treatment is available to all who need it or of adequate quality. Nicotine dependence rarely is addressed even though it is an essential part of addiction treatment. In terms of adjunct services, 22.7% of inmates with substance use disorders participated in mutual support/peer counseling and 14.2% received drug education; however, such services alone are unlikely to create lasting behavioral changes among those in need of addiction treatment.

Other conditions that frequently co-occur with substance use disorders are Hepatitis C, HIV/AIDS, and mental health disorders. Most facilities screen, test, and treat Hepatitis C and progress has been made in addressing HIV/AIDS among inmates, but significant gaps exist in the treatment of co-occurring mental health disorders.

While critical to recovery and reduced recidivism, the percentage of inmates participating in education and job training services declined between 1996 and 2006. The percentage of federal prison inmates who report participating in education or vocational programs while confined fell from 67% in 1996 to 57% in 2006. The participation rate among state inmates also declined from 57% in 1996 to 45% in 2006.

Inmate participation in religious and spiritual activities provided by volunteers has increased, but chaplain positions have declined.

Section 14.3

Substance Use Disorders in People with Disabilities

Excerpted from "Substance Use Disorders in People with Physical and Sensory Disabilities," Substance Abuse and Mental Health Services Administration (www.samhsa.gov), August 2011.

Approximately 23 million people in the United States, including people with disabilities, need treatment for substance use disorders (SUDs), a major behavioral health disorder. In addition, more than 24 million adults in the United States experienced serious psychological distress in 2006. People with and without disabilities may face many of the same barriers to substance abuse treatment, such as lacking insurance or sufficient funds for treatment services, or feeling they do not need treatment. In addition, people with disabilities may face other barriers to SUD treatment, particularly finding treatment facilities that are fully accessible. Vocational rehabilitation (VR) counselors, vocational education providers, and others who work with people with disabilities report that their clients with SUDs have less successful vocational outcomes than clients without SUDs. To improve outcomes, it is important that clients with disabilities and SUDs receive services for both conditions and that the disabilities do not prevent clients from receiving treatment for SUDs.

What is an SUD?

Substance use disorder is a broad term that encompasses abuse of and dependence on drugs or alcohol. It includes using illegal substances, such as heroin, marijuana, or methamphetamines, and using legal substances, such as prescription or over-the-counter medications, in ways not prescribed or recommended.

SUDs Harm People with Disabilities

It is difficult to estimate the number of people with physical disabilities who have SUDs. Some studies suggest that people with disabilities

153

have higher rates of legal and illegal substance use than the general population, whereas other studies show lower rates. Although debate exists among researchers about the prevalence of SUDs among people with disabilities, there is agreement that active SUDs can seriously harm the health and quality of life of individuals with disabilities. An active SUD can do the following:

- Interfere with successful engagement in rehabilitation services

- Interact with prescribed medications; alcohol, for example, can interfere with antiseizure medications

- Impede coordination and muscle control

- Impair cognition

- Reduce the ability to follow self-care regimens

- Contribute to social isolation, poor communication, and domestic strife

- Contribute to poor health, secondary disabling conditions, or the hastening of disabling diseases (e.g., cirrhosis, depression, bladder infections)

- Inhibit educational advancement

- Lead to job loss, underemployment, and housing instability

Women with Disabilities and SUDs

Across all age groups, more women than men are disabled. Women with co-occurring disabilities and SUDs are at high risk for experiencing physical abuse and domestic violence.

One study of people with disabilities and SUDs found that 47% of women reported histories of physical, sexual, or domestic violence, compared with 20% of men with disabilities reporting abuse experiences. In the same study, 37% of women reported sexual abuse, compared with 7% of men.

Another study found that 56% of women with disabilities reported abuse, with 89% of these reporting multiple abusive incidents. What is more, being a victim of physical or sexual abuse is a risk factor for SUD.

SUD Risk Factors and Warning Signs

For some people, drug or alcohol abuse is a direct or indirect cause of their disability, for example, by their becoming intoxicated and then falling or causing a car crash. Without SUD treatment, people who had SUDs before sustaining a disability will likely continue to use substances afterward. Other people may have developed SUDs after using substances such as pain medications or alcohol to cope with aspects of their disability or to cope with social isolation or depression. The following are SUD risk factors for people with disabilities:

- Pain

- Access to prescription pain medications

- Chronic medical problems

- Depression

- Social isolation

- Enabling by caregivers

- Unemployment

- Limited education

- Low socioeconomic level

- Little exposure to SUD prevention education

- History of physical or sexual abuse

Accessible SUD Treatment Facilities

Despite requirements of the Americans with Disabilities Act (ADA), studies suggest that many treatment facilities are not fully accessible to people with disabilities. Examples of physical barriers include doors and hallways too narrow for wheelchairs, uneven flooring, nonfunctioning elevators, and a reliance on signage to provide directions, which leaves people with low or no vision without a means to find their way through facilities.

Many other types of barriers exist. Some SUD treatment administrators believe that their facilities are more accessible than they actually are. Of various types of health care providers, outpatient SUD treatment providers are among the least likely to report that their services are accessible to people with disabilities or that they have had training on mobility impairments.

Comparatively little information is available on how many people with disabilities have been denied SUD treatment because of physical barriers in the treatment facility itself. One survey of 174 SUD treatment providers in Virginia found that 87% of people with multiple sclerosis, 75% of people with muscular dystrophy, and 67% of people with spinal cord injuries who sought services were denied SUD treatment services because of physical barriers at the treatment facility.

Section 14.4

Seniors and Drug Abuse

"Older Adults: Development of Substance Use Disorders in Older
Adults," Substance Abuse and Mental Health Services Administration,
Recovery Month (www.recoverymonth.gov), 2010.

From graduating high school, to landing your first job, to raising and supporting a family, life changes cause varying levels of stress. Although stress occurs at any age, older adults face distinct challenges as they transition to new stages in life. For some, this stress may contribute to a substance use disorder or a relapse in substance use after periods of abstinence.

Prevalence of Substance Use Disorders among Older Adults

Substance use disorders have become more prevalent among middle-aged and older adults and continue to become a greater public health issue as the baby boomers reach retirement age. Among people ages 50 to 59, reported use of illicit drugs has nearly doubled since 2002. The baby boomer generation is predicted to have substance use disorders at a higher rate than other groups because of the following factors:

- It was the first generation to engage in widespread recreational use of illicit drugs.

- It was the first generation where a wide variety of prescription medications were readily available.

- It is one of the last generations for which treatment and recovery is not perceived as socially acceptable.

In addition, individuals face unique stressful situations as they age that can contribute to substance use. They may encounter a jolting change of pace upon retirement, loss of a spouse or child, financial worries, health concerns, loss of control and independence, or poor social support networks.

People become more sensitive to the effects of substance use as they age. Due to physiological changes associated with aging, drinks may affect an older adult more heavily than someone in his or her early twenties.

Older adults have also been known to misuse substances both deliberately, due to increased stress and pain, and inadvertently, by mixing medications or taking them with alcohol or for purposes not originally prescribed by a doctor.

Older adults respond to alcohol and drugs differently depending on the medications they're taking and their general health. This can cause significant problems. For example:

- 50% of older adults in assisted living homes have an alcohol problem.

- 26% of assisted living home residents have misused prescription drugs.

- 70% of older adults' hospital admissions are for illness and accidents related to alcohol.

When an older person visits a doctor or hospital, addiction problems are often overlooked. Only 1% of doctors correctly diagnose alcoholism in women over 60. In addition, 10% of patients over 60 who are diagnosed with Alzheimer disease are actually suffering from brain damage caused by alcoholism.

Substance use among older adults is a problem that needs to be addressed. Avoiding the misuse of alcohol and medications contributes to lower rates of illness and disability among older adults.

Effects of Substance Use Disorders on Older Adults

Older adults who suffer from addiction are more likely to have their health deteriorate at a greater rate than those who don't have substance use disorders. Additionally, their mental health significantly declines, and they lose their ability to live independently much earlier than the average older adult.

Adults who drink excessive amounts of alcohol or use drugs put themselves at a greater risk of serious problems such as stroke, cardiovascular disease, liver disease, neurological disease, poor diabetes control, and osteoporosis. In addition, older adults are more likely to have health problems that are increased or exacerbated by alcohol, including high blood pressure, memory loss, and mood disorders.

Symptoms to Look for in Older Adults

Addiction in older adults may be difficult to detect if they live alone. Friends and family may not consider substance use problems as the issue, and may think that their loved one suffers from depression, memory or thinking problems, or anxiety.

Although alcohol and/or drugs have varied effects on an individual's overall physical and mental health, the basic patterns are similar. Symptoms of a substance use disorder in older adults include the following:

- Observable changes in sleep patterns and unusual fatigue

- Changes in mood

- Jerky eye movements

- Seizures

- Unexplained complaints about chronic pain or vision problems

- Poor hygiene and self-neglect

- Unexplained nausea or vomiting

- Slurred speech

Fortunately, abstaining from substance use can improve many health conditions in older adults. If your loved one possesses several of these warning signs, encourage him or her to seek help from a doctor or treatment program. In some cases where the person is not capable, you may need to serve as the liaison between your loved one and his or her health care provider.

Getting Help for an Older Adult

Speak with your loved ones, young and old, if you think they may have a substance use disorder. Use the following tips when speaking with older adults regarding specific addiction and treatment options:

- Talk about your worries about their substance use when they are alert.

- Share information regarding the effects of alcohol and/or drugs on their health.

- Ask to go to doctor's visits with them or contact the doctor yourself, if appropriate.

- Suggest alcohol- and drug-free activities.

- Encourage counseling and offer to drive them to and from these meetings.

- Be supportive, invite them, and encourage them to spend time with family and friends, attend family gatherings, and participate in extracurricular activities.

The initial treatment of addiction in older adults may require more intensive medical support than younger patients need, but ultimately older adults succeed in treatment more than any other age group. Inpatient treatment plans, mutual support groups, or partial hospital or day treatment programs might be appropriate for this group, especially because they encourage the interaction older adults may lack. Although it may be difficult to confront your loved one, remember that recovery is possible.

Part Three

Drugs of Abuse

Chapter 15

Anabolic Steroids and Related Drugs Used as Performance Enhancers

Chapter Contents

Section 15.1

Anabolic Steroids

"DrugFacts: Anabolic Steroids," National Institute on Drug Abuse (www.drugabuse.gov), July 2012.

"Anabolic steroids" is the familiar name for synthetic variants of the male sex hormone testosterone. The proper term for these compounds is anabolic-androgenic steroids (abbreviated AAS)—"anabolic" referring to muscle-building and "androgenic" referring to increased male sexual characteristics.

Anabolic steroids can be legally prescribed to treat conditions resulting from steroid hormone deficiency, such as delayed puberty, as well as diseases that result in loss of lean muscle mass, such as cancer and AIDS. But some athletes, bodybuilders, and others abuse these drugs in an attempt to enhance performance and/or improve their physical appearance.

How are anabolic steroids abused?

Anabolic steroids are usually either taken orally or injected into the muscles, although some are applied to the skin as a cream or gel. Doses taken by abusers may be 10 to 100 times higher than doses prescribed to treat medical conditions.

Steroids are typically taken intermittently rather than continuously, both to avert unwanted side effects and to give the body's hormonal system a periodic chance to recuperate. Continuous use of steroids can decrease the body's responsiveness to the drugs (tolerance) as well as cause the body to stop producing its own testosterone; breaks in steroid use are believed to redress these issues. "Cycling" thus refers to a pattern of use in which steroids are taken for periods of weeks or months, after which use is stopped for a period of time and then restarted.

In addition, users often combine several different types of steroids and/or incorporate other steroidal or nonsteroidal supplements in an attempt to maximize their effectiveness, a practice referred to as "stacking."

How do anabolic steroids affect the brain?

Anabolic steroids work very differently from other drugs of abuse, and they do not have the same acute effects on the brain. The most important difference is that steroids do not trigger rapid increases in the neurotransmitter dopamine, which is responsible for the rewarding "high" that drives the abuse of other substances.

However, long-term steroid use can affect some of the same brain pathways and chemicals—including dopamine, serotonin, and opioid systems—that are affected by other drugs, and thereby may have a significant impact on mood and behavior.

Abuse of anabolic steroids may lead to aggression and other psychiatric problems, for example. Although many users report feeling good about themselves while on steroids, extreme mood swings can also occur, including manic-like symptoms and anger ("roid rage") that may lead to violence. Researchers have also observed that users may suffer from paranoid jealousy, extreme irritability, delusions, and impaired judgment stemming from feelings of invincibility.

Are steroids addictive?

Even though anabolic steroids do not cause the same high as other drugs, steroids are reinforcing and can lead to addiction. Studies have shown that animals will self-administer steroids when given the opportunity, just as they do with other addictive drugs. People may persist in abusing steroids despite physical problems and negative effects on social relationships, reflecting these drugs' addictive potential. Also, steroid abusers typically spend large amounts of time and money obtaining the drug—another indication of addiction.

Individuals who abuse steroids can experience withdrawal symptoms when they stop taking them—including mood swings, fatigue, restlessness, loss of appetite, insomnia, reduced sex drive, and steroid cravings, all of which may contribute to continued abuse. One of the most dangerous withdrawal symptoms is depression—when persistent, it can sometimes lead to suicide attempts. Research has found that some steroid abusers turn to other drugs such as opioids to counteract the negative effects of steroids.

What are the other health effects of anabolic steroids?

Steroid abuse may lead to serious, even irreversible, health problems. Some of the most dangerous consequences that have been linked to steroid abuse include kidney impairment or failure; damage to the liver; and cardiovascular problems including enlargement of the heart, high blood pressure, and changes in blood cholesterol leading to an increased risk of stroke and heart attack (even in young people).

Steroid use commonly causes severe acne and fluid retention, as well as several effects that are gender- and age-specific:

- **For men:** Shrinkage of the testicles (testicular atrophy), reduced sperm count or infertility, baldness, development of breasts (gynecomastia), increased risk for prostate cancer

- **For women:** Growth of facial hair, male-pattern baldness, changes in or cessation of the menstrual cycle, enlargement of the clitoris, deepened voice

- **For adolescents:** Stunted growth due to premature skeletal maturation and accelerated puberty changes, and risk of not reaching expected height if steroid use precedes the typical adolescent growth spurt

In addition, people who inject steroids run the added risk of contracting or transmitting HIV/AIDS or hepatitis.

Section 15.2

Clenbuterol

"Clenbuterol," Drug Enforcement Administration
Office of Diversion Control, U.S. Department of Justice
(www.deadiversion.usdoj.gov), August 2011.

Clenbuterol is a potent, long-lasting bronchodilator that is prescribed for human use outside of the U.S. It is abused generally by bodybuilders and athletes for its ability to increase lean muscle mass and reduce body fat (i.e., repartitioning effects). However, clenbuterol is also associated with significant adverse cardiovascular and neurological effects.

Licit Uses

In the U.S., clenbuterol is not approved for human use; it is only approved for use in horses. In 1998, the FDA approved the clenbuterol-based Ventipulmin Syrup, manufactured by Boehringer Ingelheim Vetmedica, Inc., as a prescription-only drug for the treatment of airway obstruction in horses (0.8–3.2 g/kg twice daily). This product is not intended for human use or for use in food-producing animals.

Outside the U.S., clenbuterol is available by prescription for the treatment of bronchial asthma in humans. It is available in tablets (0.01 or 0.02 mg per tablet) and liquid preparations. The recommended dosage is 0.02–0.03 mg twice daily.

Chemistry and Pharmacology

Clenbuterol is a beta2-adrenergic agonist. Stimulation of the beta2-adrenergic receptors on bronchial smooth muscle produces bronchodilation. However, clenbuterol, like other beta-adrenergic agonists, can produce adverse cardiovascular and neurological effects, such as heart palpitations, muscle tremors, and nervousness. Activation of beta-adrenergic receptors also accounts for clenbuterol's ability to increase lean muscle mass and reduce body fat, although the downstream mechanisms by which it does so have yet to be clearly defined.

167

After ingestion, clenbuterol is readily absorbed (70%–80%) and remains in the body for awhile (25–39 hours). As a result of its long half life, the adverse effects of clenbuterol are often prolonged.

Illicit Uses

Clenbuterol is abused for its ability to alter body composition by reducing body fat and increasing skeletal muscle mass. It is typically abused by athletes and bodybuilders at a dose of 60–120 grams per day. It is often used in combination with other performance-enhancing drugs, such as anabolic steroids and growth hormone. It is also illicitly administered to livestock for its repartitioning effects. This has resulted in several outbreaks of acute illness in Spain, France, Italy, China, and Portugal one-half to three hours after individuals ingested liver and meat containing clenbuterol residues. The symptoms, which included increased heart rate, nervousness, headache, muscular tremor, dizziness, nausea, vomiting, fever, and chills, typically resolved within two to six days. Consequently, the U.S. and Europe actively monitor urine and tissue samples from livestock for the presence of clenbuterol.

There have also been reports of clenbuterol-tainted heroin and cocaine. Although no deaths were attributed to the clenbuterol exposures, the individuals were hospitalized for up to several days due to clenbuterol intoxication.

User Population

Clenbuterol is typically abused by athletes. It is thought to be more popular among female athletes as the repartitioning effects are not associated with the typical androgenic side effects (i.e., facial hair, deepening of the voice, and thickening of the skin) of anabolic steroids. Professional athletes in several different sports have tested positive for clenbuterol. Clenbuterol is also marketed and abused for weight-loss purposes.

Illicit Distribution

Clenbuterol is readily available on the internet as tablets, syrup, and an injectable formulation. The drug is purportedly obtained by illegal importation from other countries where it is approved for human use. According to the National Forensic Laboratory Information System (NFLIS) and the System to Retrieve Information from Drug Evidence (STRIDE), 21 items/exhibits were identified as clenbuterol in 2009, 24 items/exhibits were identified in 2010, and 3 items/exhibits were identified in the first quarter of 2011. The relatively small numbers of drug seizures are likely a result of low enforcement priority due to the noncontrolled status of clenbuterol in the United States.

Control Status

Clenbuterol is currently not controlled under the Controlled Substances Act (CSA). However, clenbuterol is listed by the World Anti-Doping Agency and the International Olympic Committee as a performance-enhancing drug; therefore, athletes are barred from its use.

Section 15.3

Human Growth Hormone (hGH)

"Growth Hormone Use and Abuse,"
reprinted with permission from www.hormone.org.
© Hormone Health Network, 2009. All rights reserved.

What Is Human Growth Hormone?

Human growth hormone (GH) is a substance that controls your body's growth. GH is made by the pituitary gland, located at the base of the brain. GH helps children grow taller (also called linear growth), increases muscle mass, and decreases body fat.

In both children and adults, GH also helps control the body's metabolism—the process by which cells change food into energy and make other substances that the body needs.

If children or adults have too much or too little GH, they may have health problems. Growth hormone deficiency (too little GH) and some other health problems can be treated with synthetic (manufactured) GH. Sometimes GH is used illegally for nonmedical purposes.

Did you know? Abuse of growth hormone can cause muscle pain and serious health problems.

How Is Hormone Growth Therapy Used?

The U.S. Food and Drug administration (FDA) has approved GH treatment for certain conditions. GH is available only by prescription and is injected. Synthetic GH seems to be safe and effective when used as prescribed for the FDA-approved conditions.

In children, GH is used to treat:

• growth hormone deficiency;

• conditions that cause short stature (being shorter than children of the same age), such as chronic kidney disease, turner syndrome, and Prader-Willi syndrome.

In adults, GH is used to treat:

• growth hormone deficiency;

• muscle wasting (loss of muscle tissue) from HIV;

• short bowel syndrome.

In addition to these uses, doctors outside of the U.S. sometimes prescribe GH for other health problems. (When doctors prescribe medicines for conditions other than the ones officially approved, the process is called "off-label" use.)

If you're worried about GH deficiency in yourself or a family member, talk with a doctor.

Is Growth Hormone Use Appropriate for Healthy Adults?

Studies of healthy adults taking GH have produced conflicting results. Some short-term studies showed that older adults increased their endurance and strength, with increased muscle and decreased fat mass. But other studies did not show similar benefits. More studies are needed to fully understand the benefits and risks of GH use in healthy adults.

Aside from its use in research studies, prescribing or using GH off-label is illegal in the US. Adults can achieve improved health, body composition, strength, and endurance by following a healthy diet and getting frequent exercise.

How Is Growth Hormone Abused?

People sometimes take GH illegally to stop or reverse the effects of aging or to improve athletic performance. Some athletes believe taking GH alone will not achieve the desired results, so they take it along with anabolic (tissue building) steroids in an effort to build muscle, increase strength, and decrease body fat.

Some athletes also use insulin to increase the muscular effects of GH, which is a dangerous practice because it lowers blood sugar.

What Are the Risks of Growth Hormone Abuse?

People can experience harmful side effects when they abuse GH. Side effects of short-term use include joint and muscle pain, fluid build-up, and swelling in the joints. If GH is injected with shared needles, people may be exposed to HIV, AIDS, or hepatitis.

Taking high doses of GH over a long time may contribute to heart disease. GH sold illegally may contain unknown and potentially harmful ingredients. For instance, if people take GH derived from human tissue, they risk developing a fatal brain disease called Creutzfeldt-Jakob disease, which is similar to mad cow disease.

Growth Hormone Sold without a Prescription

Some companies sell human GH pills or GH releasers, claiming that the pills are "anti-aging" substances. But these substances have not been proven to increase the body's production of GH or to fight aging, increase muscle, or provide other benefits. GH has no effect if it is taken as a pill because it is inactivated (loses its action) during digestion.

Questions to Ask Your Doctor

- Do I (or my child) need human growth hormone treatment for medical reasons?
- What are the benefits and risks of growth hormone treatment?
- What are the signs of growth hormone abuse?
- Should I see an endocrinologist about my condition?

Chapter 16

Cannabinoids

Chapter Contents

Section 16.1

Hashish

When the leaves and flowers of the cannabis plant are dried and crumbled, this is called marijuana in the U.S. and cannabis elsewhere. When the resins from the cannabis plant are collected and compressed into sticks, balls, or blocks, it is called hashish. Hashish is most often a hard, dry, crumbly substance that is usually brown but can also be a dark yellow. It can also be an oily, almost black block of material.

In this form, the tetrahydrocannabinol (THC), the intoxicating ingredient in cannabis, is concentrated. Therefore smaller amounts are needed to produce similar or stronger effects to those of cannabis/marijuana.

Hash oil is also available. It may be found in small glass bottles and may range in color from amber to dark brown. A drop or two is dropped on a cigarette before it is smoked.

Hashish is not in widespread use in the U.S., but there are signs of heavy use in some parts of Canada and Europe. In fact, in 2011, the Royal Canadian Mounted Police reported that they had participated in a worldwide operation that seized 43 metric tonnes of hashish that were destined for Montreal and Halifax.

In Asia and Northern Africa, hashish has been used since ancient times in Asia and is still used today. The majority of the world's hashish originates from Morocco.

Using Hashish

Hashish is mostly smoked, so a person who abuses hashish may leave behind crumbly brown or almost black powder or a gummy resinous substance, small pipes, or other paraphernalia. Some people roll hashish into cigarettes, heating hash with a flame and then breaking it up into a fine consistency. It is then mixed with herbs or tobacco and smoked. So a person abusing hashish this way could leave behind lighters, rolling papers, and small unsmoked ends of the hand-rolled cigarettes.

Hashish can also be eaten, but some people consider it is easier to get the correct dose and therefore the desired effect when it is smoked. It can be mixed into baked items, particularly brownies.

Common Signs of Hashish Use

Like cannabis, hashish acts somewhat as a sedative, causing a mellow, relaxed feeling. Unfortunately for those who habitually abuse this drug, it is also addictive and causes other symptoms that are undesirable.

Other signs include:

- drowsiness;

- loss of an accurate time sense;

- partial loss of or reduction in short-term memory;

- loss of ability to concentrate and complete tasks;

- lowered coordination;

- impaired ability to carry out complex tasks such as driving due to distortions in time and space perceptions;

- reduced comprehension and ability to learn;

- lowered inhibitions;

- impaired judgment;

- lowered ability to listen accurately and think clearly;

- an "I don't care" attitude;

- slow speech;

- lowered motivation.

This last sign is one of the most defining characteristics of cannabis or hashish use. When young people abuse cannabis or hashish, they tend to drop their prior interests, such as clubs and educational and career goals, in favor of the dreamy relaxation of cannabis intoxication.

Hashish can make it difficult to learn and solve problems, and the alteration of time and space perceptions can impair a person's ability to be successful at sports. As a result, a young person who was an athlete and scholar before hashish use may drop out of his sports activities. His grades may drop markedly as well.

See also our page about the effects of hashish [at www.narconon .org/drug-abuse/effects-of-hashish.html].

When looking for physical signs of hashish use, you would look for bloodshot eyes, dry mouth, cravings for snacks or drinks.

A person who is a heavy user of hashish or cannabis can develop paranoia and hallucinations. Long-term users can become dependent on the drug. If a person continues to abuse any substance despite suffering damage to life, health, or relationships, they can be considered abusers of the drug. If they also develop a tolerance (meaning that more of the drug must be consumed to get the same effects as before) and withdrawal symptoms when they quit using it, they are considered dependent. Cannabis does have withdrawal symptoms if the drug is discontinued.

These include:

- disturbed sleep;

- hyperactivity;

- reduced appetite;

- irritability;

- stomach problems and pain;

- sweating and shakes.

When a person takes too much hashish, they can experience aggression, anxiety, confusion, panic, immobility, and heavy sedation.

Eliminating Hashish Addiction

For many people, cannabis products are stepping stones to heavier drug use. If a person becomes addicted to any form of cannabis, immediately recovery through an effective rehabilitation program can prevent the need for rehabilitation from addiction to heroin, prescription painkillers, cocaine, or other drugs.

At the Narconon drug and alcohol recovery centers across the world, 7 out of 10 of those who come from rehab stay sober after they go home. Learn about the sauna detoxification program that enables a person to flush out stored drug toxins that can be involved in triggering cravings. For cannabis in particular, intoxicating components can become stored in fatty tissue, causing lingering symptoms of marijuana or hashish use, even weeks or months after use stopped. By combining time in a sauna with nutritional supplements and moderate exercise, the body's ability to get rid of old drug residues is activated. A person who craved the drug so badly that continued abuse was a necessity can find sobriety at last, after completion of this rehab program.

If you want to help someone who is addicted to hashish or cannabis, contact Narconon at 800-775-8750.

Section 16.2

Marijuana

"DrugFacts: Marijuana," National Institute on Drug Abuse (www.drugabuse.gov), December 2012.

Marijuana is a dry, shredded green and brown mix of leaves, flowers, stems, and seeds from the hemp plant *Cannabis sativa*. In a more concentrated, resinous form, it is called hashish, and as a sticky black liquid, hash oil. The main psychoactive (mind-altering) chemical in marijuana is delta-9-tetrahydrocannabinol, or THC.

Marijuana is the most common illicit drug used in the United States. After a period of decline in the last decade, its use has generally increased among young people since 2007, corresponding to a diminishing perception of the drug's risks. More teenagers are now current (past-month) smokers of marijuana than of cigarettes, according to annual survey data.

How is marijuana abused?

Marijuana is usually smoked in hand-rolled cigarettes (joints) or in pipes or water pipes (bongs). It is also smoked in blunts—cigars that have been emptied of tobacco and refilled with a mixture of marijuana and tobacco. Marijuana smoke has a pungent and distinctive, usually sweet-and-sour, odor. Marijuana can also be mixed in food or brewed as a tea.

How does marijuana affect the brain?

When marijuana is smoked, THC rapidly passes from the lungs into the bloodstream, which carries the chemical to the brain and other organs throughout the body. It is absorbed more slowly when ingested in food or drink.

However it is ingested, THC acts upon specific molecular targets on brain cells, called cannabinoid receptors. These receptors are ordinarily activated by chemicals similar to THC called endocannabinoids, such as anandamide. These are naturally occurring in the body and are part of a neural communication network (the endocannabinoid system) that plays an important role in normal brain development and function.

The highest density of cannabinoid receptors is found in parts of the brain that influence pleasure, memory, thinking, concentration, sensory and time perception, and coordinated movement. Marijuana overactivates the endocannabinoid system, causing the high and other effects that users experience. These include distorted perceptions, impaired coordination, difficulty with thinking and problem solving, and disrupted learning and memory.

What are marijuana's effects on daily life?

Research clearly demonstrates that marijuana has the potential to cause problems in daily life or make a person's existing problems worse. In fact, heavy marijuana users generally report lower life satisfaction, poorer mental and physical health, relationship problems, and less academic and career success compared to their peers who came from similar backgrounds. For example, marijuana use is associated with a higher likelihood of dropping out from school. Several studies also associate workers' marijuana smoking with increased absences, tardiness, accidents, workers' compensation claims, and job turnover.

Research has shown that, in chronic users, marijuana's adverse impact on learning and memory persists after the acute effects of the drug wear off; when marijuana use begins in adolescence, the effects may persist for many years. Research from different areas is converging on the fact that regular marijuana use by young people can have long-lasting negative impact on the structure and function of their brains.

A recent study of marijuana users who began using in adolescence revealed a profound deficit in connections between brain areas responsible for learning and memory. And a large prospective study (following individuals across time) showed that people who began smoking marijuana heavily in their teens lost as much as 8 points in IQ between age 13 and age 38; importantly, the lost cognitive abilities were not restored in those who quit smoking marijuana as adults. (Individuals who started smoking marijuana in adulthood did not show significant IQ declines.)

What are the other health effects of marijuana?

Marijuana use can have a variety of adverse, short- and long-term effects, especially on cardiopulmonary and mental health.

Marijuana raises heart rate by 20%–100% shortly after smoking; this effect can last up to three hours. In one study, it was estimated that marijuana users have a 4.8-fold increase in the risk of heart attack in the first hour after smoking the drug. This may be due to increased heart rate as well as the effects of marijuana on heart rhythms, causing palpitations and arrhythmias. This risk may be greater in older individuals or in those with cardiac vulnerabilities.

Marijuana smoke is an irritant to the lungs, and frequent marijuana smokers can have many of the same respiratory problems experienced by tobacco smokers, such as daily cough and phlegm production, more frequent acute chest illness, and a heightened risk of lung infections. One study found that people who smoke marijuana frequently but do not smoke tobacco have more health problems and miss more days of work than nonsmokers, mainly because of respiratory illnesses.

A number of studies have shown an association between chronic marijuana use and mental illness. High doses of marijuana can produce a temporary psychotic reaction (involving hallucinations and paranoia) in some users, and using marijuana can worsen the course of illness in patients with schizophrenia. A series of large prospective studies also showed a link between marijuana use and later development of psychosis. This relationship was influenced by genetic variables as well as the amount of drug used and the age at which it was first taken—those who start young are at increased risk for later problems.

Associations have also been found between marijuana use and other mental health problems, such as depression, anxiety, suicidal thoughts among adolescents, and personality disturbances, including a lack of motivation to engage in typically rewarding activities. More research is still needed to confirm and better understand these linkages.

Marijuana use during pregnancy is associated with increased risk of neurobehavioral problems in babies. Because THC and other compounds in marijuana mimic the body's own cannabinoid-like chemicals, marijuana use by pregnant mothers may alter the developing endocannabinoid system in the brain of the fetus. Consequences for the child may include problems with attention, memory, and problem solving.

In addition, marijuana use has been linked in a few recent studies to an increased risk of an aggressive type of testicular cancer in young men, although further research is needed to establish whether there is a direct causal connection.

Marijuana and driving: Because it seriously impairs judgment and motor coordination, marijuana also contributes to accidents while driving. A recent analysis of data from several studies found that marijuana use more than doubles a driver's risk of being in an accident. Further, the combination of marijuana and alcohol is worse than either substance alone with respect to driving impairment.

Is marijuana medicine?

Although many have called for the legalization of marijuana to treat conditions including pain and nausea caused by HIV/AIDS, cancer, and other conditions, the scientific evidence to date is not sufficient for the marijuana plant to gain U.S. Food and Drug Administration (FDA) approval, for two main reasons.

First, there have not been enough clinical trials showing that marijuana's benefits outweigh its health risks in patients with the symptoms it is meant to treat. The FDA requires carefully conducted studies in large numbers of patients (hundreds to thousands) to accurately assess the benefits and risks of a potential medication.

Also, to be considered a legitimate medicine, a substance must have well-defined and measureable ingredients that are consistent from one unit (such as a pill or injection) to the next. This consistency allows doctors to determine the dose and frequency. As the marijuana plant contains hundreds of chemical compounds that may have different effects and that vary from plant to plant, its use as a medicine is difficult to evaluate.

However, THC-based drugs to treat pain and nausea are already FDA approved and prescribed, and scientists continue to investigate the medicinal properties of cannabinoids.

Is marijuana addictive?

Contrary to common belief, marijuana is addictive. Estimates from research suggest that about 9% of users become addicted to marijuana; this number increases among those who start young (to about 17%, or one in six) and among daily users (to 25%–50%). Thus, many of the nearly 7% of high-school seniors who (according to annual survey data) report smoking marijuana daily or almost daily are well on their way to addiction, if not already addicted (besides functioning at a suboptimal level all the time).

Long-term marijuana users trying to quit report withdrawal symptoms including irritability, sleeplessness, decreased appetite, anxiety, and drug craving, all of which can make it difficult to remain abstinent.

Behavioral interventions, including cognitive-behavioral therapy and motivational incentives (i.e., providing vouchers for goods or services to patients who remain abstinent), have proven to be effective in treating marijuana addiction. Although no medications are currently available, recent discoveries about the workings of the endocannabinoid system offer promise for the development of medications to ease withdrawal, block the intoxicating effects of marijuana, and prevent relapse.

Rising potency: The amount of THC in marijuana samples confiscated by police has been increasing steadily over the past few decades. In 2009, THC concentrations in marijuana averaged close to 10%, compared to around 4% in the 1980s. For a new user, this may mean exposure to higher concentrations of THC, with a greater chance of an adverse or unpredictable reaction. Increases in potency may account for the rise in emergency department visits involving marijuana use. For experienced users, it may mean a greater risk for addiction if they are exposing themselves to high doses on a regular basis. However, the full range of consequences associated with marijuana's higher potency is not well understood, nor is it known whether experienced marijuana users adjust for the increase in potency by using less.

Learn More

For additional information on marijuana and marijuana abuse, please see NIDA's Research Report *Marijuana Abuse* (at www.drugabuse.gov/publications/research-reports/marijuana-abuse).

Chapter 17

Date Rape Drugs

Chapter Contents

Section 17.1

Gamma Hydroxybutyrate (GHB)

Excerpted from "Drugs of Abuse," Drug Enforcement Administration, U.S. Department of Justice (www.justice.gov/dea), 2011.

What is GHB?

Gamma-hydroxybutyric acid (GHB) is another name for the generic drug sodium oxybate. Xyrem (which is sodium oxybate) is the trade name of the Food and Drug Administration (FDA)-approved prescription medication.

Analogues that are often substituted for GHB include GBL (gamma butyrolactone) and 1,4 BD (also called just "BD"), which is 1,4-butanediol. These analogues are available legally as industrial solvents used to produce polyurethane, pesticides, elastic fibers, pharmaceuticals, coatings on metal or plastic, and other products. They are also are sold illicitly as supplements for bodybuilding, fat loss, reversal of baldness, improved eyesight, and to combat aging, depression, drug addiction, and insomnia.

GBL and BD are sold as "fish tank cleaner," "ink stain remover," "ink cartridge cleaner," and "nail enamel remover" for approximately $100 per bottle—much more expensive than comparable products. Attempts to identify the abuse of GHB analogues are hampered by the fact that routine toxicological screens do not detect the presence of these analogues.

What is its origin?

GHB is produced illegally in both domestic and foreign clandestine laboratories. The major source of GHB on the street is through clandestine synthesis by local operators. At bars or "rave" parties, GHB is typically sold in liquid form by the capful or "swig" for $5 to $25 per cap. Xyrem has the potential for diversion and abuse like any other pharmaceutical containing a controlled substance. GHB has been encountered in nearly every region of the country.

What are common street names?

Common street names include Easy Lay, G, Georgia Home Boy, GHB, Goop, Grievous Bodily Harm, Liquid Ecstasy, Liquid X, and Scoop.

What does it look like?

GHB is usually sold as a liquid or as a white powder that is dissolved in a liquid, such as water, juice, or alcohol. GHB dissolved in liquid has been packaged in small vials or small water bottles. In liquid form, GHB is clear and colorless and slightly salty in taste.

How is it abused?

GHB and its analogues are abused for their euphoric and calming effects and because some people believe they build muscles and cause weight loss.

GHB and its analogues are also misused for their ability to increase libido, suggestibility, passivity, and to cause amnesia (no memory of events while under the influence of the substance)—traits that make users vulnerable to sexual assault and other criminal acts.

GHB abuse became popular among teens and young adults at dance clubs and "raves" in the 1990s and gained notoriety as a date rape drug. GHB is taken alone or in combination with other drugs, such as alcohol (primarily), other depressants, stimulants, hallucinogens, and marijuana.

The average dose ranges from one to five grams (depending on the purity of the compound, this can be one to two teaspoons mixed in a beverage). However, the concentrations of these "home brews" have varied so much that users are usually unaware of the actual dose they are drinking.

What is its effect on the mind?

GHB occurs naturally in the central nervous system in very small amounts. Use of GHB produces central nervous system (CNS) depressant effects including euphoria, drowsiness, decreased anxiety, confusion, and memory impairment.

GHB can also produce both visual hallucinations and—paradoxically—excited and aggressive behavior. GHB greatly increases the CNS depressant effects of alcohol and other depressants.

What is its effect on the body?

GHB takes effect in 15 to 30 minutes, and the effects last three to six hours. Low doses of GHB produce nausea. At high doses, GHB overdose can result in unconsciousness, seizures, slowed heart rate, greatly slowed breathing, lower body temperature, vomiting, nausea, coma, and death.

Regular use of GHB can lead to addiction and withdrawal that includes insomnia, anxiety, tremors, increased heart rate and blood pressure, and occasional psychotic thoughts. Currently, there is no antidote available for GHB intoxication.

GHB analogues are known to produce side effects such as topical irritation to the skin and eyes, nausea, vomiting, incontinence, loss of consciousness, seizures, liver damage, kidney failure, respiratory depression, and death.

GHB overdose can cause death.

Which drugs cause similar effects?

GHB analogues are often abused in place of GHB. Both GBL and BD metabolize to GHB when taken and produce effects similar to GHB.

CNS depressants such as barbiturates and methaqualone also produce effects similar to GHB.

What is its legal status in the United States?

GHB is a schedule I controlled substance, meaning that it has a high potential for abuse, no currently accepted medical use in treatment in the United States, and a lack of accepted safety for use under medical supervision. GHB products are schedule III substances under the Controlled Substances Act. In addition, GBL is a list I chemical. It was placed on schedule I of the Controlled Substances Act in March 2000. However, when sold as GHB products (such as Xyrem), it is considered schedule III, one of several drugs that are listed in multiple schedules.

Section 17.2

Ketamine

Excerpted from "Drugs of Abuse," Drug Enforcement
Administration, U.S. Department of Justice
(www.justice.gov/dea), 2011.

What is ketamine?

Ketamine is a dissociative anesthetic that has some hallucinogenic effects. It distorts perceptions of sight and sound and makes the user feel disconnected and not in control. It is an injectable, short-acting anesthetic for use in humans and animals. It is referred to as a "dissociative anesthetic" because it makes patients feel detached from their pain and environment.

Ketamine can induce a state of sedation (feeling calm and relaxed), immobility, relief from pain, and amnesia (no memory of events while under the influence of the drug). It is abused for its ability to produce dissociative sensations and hallucinations. Ketamine has also been used to facilitate sexual assault.

What is its origin?

Ketamine is produced commercially in a number of countries, including the United States. Most of the ketamine illegally distributed in the United States is diverted or stolen from legitimate sources, particularly veterinary clinics, or smuggled into the United States from Mexico.

Distribution of ketamine typically occurs among friends and acquaintances, most often at raves, nightclubs, and at private parties; street sales of ketamine are rare.

What are common street names?

Common street names include Cat Tranquilizer, Cat Valium, Jet K, Kit Kat, Purple, Special K, Special La Coke, Super Acid, Super K, and Vitamin K.

What does it look like?

Ketamine comes in a clear liquid and a white or off-white powder. Powdered ketamine (100 to 200 milligrams) typically is packaged in small glass vials, small plastic bags, and capsules as well as paper, glassine, or aluminum foil folds.

How is it abused?

Ketamine, along with the other "club drugs," has become popular among teens and young adults at dance clubs and "raves." Ketamine is manufactured commercially as a powder or liquid. Powdered ketamine is also formed from pharmaceutical ketamine by evaporating the liquid using hot plates, warming trays, or microwave ovens, a process that results in the formation of crystals, which are then ground into powder.

Powdered ketamine is cut into lines known as bumps and snorted, or it is smoked, typically in marijuana or tobacco cigarettes. Liquid ketamine is injected or mixed into drinks. Ketamine is found by itself or often in combination with MDMA, amphetamine, methamphetamine, or cocaine.

What is its effect on the mind?

Ketamine produces hallucinations. It distorts perceptions of sight and sound and makes the user feel disconnected and not in control. A "Special K" trip is touted as better than that of LSD (lysergic acid diethylamide) or PCP (phencyclidine) because its hallucinatory effects are relatively short in duration, lasting approximately 30 to 60 minutes as opposed to several hours.

Slang for experiences related to ketamine or effects of ketamine include the following:

- "K-land" (refers to a mellow and colorful experience)

- "K-hole" (refers to the out-of-body, near death experience)

- "Baby food" (users sink in to blissful, infantile inertia)

- "God" (users are convinced that they have met their maker)

The onset of effects is rapid and often occurs within a few minutes of taking the drug, though taking it orally results in a slightly slower onset of effects. Flashbacks have been reported several weeks after ketamine is used. Ketamine may also cause agitation, depression, cognitive difficulties, unconsciousness, and amnesia.

What is its effect on the body?

A couple of minutes after taking the drug, the user may experience an increase in heart rate and blood pressure that gradually decreases over the next 10 to 20 minutes. Ketamine can make users unresponsive to stimuli. When in this state, users experience involuntarily rapid eye movement, dilated pupils, salivation, tear secretions, and stiffening of the muscles. This drug can also cause nausea.

An overdose can cause unconsciousness and dangerously slowed breathing.

Which drugs cause similar effects?

Other hallucinogenic drugs such as LSD, PCP, and mescaline can cause hallucinations. There are also several drugs such as GHB, Rohypnol, and other depressants that are misused for their amnesiac or sedative properties to facilitate sexual assault.

What is its legal status in the United States?

Since the 1970s, ketamine has been marketed in the United States as an injectable, short-acting anesthetic for use in humans and animals. In 1999, ketamine including its salts, isomers, and salts of isomers, became a schedule III nonnarcotic substance under the Federal Controlled Substances Act. It has a currently acceptable medical use but some potential for abuse, which may lead to moderate or low physical dependence or high psychological dependence.

Section 17.3

Rohypnol

Excerpted from "Drugs of Abuse," Drug Enforcement Administration,
U.S. Department of Justice (www.justice.gov/dea), 2011.

What is Rohypnol?

Rohypnol is a trade name for flunitrazepam, a central nervous
system depressant that belongs to a class of drugs known as benzodiazepines. Flunitrazepam is also marketed as generic preparations and
other trade name products outside of the United States.

Like other benzodiazepines, Rohypnol produces sedative-hypnotic,
antianxiety, and muscle relaxant effects. This drug has never been
approved for medical use in the United States by the Food and Drug
Administration. Outside the United States, Rohypnol is commonly
prescribed to treat insomnia. Rohypnol is also referred to as a "date
rape" drug.

What is its origin?

Rohypnol is smuggled into the United States from other countries,
such as Mexico.

What are common street names?

Common street names include Circles, Forget Pill, Forget-Me-Pill,
La Rocha, Lunch Money Drug, Mexican Valium, Pingus, R2, Reynolds,
Roach, Roach 2, Roaches, Roachies, Roapies, Robutal, Rochas Dos,
Rohypnol, Roofies, Rophies, Ropies, Roples, Row-Shay, Ruffies, and
Wolfies.

What does it look like?

Prior to 1997, Rohypnol was manufactured as a white tablet (0.5–2
milligrams per tablet), and when mixed in drinks, was colorless, tasteless, and odorless. In 1997, the manufacturer responded to concerns
about the drug's role in sexual assaults by reformulating the drug.

Rohypnol is now manufactured as an oblong olive green tablet with a speckled blue core that when dissolved in light-colored drinks will dye the liquid blue. However, generic versions of the drug may not contain the blue dye.

How is it abused?

The tablet can be swallowed whole, crushed and snorted, or dissolved in liquid. Adolescents may abuse Rohypnol to produce a euphoric effect often described as a "high." While high, they experience reduced inhibitions and impaired judgment. Rohypnol is also abused in combination with alcohol to produce an exaggerated intoxication.

In addition, abuse of Rohypnol may be associated with multiple-substance abuse. For example, cocaine addicts may use benzodiazepines such as Rohypnol to relieve the side effects (e.g., irritability and agitation) associated with cocaine binges.

Rohypnol is also misused to physically and psychologically incapacitate women targeted for sexual assault. The drug is usually placed in the alcoholic drink of an unsuspecting victim to incapacitate them and prevent resistance to sexual assault. The drug leaves the victim unaware of what has happened to them.

What is its effect on the mind?

Like other benzodiazepines, Rohypnol slows down the functioning of the CNS, producing drowsiness (sedation), sleep (pharmacological hypnosis), decreased anxiety, and amnesia (no memory of events while under the influence of the substance). Rohypnol can also cause increased or decreased reaction time, impaired mental functioning and judgment, confusion, aggression, and excitability.

What is its effect on the body?

Rohypnol causes muscle relaxation. Adverse physical effects include slurred speech, loss of motor coordination, weakness, headache, and respiratory depression. Rohypnol also can produce physical dependence when taken regularly over a period of time.

What are its overdose effects?

High doses of Rohypnol, particularly when combined with CNS depressant drugs such as alcohol and heroin, can cause severe sedation, unconsciousness, slow heart rate, and suppression of respiration that may be sufficient to result in death.

Which drugs cause similar effects?

Drugs that cause similar effects include GHB (gamma hydroxybutyrate) and other benzodiazepines such as alprazolam (e.g., Xanax), clonazepam (e.g., Klonopin), and diazepam (e.g., Valium).

What is its legal status in the United States?

Rohypnol is a schedule IV substance under the Controlled Substance Act. Rohypnol is not approved for manufacture, sale, use, or importation to the United States. It is legally manufactured and marketed in many countries. Penalties for possession, trafficking, and distribution involving one gram or more are the same as those of a schedule I drug.

Chapter 18

Dissociative Drugs

Chapter Contents

193

Section 18.1

Dextromethorphan (DXM)

Excerpted from "Drugs of Abuse," Drug Enforcement Administration,
U.S. Department of Justice (www.justice.gov/dea), 2011.

What is dextromethorphan (DXM)?

DXM is a cough suppressor found in more than 120 over-the-counter
(OTC) cold medications, either alone or in combination with other
drugs such as analgesics (e.g., acetaminophen), antihistamines (e.g.,
chlorpheniramine), decongestants (e.g., pseudoephedrine), and/or expectorants (e.g., guaifenesin). The typical adult dose for cough is 15 or
30 milligrams taken three to four times daily. The cough-suppressing
effects of DXM persist for 5 to 6 hours after ingestion. When taken as
directed, side effects are rarely observed.

What is its origin?

DXM abusers can obtain the drug at almost any pharmacy or
supermarket, seeking out the products with the highest concentration of the drug from among all the OTC cough and cold remedies
that contain it. DXM products and powder can also be purchased on
the internet.

What are common street names?

Common street names include CCC, Dex, DXM, Poor Man's PCP,
Robo, Rojo, Skittles, Triple C, and Velvet.

What does it look like?

DXM can come in the form of cough syrup, tablets, capsules, or
powder.

How is it abused?

DXM is abused in high doses to experience euphoria and visual and
auditory hallucinations. Abusers take various amounts depending on

their body weight and the effect they are attempting to achieve. Some abusers ingest 250 to 1,500 milligrams in a single dosage, far more than the recommended therapeutic dosages.

Illicit use of DXM is referred to on the street as "Robotripping," "skittling," or "dexing." The first two terms are derived from the products that are most commonly abused, Robitussin and Coricidin HBP. DXM abuse has traditionally involved drinking large volumes of the OTC liquid cough preparations. More recently, however, abuse of tablet and gel capsule preparations has increased.

These newer, high-dose DXM products have particular appeal for abusers. They are much easier to consume, eliminate the need to drink large volumes of unpleasant-tasting syrup, and are easily portable and concealed, allowing an abuser to continue to abuse DXM throughout the day, whether at school or work.

DXM powder, sold over the internet, is also a source of DXM for abuse. (The powdered form of DXM poses additional risks to the abuser due to the uncertainty of composition and dose.)

DXM is also distributed in illicitly manufactured tablets containing only DXM or mixed with other drugs such as pseudoephedrine and/ or methamphetamine.

DXM is abused by individuals of all ages, but its abuse by teenagers and young adults is of particular concern. This abuse is fueled by DXM's OTC availability and extensive "how to" abuse information on various websites.

What is its effect on the mind?

Some of the many psychoactive effects associated with high-dose DXM include confusion, inappropriate laughter, agitation, paranoia, and hallucinations.

Other sensory changes can occur, including the feeling of floating and changes in hearing and touch.

Long-term abuse of DXM is associated with severe psychological dependence. Abusers of DXM describe the following four dose-dependent "plateaus":

- **First plateau (100–200 mg):** Mild stimulation

- **Second plateau (200–400 mg):** Euphoria and hallucinations

- **Third plateau (300–600 mg):** Distorted visual perceptions, loss of motor coordination

- **Fourth plateau (500–1,500 mg):** Out-of-body sensations

What is its effect on the body?

DXM intoxication involves over-excitability, lethargy, loss of co-ordination, slurred speech, sweating, hypertension, and involuntary spasmodic movement of the eyeballs.

The use of high doses of DXM in combination with alcohol or other drugs is particularly dangerous, and deaths have been reported. Approximately 5%–10% of Caucasians are poor DXM metabolizers and at increased risk for overdoses and deaths. DXM taken with antidepressants can be life threatening. OTC products that contain DXM often contain other ingredients such as acetaminophen, chlorpheniramine, and guaifenesin that have their own effects, such as liver damage, rapid heart rate, lack of coordination, vomiting, seizures, and coma.

To circumvent the many side effects associated with these other ingredients, a simple chemical extraction procedure has been developed and published on the internet that removes most of these other ingredients in cough syrup.

What are its overdose effects?

DXM overdose can be treated in an emergency room setting and generally does not result in severe medical consequences or death. Most DXM-related deaths are caused by ingesting the drug in combination with other drugs. DXM-related deaths also occur from impairment of the senses, which can lead to accidents.

In 2003, a 14-year-old boy in Colorado who abused DXM died when he was hit by two cars as he attempted to cross a highway. State law enforcement investigators suspect that the drug affected the boy's depth perception and caused him to misjudge the distance and speed of the oncoming vehicles.

Which drugs cause similar effects?

Depending on the dose, DXM can have effects similar to marijuana or ecstasy. In high doses its out-of-body effects are similar to those of ketamine or PCP.

What is its legal status in the United States?

DXM is a legally marketed cough suppressant that is neither a controlled substance nor a regulated chemical under the Controlled Substances Act.

Section 18.2

PCP and Analogs

"Phencyclidine," Drug Enforcement Administration
Office of Diversion Control, U.S. Department of Justice
(www.deadiversion.usdoj.gov), January 2013.

After a decline in abuse during the late 1980s and 1990s, the abuse of phencyclidine (PCP) has increased slightly in recent years.

Street names include Angel Dust, Hog, Ozone, Rocket Fuel, Shermans, Wack, Crystal, and Embalming Fluid. Street names for PCP combined with marijuana include Killer Joints, Super Grass, Fry, Lovelies, Wets, and Waters.

Licit Uses

PCP was developed in the 1950s to be used as an intravenous anesthetic in the United States, but its use was discontinued due to the high incidence of patients experiencing postoperative delirium with hallucinations. PCP is no longer produced or used for medical purposes in the United States.

Chemistry and Pharmacology:

Phencyclidine, 1-(1-phencyclohexyl) piperidine, is a white crystalline powder readily soluble in water or alcohol. PCP is classified as a hallucinogen. PCP is a "dissociative" drug; it induces distortion of sight and sound and produces feelings of detachment. PCP's effects include sedation, immobility, amnesia, and marked analgesia. The effects of PCP vary by the route of administration and dose. The intoxicating effects can be produced within 2 to 5 minutes after smoking and 30 to 60 minutes after swallowing. PCP intoxication may last from 4 to 8 hours; some users report experiencing subjective effects from 24 to 48 hours after using PCP. Low to moderate doses (one to five milligrams) induce feelings of detachment from surroundings and self, numbness, slurred speech, and loss of coordination accompanied by a sense of strength and invulnerability. A blank stare and rapid and involuntary eye movements are the more observable effects. Catatonic posturing, resembling that observed with schizophrenia, is also produced. Higher doses of PCP produce hallucinations. Physiological effects include increased blood pressure, rapid and shallow breathing, elevated heart rate, and elevated temperature.

Chronic use of PCP can result in dependency with a withdrawal syndrome upon cessation of the drug. Chronic abuse of PCP can impair memory and thinking. Other effects of long-term use include persistent speech difficulties, suicidal thoughts, anxiety, depression, and social withdrawal.

Illicit Uses

PCP is abused for its mind altering effects. It can be abused by snorting, smoking, or swallowing. Smoking is the most common method of abusing PCP. Leafy material such as mint, parsley, oregano, tobacco, or marijuana is saturated with PCP and subsequently rolled into a cigarette and smoked. A marijuana joint or cigarette dipped in liquid PCP is known as a "dipper." PCP is typically used in small quantities; 5 to 10 mg is an average dose.

User Population

PCP is predominantly abused by young adults and high school students. In 2010, there was an estimated 53,542 emergency department visits associated with PCP use, according to the Drug Abuse Warning Network (DAWN). This is a significant increase from an estimated 37,266 PCP-associated visits in 2008. The American Association of Poison Control Centers (AAPCC) National Poison Data System reports 747 PCP exposure case mentions and 350 single exposures in 2010. According to the 2011 National Survey on Drug Use and Health (NSDUH), 6.1 million (2.4%) individuals in the U.S., aged 12 and older, reported using PCP in their lifetime. The Monitoring the Future (MTF) survey indicates that PCP use among 12th graders in the past year increased from 1.0% in 2010 to 1.3% in 2011 and then decreased to 0.9% in 2012.

Illicit Distribution

PCP is available in powder, crystal, tablet, capsule, and liquid forms. It is most commonly sold in powder and liquid forms. Tablets sold as MDMA (ecstasy) occasionally are found to contain PCP. Prices for PCP range from $5–$15 per tablet, $20–$30 for a gram of powder PCP, and $200–$300 for an ounce of liquid PCP. The "dipper" sells for $10–$20 each.

According to the System to Retrieve Information from Drug Evidence (STRIDE) and the National Forensic Laboratory Information System (NFLIS), 5,374 PCP reports were from federal, state, and local forensic laboratories in 2011. In the first six months of 2012, there were 2,748 PCP reports from forensic laboratories.

Control Status

On January 25, 1978, PCP was transferred from schedule III to schedule II under the Controlled Substances Act.

Section 18.3

Salvia Divinorum

Excerpted from "Drugs of Abuse," Drug Enforcement Administration, U.S. Department of Justice (www.justice.gov/dea), 2011.

What is Salvia divinorum*?*

Salvia divinorum is a perennial herb in the mint family that is abused for its hallucinogenic effects.

What is its origin?

Salvia is native to certain areas of the Sierra Mazaleca region of Oaxaca, Mexico. It is one of several plants that are used by Mazatec indians for ritual divination. *Salvia divinorum* plants can be grown successfully outside of this region. They can be grown indoors and outdoors, especially in humid semitropical climates.

What are common street names?

Common street names include Maria Pastora, Sally-D, and *Salvia*.

What does it look like?

The plant has spade-shaped variegated green leaves that look similar to mint. The plants themselves grow to more than three feet high and have large green leaves, hollow square stems, and white flowers with purple calyces.

How is it abused?

Salvia can be chewed, smoked, or vaporized.

What is its effect on the mind?

Psychic effects include perceptions of bright lights, vivid colors, shapes, and body movement, as well as body or object distortions. *Salvia divinorum* may also cause fear and panic, uncontrollable laughter, a sense of overlapping realities, and hallucinations.

Salvinorin A is believed to be the ingredient responsible for the psychoactive effects of *Salvia divinorum*.

What is its effect on the body?

Adverse physical effects may include loss of coordination, dizziness, and slurred speech.

Which drugs cause similar effects?

When *Salvia divinorum* is chewed or smoked, the hallucinogenic effects elicited are similar to those induced by other schedule hallucinogenic substances.

What is its legal status in the United States?

Neither *Salvia divinorum* nor its active constituent Salvinorin A has an approved medical use in the United States. Salvia is not controlled under the Controlled Substances Act. *Salvia divinorum* is, however, controlled by a number of states. Since *Salvia* is not controlled by the CSA, some online botanical companies and drug promotional sites have advertised *Salvia* as a legal alternative to other plant hallucinogens like mescaline.

Chapter 19

Hallucinogenic Drugs

Chapter Contents

Section 19.1

Introduction to Hallucinogens

Excerpted from "Drugs of Abuse," Drug Enforcement Administration,
U.S. Department of Justice (www.justice.gov/dea), 2011.

What are hallucinogens?

Hallucinogens are found in plants and fungi or are synthetically
produced and are among the oldest known group of drugs used for
their ability to alter human perception and mood.

What is their origin?

Hallucinogens can be synthetically produced in illicit laboratories
or are found in plants.

What do they look like?

Hallucinogens come in a variety of forms. MDMA, or ecstasy, tablets
are sold in many colors with a variety of logos to attract young abusers.
LSD (lysergic acid diethylamide) is sold in the form of impregnated
paper (blotter acid), typically imprinted with colorful graphic designs.

How are they abused?

The most commonly abused hallucinogens among junior and senior
high school students are hallucinogenic mushrooms, LSD, and MDMA
or ecstasy. Hallucinogens are typically taken orally or can be smoked.

What is their effect on the mind?

Sensory effects include perceptual distortions that vary with dose,
setting, and mood. Psychic effects include distortions of thought associated with time and space. Time may appear to stand still, and forms
and colors seem to change and take on new significance. Weeks or even
months after some hallucinogens have been taken, the user may experience flashbacks—fragmentary recurrences of certain aspects of the drug

experience in the absence of actually taking the drug. The occurrence of a flashback is unpredictable but is more likely to occur during times of stress and seems to occur more frequently in younger individuals. With time, these episodes diminish and become less intense.

What is their effect on the body?

Physiological effects include elevated heart rate, increased blood pressure, and dilated pupils.

Deaths exclusively from acute overdose of LSD, magic mushrooms, and mescaline are extremely rare. Deaths generally occur due to suicide, accidents, and dangerous behavior, or due to the person inadvertently eating poisonous plant material.

A severe overdose of PCP (phencyclidine) and ketamine can result in respiratory depression, coma, convulsions, seizures, and death due to respiratory arrest.

What is their legal status in the United States?

Many hallucinogens are schedule I under the Controlled Substances Act (CSA), meaning that they have a high potential for abuse, no currently accepted medical use in treatment in the United States, and a lack of accepted safety for use under medical supervision.

Section 19.2

2C-I

"4-Iodo-2,5-Dimethoxyphenethylamine,"
Drug Enforcement Administration Office of Diversion Control, U.S.
Department of Justice (www.deadiversion.usdoj.gov), May 2013.

4-Iodo-2,5-dimethoxyphenethylamine (2C-I, 4-iodo-2,5-DMPEA)
is a synthetic drug abused for its hallucinogenic effects. It has been
encountered in a number of states by federal, state, and local law
enforcement agencies.

Licit Uses

2C-I has no approved medical uses in the United States.

Chemistry and Pharmacology

4-Iodo-2,5-dimethoxyphenethylamine is closely related to the
phenethylamine hallucinogens, 1-(4-bromo-2,5-dimethoxyphenyl)-
2-aminopropane (DOB) and 2,5-dimethoxy-4-methylamphetamine
(DOM). Like DOM and DOB, 2C-I displays high affinity for central
serotonin receptors. 2C-I selectively binds to the 5-HT receptor system.

Drug discrimination studies in animals indicate that 2C-I produces
discriminative stimulus effects that are similar to those of several
schedule I hallucinogens such as LSD, N,N-dimethyltryptamine (DMT)
and 3,4-methylenedioxymethamphetamine (MDMA). In rats trained to
discriminate LSD, DMT, or MDMA from saline, 2C-I fully substituted
for these schedule I hallucinogens.

In humans, 2C-I produces dose-dependent psychoactive effects.
User reports have mentioned oral doses between 3 and 25 mg producing LSD-like hallucinations and visual distortions and MDMA-like
empathy. Onset of subjective effects following 2C-I ingestion is around
40 minutes with peak effects occurring at approximately two hours. Effects of 2C-I can last up to eight hours. Various users reported delayed
desired effects compared to related drugs, which may result in some
users taking additional doses or other drugs which may increase the
risk of toxicity or accidental overdosage.

Radioimmunoassay detection system that is commonly used for testing amphetamine and hallucinogens is not expected to detect 2C-I. In the Marquis Reagent Field Test, 2C-I produces a dark green to black color.

Illicit Uses

2C-I is abused for its hallucinogenic effects. 2C-I is taken orally in tablet or capsule forms or snorted in its powder form. It has also been found impregnated on small squares of blotter paper for oral administration, which is a technique often seen for the distribution and abuse of LSD. The drug has been misrepresented by distributors and sold as other hallucinogens such as MDMA and LSD.

User Population

2C-I is used by the same population as those using "ecstasy" and other club drugs, high school and college students, and other young adults in dance and nightlife settings.

Illicit Distribution

2C-I is distributed as capsules, tablets, in powder form, or in liquid form. DEA identified occurrences of the drug being purchased through internet retailers. In one instance, it was purchased in powder form through the internet and encapsulated for retail, at a street value of $6 per capsule. In Europe, 2C-I has often been seized in tablet form with an "i" logo which may be to signify that it is not ecstasy (MDMA).

The National Forensic Laboratory Information System (NFLIS) is a DEA database that collects scientifically verified data on drug items and cases submitted to and analyzed by state and local forensic laboratories. The System to Retrieve Information from Drug Evidence (STRIDE) provides information on drug seizures reported to and analyzed by DEA laboratories. From 2007 to 2012, 353 exhibits have been identified as 2C-I by federal, state, and local forensic laboratories in 33 states. In 2010, there were 61 2C-I reports. There were 95 2C-I reports in 2011 and 73 reports in 2012.

Control Status

The Controlled Substances Act lists 2C-I in schedule I.

Section 19.3

AMT (Spirals)

"Alpha-Methyltryptamine," Drug Enforcement Administration Office of Diversion Control, U.S. Department of Justice (www.deadiversion.usdoj.gov), April 2013.

Alpha-methyltryptamine (AMT) is a tryptamine derivative and shares many pharmacological similarities with those of schedule I hallucinogens such as alpha-ethyltryptamine, N,N-dimethyltryptamine, psilocybin, and LSD. Since 1999, AMT has become popular among drug abusers for its hallucinogenic-like effects. In the 1960s, following extensive clinical studies on AMT as a possible antidepressant drug, the Upjohn Company concluded that AMT was a toxic substance and produces psychosis.

Licit Uses

AMT has no currently accepted medical uses in treatment in the United States.

Chemistry/Pharmacology

The hydrochloride salt of AMT is a white crystalline powder. AMT, similar to several other schedule I hallucinogens, binds with moderate affinities to serotonin (5-HT) receptors (5-HT1 and 5-HT2). AMT inhibits the uptake of monoamines especially 5-HT and is a potent inhibitor of monoamine oxidase (MAO) (especially MAO-A), an enzyme critical for the metabolic degradation of monoamines, the brain chemicals important for sensory, emotional, and other behavioral functions. AMT has been shown to produce locomotor stimulant effects in animals. It has been hypothesized that both 5-HT and dopamine systems mediate the stimulant effects of AMT. In animals, AMT produces behavioral effects that are substantially similar to those of 1-(2,5-dimethoxy-4-methylphenyl)-2-aminopropane (DOM) and MDMA, both schedule I hallucinogens, in animals.

In humans, AMT elicits subjective effects including hallucinations. It has an onset of action of about 3 to 4 hours and duration of about

12 to 24 hours, but may produce an extended duration of two days in some subjects. Subjects report uncomfortable feelings, muscular tension, nervous tension, irritability, restlessness, unsettled feeling in stomach, and the inability to relax and sleep. AMT can alter sensory perception and judgment and can pose serious health risks to the user and the general public. Abuse of AMT led to two emergency department admissions and one death. AMT increases blood pressure and heart rate, dilates pupils, and causes deep tendon reflexes and impairs coordination.

Illicit Uses

AMT is abused for its hallucinogenic effects and is used as substitute for MDMA. It is often administered orally as either powder or capsules at doses ranging from 15–40 mg. Other routes of administration include smoking and snorting.

User Population

Youth and young adults are the main abusers of AMT. Internet websites are a source that high school students and United States soldiers have used to obtain and abuse AMT.

Illicit Distribution

The National Forensic Laboratory Information System is a DEA database that collects scientifically verified data on drug items and cases submitted to and analyzed by state and local forensic laboratories. STRIDE provides information on drug seizures reported to and analyzed by DEA laboratories. According to STRIDE data, the first recorded submission by law enforcement to DEA laboratories of a drug exhibit containing AMT occurred in 1999.

NFLIS and STRIDE indicate that reports of AMT by federal, state, and local forensic laboratories increased from 10 in 2002 to 31 in 2003. In the years after temporary scheduling of AMT in 2003, the number of reports declined. In 2004, there were six reports and in 2005, there were two reports. From 2006 to 2011, NFLIS and STRIDE indicated a total of five AMT reports in those databases. However, in 2012, the number of AMT reports in NFLIS and STRIDE increased to 25. AMT has been illicitly available from United States and foreign chemical companies and from internet websites. Additionally, there is evidence of attempted clandestine production of AMT.

Control Status

The DEA placed AMT temporarily in schedule I of the Controlled Substances Act on April 4, 2003, pursuant to the temporary scheduling provisions of the CSA (68 FR 16427). On September 29, 2004, AMT was permanently controlled as a schedule I substance under the CSA (69 FR 58050).

Section 19.4

Blue Mystic (2C-T-7)

"2,5-Dimethoxy-4-(N)-Propylthiophenethylamine," Drug Enforcement Administration Office of Diversion Control, U.S. Department of Justice (www.deadiversion.usdoj.gov), May 2013.

In the fall of 2000, a young healthy male died following snorting an excessive amount of 2C-T-7. Since this initial 2C-T-7-related death, two additional deaths reported in April 2001 have been linked to 2C-T-7. These two deaths resulted from the co-abuse of 2C-T-7 with MDMA.

Licit Uses

2C-T-7 is not approved for marketing by the Food and Drug Administration and is not sold legally in the United States.

Chemistry and Pharmacology

2,5-Dimethoxy-4-(n)-propylthiophenethylamine (2C-T-7) is a phenethylamine hallucinogen that is structurally related to the schedule I phenethylamine hallucinogens, 4-bromo-2,5-dimethoxyphenethylamine (2C-B, Nexus) and mescaline. Based on structural similarly to these compounds, the pharmacological profile of 2C-T-7 is expected to be qualitatively similar to these hallucinogens.

Drug discrimination studies in animals indicate that 2C-T-7 produces discriminative stimulus effects similar to those of several schedule I hallucinogens. In rats trained to discriminate 2,5-dimethoxy-4-methyl-amphetamine (DOM), 2C-T-7 fully substituted for DOM and was slightly less potent than 2C-B in eliciting DOM-like effects. 2C-T-7 was also shown to share some commonality with LSD; it partially substituted for LSD up to doses that severely disrupted performance in rats trained to discriminate LSD. 2C-T-7 can also function as a discriminative stimulus in rats. Rats readily learned to discriminate 2C-T-7 from saline. When either 2C-B or LSD was substituted for 2C-T-7, each elicited 2C-T-7-like discriminative stimulus effects.

The subjective effects of 2C-T-7, like those of 2C-B and DOM, appear to be mediated through central serotonin receptors. 2C-T-7 selectively binds to the 5-HT receptor system.

According to one published case report, 2C-T-7 abuse has been associated with convulsions in humans.

Illicit Uses

2C-T-7 is abused orally and intranasally for its hallucinogenic effects. Information from a website about a variety of illicit drugs has suggested that 2C-T-7 produces effects similar to those of 2C-B. This information is based on individuals self-administering 2C-T-7 illicitly and self-reporting the effects. Its effects include visual hallucination, mood lifting, sense of well-being, emotionality, volatility, increased appreciation of music, and psychedelic ideation. The oral and intranasal doses recommended on this website are 10–50 mg and 5–10 mg, respectively. 2C-T-7's onset and duration of actions are dependent upon the route of administration. Following oral administration, onset and duration of effects are one to two and one-half hours and five to seven hours, respectively. After intranasal administration, the onset of action and duration of effects are 5 to 15 minutes and two to four hours, respectively.

User Population

Young adults are the main abusers of 2C-T-7.

Illicit Distribution

NFLIS is a DEA database that collects scientifically verified data on drug items and cases submitted to and analyzed by state and local forensic laboratories. STRIDE provides information on drug seizures reported to and analyzed by DEA laboratories. From January 2007 to December 2012, 51 reports, identified as 2C-T-7, were submitted to forensic laboratories. During this time, law enforcement officials encountered 2C-T-7 in 13 states; 28 of the 51 exhibits were encountered in the state of Florida.

2C-T-7 was being purchased over the internet from a company located in Indiana. This site was traced to an individual who had been selling large quantities of this substance since January 2000. Sales through this internet site were thought to be the major sources of 2C-T-7 in the United States. One clandestine laboratory was identified in Las Vegas, Nevada, as the supplier of 2C-T-7 to the individual in Indiana. 2C-T-7 has been sold under the street names Blue Mystic, T7, Beautiful, Tweety-Bird Mescaline, or Tripstay.

Control Status

2C-T-7 has been placed in schedule I of the Controlled Substances Act.

Section 19.5

DMT

Excerpted from "N,N-Dimethyltryptamine," Drug Enforcement Administration Office of Diversion Control, U.S. Department of Justice (www.deadiversion.usdoj.gov), January 2013.

N,N-dimethyltryptamine (DMT) is the prototypical indolethylamine hallucinogen. The history of human experience with DMT probably goes back several hundred years since DMT usage is associated with a number of religious practices and rituals. As a naturally occurring substance in many species of plants, DMT is present in a number of South American snuffs and brewed concoctions, like Ayahuasca. In addition, DMT can be produced synthetically. The original synthesis was conducted by a British chemist, Richard Manske, in 1931.

DMT gained popularity as a drug of abuse in the 1960s and was placed under federal control in schedule I when the Controlled Substances Act was passed in 1971. Today, it is still encountered on the illicit market along with a number of other tryptamine hallucinogens.

Licit Use

DMT has no approved medical use in the United States but can be used by researchers under a schedule I research registration that requires approval from both DEA and the Food and Drug Administration.

Pharmacology

Administered alone, DMT is usually snorted, smoked, or injected because the oral bioavailability of DMT is very poor unless it is combined with a substance that inhibits its metabolism. For example, in Ayahuasca, the presence of harmala alkaloids (harmine, harmaline, tetrahydro-harmaline) inhibits the enzyme, monoamine oxidase, which normally metabolizes DMT. As a consequence, DMT remains intact long enough to be absorbed in sufficient amounts to affect brain function and produce psychoactive effects.

In clinical studies, DMT was fully hallucinogenic at doses between 0.2 and 0.4 mg/kg. The onset of DMT effects is very rapid but usually resolves within 30 to 45 minutes. Psychological effects include intense visual hallucinations, depersonalization, auditory distortions, and an altered sense of time and body image. Physiological effects include hypertension, increased heart rate, agitation, seizures, dilated pupils, nystagmus (involuntary rapid rhythmic movement of the eye), dizziness, and ataxia (muscular incoordination). At high doses, coma and respiratory arrest have occurred.

Illicit Use

DMT is used for its psychoactive effects. The intense effects and short duration of action are attractive to individuals who want the psychedelic experience but do not choose to experience the mind-altering perceptions over an extended period of time as occurs with other hallucinogens, like LSD.

DMT is generally smoked or consumed orally in brews like Ayahuasca.

Illicit Distribution

DMT is found in a number of plant materials and can be extracted or synthetically produced in clandestine labs. Like other hallucinogens, internet sales and distribution have served as the source of drug supply in this country. According to the National Forensic Laboratory Information System and the System to Retrieve Information from

Drug Evidence, there were 540 DMT reports from federal, state, and local forensic laboratories in 2011. From January to June 2012, there were 338 DMT reports. According to STRIDE and NFLIS, illicit use of DMT has been encountered in most states and the District of Columbia.

Control Status

DMT is controlled in schedule I of the Controlled Substances Act.

Section 19.6

Ecstasy (MDMA)

"DrugFacts: MDMA (Ecstasy)," National Institute on Drug Abuse (www.drugabuse.gov), December 2012.

MDMA (3,4-methylenedioxy-methamphetamine), popularly known as ecstasy, is a synthetic, psychoactive drug that has similarities to both the stimulant amphetamine and the hallucinogen mescaline. It produces feelings of increased energy, euphoria, emotional warmth, and empathy toward others and distortions in sensory and time perception.

MDMA was initially popular among white adolescents and young adults in the nightclub scene or at "raves" (long dance parties), but the drug now affects a broader range of users and ethnicities.

How is MDMA abused?

MDMA is taken orally, usually as a capsule or tablet. Its effects last approximately three to six hours, although it is not uncommon for users to take a second dose of the drug as the effects of the first dose begin to fade. It is commonly taken in combination with other drugs. For example some urban gay and bisexual men report using MDMA as part of a multiple-drug experience that includes cocaine, GHB, methamphetamine, ketamine, and the erectile-dysfunction drug sildenafil (Viagra).

How does MDMA affect the brain?

MDMA acts by increasing the activity of three neurotransmitters, serotonin, dopamine, and norepinephrine. The emotional and pro-social effects of MDMA are likely caused directly or indirectly by the release of large amounts of serotonin, which influences mood (as well as other functions such as appetite and sleep). Serotonin also triggers the release of the hormones oxytocin and vasopressin, which play important roles in love, trust, sexual arousal, and other social experiences. This may account for the characteristic feelings of emotional closeness and empathy produced by the drug; studies in both rats and humans have shown that MDMA raises the levels of these hormones.

The surge of serotonin caused by taking MDMA depletes the brain of this important chemical, however, causing negative aftereffects— including confusion, depression, sleep problems, drug craving, and anxiety—that may occur soon after taking the drug or during the days or even weeks thereafter.

Some heavy MDMA users experience long-lasting confusion, depression, sleep abnormalities, and problems with attention and memory, although it is possible that some of these effects may be due to the use of other drugs in combination with MDMA (especially marijuana).

Is MDMA addictive?

Research thus far on MDMA's addictive properties has shown varying results, but we do know that some users report symptoms of dependence, including continued use despite knowledge of physical or psychological harm, tolerance (or diminished response), and withdrawal effects.

The neurotransmitter systems targeted by MDMA are the same as those targeted by other addictive drugs. Experiments have shown that animals will self-administer MDMA—an important indicator of a drug's abuse potential—although the degree of self-administration is less than some other drugs of abuse such as cocaine

What are other health effects of MDMA?

MDMA can have many of the same physical effects as other stimulants like cocaine and amphetamines. These include increases in heart rate and blood pressure, which are particularly risky for people with circulatory problems or heart disease. MDMA users may experience other symptoms such as muscle tension, involuntary teeth clenching, nausea, blurred vision, faintness, and chills or sweating.

In high doses, MDMA can interfere with the body's ability to regulate temperature. On rare but unpredictable occasions, this can lead to a sharp increase in body temperature (hyperthermia), which can result in liver, kidney, or cardiovascular system failure or even death. MDMA can interfere with its own metabolism (breakdown within the body), causing potentially harmful levels to build up in the body if it is taken repeatedly within short periods of time.

Compounding the risks of ecstasy use is the fact that other potentially harmful drugs (including synthetic cathinones, the psychoactive ingredients in "bath salts") are sometimes sold as ecstasy. These drugs can be neurotoxic or pose other unpredictable health risks. And ecstasy tablets that do contain MDMA may contain additional substances such as ephedrine (a stimulant), dextromethorphan (a cough suppressant), ketamine, caffeine, cocaine, or methamphetamine. The combination of MDMA with one or more of these drugs may be hazardous. Users who intentionally or unknowingly combine such a mixture with additional substances such as marijuana and alcohol may be putting themselves at even higher risk for adverse health effects.

Additionally, the closeness-promoting effects of MDMA and its use in sexually charged contexts (and especially in combination with sildenafil) may encourage unsafe sex, which is a risk factor for contracting or spreading HIV and hepatitis.

Does MDMA have therapeutic value?

MDMA was first used in the 1970s, not as a recreational drug but as an aid in psychotherapy—although without the support of clinical trial research or FDA approval. In 1985, the DEA labeled MDMA a schedule I substance, or a drug with high abuse potential and no recognized medicinal use. Some researchers remain interested in its potential therapeutic value when administered under carefully monitored conditions. It is currently in clinical trials as a possible pharmacotherapy aid to treat posttraumatic stress disorder (PTSD) and anxiety in terminal cancer patients.

Section 19.7

Foxy

"5-Methoxy-N,N-Diisopropyltryptamine," Drug Enforcement Administration Office of Diversion Control, U.S. Department of Justice (www.deadiversion.usdoj.gov), April 2013.

5-methoxy-N,N-diisopropyltryptamine (5-MeO-DIPT) is a tryptamine derivative and shares many similarities with schedule I tryptamine hallucinogens such as alpha-ethyltryptamine, N,N-dimethyltryptamine, N,N-diethyltryptamine, bufotenine, psilocybin, and psilocin. Since 1999, 5-MeO-DIPT has become popular among drug abusers. This substance is abused for its hallucinogenic effects.

Licit Uses

5-MeO-DIPT has no accepted medical uses in treatment in the United States.

Chemistry/Pharmacology

5-MeO-DIPT is a tryptamine derivative. The hydrochloride salt of 5-MeO-DIPT is a white crystalline powder. In animal behavioral studies, 5-MeO-DIPT has been shown to produce behavioral effects that are substantially similar to those of 1-(2,5-dimethoxy-4-methylphenyl)-2-aminopropane (DOM) and lysergic acid diethylamide (LSD), both schedule I hallucinogens.

In humans, 5-MeO-DIPT elicit s subjective effects including hallucinations similar to those produced by several schedule I hallucinogens such as 2C-B and 4-ethyl-2,5-dimethoxyphenyl-isopropylamine (DOET). The threshold dose of 5-MeO-DIPT to produce psychoactive effects is 4 mg, while effective doses range from 6 to 20 mg. 5-MeO-DIPT produces effects with an onset of 20 to 30 minutes and with peak effects occurring between one and one and one-half hours after administration. Effects last about three to six hours. Initial effects include mild nausea, muscular hyperreflexia, and dilation of pupils. Other effects include relaxation associated with emotional enhancement, talkativeness, and behavioral disinhibition. High doses of 5-MeO-DIPT produce abstract eyes-closed imagery. 5-MeO-DIPT alters sensory perception and judgment and can pose serious health risks to the user and the general public. Abuse of 5-MeO-DIPT led to at least one emergency department admission.

Illicit Uses

5-MeO-DIPT is abused for its hallucinogenic-like effects and is used as a substitute for MDMA. It is often administered orally as either powder, tablets, or capsules at doses ranging from 6–20 mg. Other routes of administration include smoking and snorting. Tablets often bear imprints commonly seen on MDMA tablets (spider and alien head logos) and vary in color. Powder in capsules was found to vary in colors.

User Population

Youth and young adults are the main abusers of 5-MeO-DIPT.

Illicit Distribution

NFLIS is a DEA database that collects scientifically verified data on drug items and cases submitted to and analyzed by state and local forensic laboratories. STRIDE provides information on drug seizures reported to and analyzed by DEA laboratories. According to NFLIS and STRIDE, 5-MeO-DIPT drug reports increased sharply from 72 in 2010 to 3,271 in 2011 and then decreased to 1,525 in 2012.

5-MeO-DIPT has been illicitly available from United States and foreign chemical companies and from individuals through the internet. There is some evidence of the attempted clandestine production of 5-MeO-DIPT.

Control Status

The DEA placed 5-MeO-DIPT temporarily in schedule I of the Controlled Substances Act on April 4, 2003, pursuant to the temporary scheduling provisions of the CSA (68 FR 16427). On September 29, 2004, 5-MeO-DIPT was permanently controlled as schedule I substance under the CSA (69 FR 58050).

Section 19.8

LSD

Excerpted from "DrugFacts: Hallucinogens - LSD, Peyote, Psilocybin, and PCP," National Institute on Drug Abuse (www.drugabuse.gov), June 2009.

Hallucinogenic compounds found in some plants and mushrooms (or their extracts) have been used—mostly during religious rituals—for centuries. Almost all hallucinogens contain nitrogen and are classified as alkaloids. Many hallucinogens have chemical structures similar to those of natural neurotransmitters (e.g., acetylcholine-, serotonin-, or catecholamine-like). While the exact mechanisms by which hallucinogens exert their effects remain unclear, research suggests that these drugs work, at least partially, by temporarily interfering with neurotransmitter action or by binding to their receptor sites.

LSD (d-lysergic acid diethylamide) is one of the most potent mood-changing chemicals. It was discovered in 1938 and is manufactured from lysergic acid, which is found in ergot, a fungus that grows on rye and other grains.

How is LSD abused?

The very same characteristics that led to the incorporation of hallucinogens into ritualistic or spiritual traditions have also led to their propagation as drugs of abuse. Importantly, and unlike most other drugs, the effects of hallucinogens are highly variable and unreliable, producing different effects in different people at different times. This is mainly due to the significant variations in amount and composition of active compounds, particularly in the hallucinogens derived from plants and mushrooms. Because of their unpredictable nature, the use of hallucinogens can be particularly dangerous.

LSD is sold in tablets, capsules, and, occasionally, liquid form; thus, it is usually taken orally. LSD is often added to absorbent paper, which is then divided into decorated pieces, each equivalent to one dose. The experiences, often referred to as "trips," are long; typically, they end after about 12 hours.

How does LSD affect the brain?

LSD, peyote, psilocybin, and PCP are drugs that cause hallucinations, which are profound distortions in a person's perception of reality. Under the influence of hallucinogens, people see images, hear sounds, and feel sensations that seem real but are not. Some hallucinogens also produce rapid, intense emotional swings. LSD, peyote, and psilocybin cause their effects by initially disrupting the interaction of nerve cells and the neurotransmitter serotonin. Distributed throughout the brain and spinal cord, the serotonin system is involved in the control of behavioral, perceptual, and regulatory systems, including mood, hunger, body temperature, sexual behavior, muscle control, and sensory perception.

There have been no properly controlled research studies on the specific effects of these drugs on the human brain, but smaller studies and several case reports have been published documenting some of the effects associated with the use of hallucinogens.

Sensations and feelings change much more dramatically than the physical signs in people under the influence of LSD. The user may feel several different emotions at once or swing rapidly from one emotion to another. If taken in large enough doses, the drug produces delusions and visual hallucinations. The user's sense of time and self is altered. Experiences may seem to "cross over" different senses, giving the user the feeling of hearing colors and seeing sounds. These changes can be frightening and can cause panic. Some LSD users experience severe, terrifying thoughts and feelings of despair, fear of losing control, or fear of insanity and death while using LSD.

LSD users can also experience flashbacks, or recurrences of certain aspects of the drug experience. Flashbacks occur suddenly, often without warning, and may do so within a few days or more than a year after LSD use. In some individuals, the flashbacks can persist and cause significant distress or impairment in social or occupational functioning, a condition known as hallucinogen-induced persisting perceptual disorder (HPPD).

Most users of LSD voluntarily decrease or stop its use over time. LSD is not considered an addictive drug since it does not produce compulsive drug-seeking behavior. However, LSD does produce tolerance, so some users who take the drug repeatedly must take progressively higher doses to achieve the state of intoxication that they had previously achieved. This is an extremely dangerous practice, given the unpredictability of the drug. In addition, cross-tolerance between LSD and other hallucinogens has been reported.

What other adverse effects does LSD have on health?

Unpleasant adverse effects as a result of the use of hallucinogens are not uncommon. These may be due to the large number of psychoactive ingredients in any single source of hallucinogen.

The effects of LSD depend largely on the amount taken. LSD causes dilated pupils; can raise body temperature and increase heart rate and blood pressure; and can cause profuse sweating, loss of appetite, sleeplessness, dry mouth, and tremors.

How widespread is the abuse of LSD?

According to the National Survey on Drug Use and Health (NSDUH), there were approximately 1.1 million persons aged 12 or older in 2007 who reported using hallucinogens for the first time within the past 12 months. Also in 2007, more than 22.7 million persons aged 12 or older reported they had used LSD in their lifetime (9.1%); however, fewer than 620,000 had used the drug in the past year. There was no change between 2006 and 2007 in the number of past-year initiates of LSD.

According to the Monitoring the Future Survey (MTF), there were no significant changes in LSD use from 2007 to 2008 for most prevalence periods among the 8th, 10th, and 12th graders surveyed; however, there was a significant increase in past-month use of LSD among 12th graders. Perceived risk of harm from taking LSD regularly decreased among 12th graders (from 67.3% in 2007 to 63.6% in 2008). No other changes were significant, but longer-term trends indicate a steady decline in perceived harmfulness of LSD in all three grades. Such changes in attitude could signal a subsequent increase in use, an outcome that would be of great concern after the large decreases seen since the mid-1990s, when LSD use peaked among youth.

Section 19.9

Mescaline (Peyote)

Excerpted from "Drugs of Abuse," Drug Enforcement Administration, U.S. Department of Justice (www.justice.gov/dea), 2011.

What are peyote and mescaline?

Peyote is a small, spineless cactus. The active ingredient in peyote is the hallucinogen mescaline.

What is its origin?

From earliest recorded time, peyote has been used by natives in northern Mexico and the southwestern United States as a part of their religious rites. Mescaline can be extracted from peyote or produced synthetically.

What are common street names?

Common street names include Buttons, Cactus, Mesc, and Peyoto.

What does it look like?

The top of the peyote cactus is referred to as the "crown" and consists of disc-shaped buttons that are cut off.

How is it abused?

The fresh or dried buttons are chewed or soaked in water to produce an intoxicating liquid. Peyote buttons may also be ground into a powder that can be placed inside gelatin capsules to be swallowed, or smoked with a leaf material such as cannabis or tobacco.

What is its effect on the mind?

Abuse of peyote and mescaline will cause varying degrees of illusions, hallucinations, altered perception of space and time, and altered body image. Users may also experience euphoria, which is sometimes followed by feelings of anxiety.

What is its effect on the body?

Following the consumption of peyote and mescaline, users may experience intense nausea, vomiting, dilation of the pupils, increased heart rate, increased blood pressure, a rise in body temperature that causes heavy perspiration, headaches, muscle weakness, and impaired motor coordination.

Which drugs cause similar effects?

Other hallucinogens like LSD, psilocybin (mushrooms), and PCP cause similar effects.

What is its legal status in the United States?

Peyote and mescaline are schedule I substances under the Controlled Substances Act, meaning that they have a high potential for abuse, no currently accepted medical use in treatment in the United States, and a lack of accepted safety for use under medical supervision.

Section 19.10

Psilocybin

Excerpted from "Drugs of Abuse," Drug Enforcement Administration,
U.S. Department of Justice (www.justice.gov/dea), 2011.

What is psilocybin?

Psilocybin is a chemical obtained from certain types of fresh or
dried mushrooms.

What is its origin?

Psilocybin mushrooms are found in Mexico, Central America, and
the United States.

What are common street names?

Common street names include Magic Mushrooms, Mushrooms, and
Shrooms.

What does it look like?

Mushrooms containing psilocybin are available fresh or dried and
have long, slender stems topped by caps with dark gills on the underside.
Fresh mushrooms have white or whitish-gray stems; the caps are dark
brown around the edges and light brown or white in the center. Dried
mushrooms are usually rusty brown with isolated areas of off-white.

How is it abused?

Psilocybin mushrooms are ingested orally. They may also be brewed
as a tea or added to other foods to mask their bitter flavor.

What is its effect on the mind?

The psychological consequences of psilocybin use include hallucinations and an inability to discern fantasy from reality. Panic reactions
and psychosis also may occur, particularly if a user ingests a large dose.

What is its effect on the body?

The physical effects include nausea, vomiting, muscle weakness, and lack of coordination.

Effects of overdose include longer, more intense "trip" episodes, psychosis, and possible death.

Abuse of psilocybin mushrooms could also lead to poisoning if one of the many varieties of poisonous mushrooms is incorrectly identified as a psilocybin mushroom.

Which drugs cause similar effects?

Psilocybin effects are similar to other hallucinogens, such as mescaline and peyote.

What is its legal status in the United States?

Psilocybin is a schedule I substance under the Controlled Substances Act, meaning that it has a high potential for abuse, no currently accepted medical use in treatment in the United States, and a lack of accepted safety for use under medical supervision.

Section 19.11

Toonies (Nexus, 2C-B)

"4-Bromo-2,5-Dimethoxyphenethylamine," Drug Enforcement
Administration Office of Diversion Control, U.S. Department of Justice
(www.deadiversion.usdoj.gov), May 2013.

4-Bromo-2,5-dimethoxyphenethylamine (2C-B, 4-bromo-2,5-DMPEA)
is a synthetic schedule I hallucinogen. It is abused for its hallucinogenic effects primarily as a club drug in the rave culture and "circuit"
party scene.

Licit Uses

2C-B has no approved medical uses in the United States.

Chemistry and Pharmacology

4-Bromo-2,5-dimethoxyphenethylamine is closely related to the
phenylisopropylamine hallucinogen 1-(4-bromo-2,5-dimethoxyphenyl)-
2-aminopropane (DOB) and is referred to as alpha-desmethyl DOB. 2C-B
produces effects similar to 2,5-dimethoxy-4-methylamphetamine (DOM)
and DOB. 2C-B displays high affinity for central serotonin receptors.
2C-B produces dose-dependent psychoactive effects. Threshold effects
are noted at approximately 4 mg of an oral dose; the user becomes passive and relaxed and is aware of an integration of sensory perception
with emotional states. There is euphoria with increased body awareness
and enhanced receptiveness of visual, auditory, olfactory, and tactile
sensation. Oral doses of 8 to 10 mg produce stimulant effects and cause
a full intoxicated state. Doses in the range of 20 to 40 mg produce LSD-
like hallucinations. Doses greater than 50 mg have produced extremely
fearful hallucinations and morbid delusions. Onset of subjective effects
following 2C-B ingestion is between 20 to 30 minutes with peak effects
occurring at one and one-half to two hours. Effects of 2C-B can last up
to eight hours.

Radioimmunoassay detection system that is commonly used for testing
amphetamine and hallucinogens does not detect 2C-B. In the Marquis

Reagent Field Test-902, 2C-B produces a bright green color. 2C-B is the only known drug to produce a bright green color when using this test.

Illicit Uses

2C-B is abused for its hallucinogenic effects. 2C-B is abused orally in tablet or capsule forms or snorted in its powder form. The drug has been misrepresented by distributors and sold as other hallucinogens such as MDMA and LSD. Some users abuse 2C-B in combination with LSD (referred to as a "banana split") or MDMA (called a "party pack").

User Population

2C-B is used by the same population as those using "ecstasy" and other club drugs, high school and college students, and other young adults who frequent "rave" or "techno" parties.

Illicit Distribution

2C-B is distributed as tablets, capsules, or in powder form. Usually sold as MDMA, a single dosage unit of 2C-B typically sells for $10 to $30 per tablet. The illicit source of 2C-B currently available on the street has not been identified by DEA. Prior to its control, DEA seized both clandestine laboratories and illicit "repacking shops." As the name implies, these shops would repackage and reformulate the doses of the tablets prior to illicit sales.

According to STRIDE data, the first recorded submission by law enforcement to DEA forensic laboratories of a drug exhibit containing 2C-B occurred in 1986.

NFLIS is a DEA database that collects scientifically verified data on drug items and cases submitted to and analyzed by state and local forensic laboratories. The STRIDE database provides information on drug seizures reported to and analyzed by DEA laboratories. From 2007 to 2012, 2C-B has been encountered by law enforcement in 37 states. Law enforcement officials submitted 89 exhibits identified as 2C-B to federal, state, and local forensic laboratories in 2010, 66 exhibits in 2011, and 74 exhibits in 2012.

Control Status

The Drug Enforcement Administration placed 2C-B in schedule I of the Controlled Substances Act.

Chapter 20

Inhalants

Many products readily found in the home or workplace—such as spray paints, markers, glues, and cleaning fluids—contain volatile substances that have psychoactive (mind-altering) properties when inhaled. People do not typically think of these products as drugs because they were never intended for that purpose. However, these products are sometimes abused in that way. They are especially (but not exclusively) abused by young children and adolescents and are the only class of substance abused more by younger than by older teens.

According to the 2011 Monitoring the Future survey, 13% of 8th graders, 10% of 10th graders, and 8% of 12th graders report ever having used inhalants.

Definition: Although other abused drugs can be inhaled, the term *inhalants* is reserved for the wide variety of substances—including solvents, aerosols, gases, and nitrites—that are rarely, if ever, taken via any other route of administration.

How are inhalants abused?

Abusers of inhalants breathe them in through the nose or mouth in a variety of ways (known as "huffing"). They may sniff or snort fumes from a container or dispenser (such as a glue bottle or a marking pen), spray aerosols (such as computer cleaning dusters) directly into

"DrugFacts: Inhalants," National Institute on Drug Abuse (www.drugabuse.gov), September 2012.

their nose or mouth, or place a chemical-soaked rag in their mouth. Abusers may also inhale fumes from a balloon or a plastic or paper bag. Although the high produced by inhalants usually lasts just a few minutes, abusers often try to prolong it by continuing to inhale repeatedly over several hours.

People tend to abuse different inhalant products at different ages. New users ages 12–15 most commonly abuse glue, shoe polish, spray paints, gasoline, and lighter fluid. New users ages 16–17 most commonly abuse nitrous oxide or "whippets." Adults most commonly abuse a class of inhalants known as nitrites (such as amyl nitrites or "poppers").

How do inhalants affect the brain?

Most abused inhalants other than nitrites depress the central nervous system in a manner not unlike alcohol. The effects are similar—including slurred speech, lack of coordination, euphoria, and dizziness. Inhalant abusers may also experience light-headedness, hallucinations, and delusions. With repeated inhalations, many users feel less inhibited and less in control. Some may feel drowsy for several hours and experience a lingering headache.

Unlike other types of inhalants, nitrites enhance sexual pleasure by dilating and relaxing blood vessels.

Although it is not very common, addiction to inhalants can occur with repeated abuse.

What are the other health effects of inhalants?

Chemicals found in different types of inhaled products may produce a variety of other short-term effects, such as nausea or vomiting, as well as more serious long-term consequences. These may include liver and kidney damage, hearing loss, or bone marrow damage. Effects may also include loss of coordination and limb spasms due to damage to myelin—a protective sheathing around nerve fibers that helps nerves transmit messages in the brain and peripheral nervous system. Inhalants can also cause brain damage by cutting off oxygen flow to the brain.

Inhalants can even be lethal. Sniffing highly concentrated amounts of the chemicals in solvents or aerosol sprays can directly cause heart failure within minutes. This syndrome, known as "sudden sniffing death," can result from a single session of inhalant use by an otherwise healthy young person. High concentrations of inhalants may also cause death from suffocation, especially when inhaled from a paper or plastic bag or in a closed area. Even when using aerosols or volatile products for their legitimate purposes like painting or cleaning, it is wise to do so in a well-ventilated room or outdoors.

Nitrites are a special class of inhalants that are abused to enhance sexual pleasure and performance. They can be associated with unsafe sexual practices that increase the risk of contracting and spreading infectious diseases like HIV/AIDS and hepatitis.

What products are abused as inhalants?

Volatile solvents are liquids that vaporize at room temperature:

- Industrial or household products, including paint thinners or removers, degreasers, dry-cleaning fluids, gasoline, and lighter fluid

- Art or office supply solvents, including correction fluids, felt-tip marker fluid, electronic contact cleaners, and glue

Aerosols are sprays that contain propellants and solvents:

- Household aerosol propellants in items such as spray paints, hair or deodorant sprays, fabric protector sprays, aerosol computer cleaning products, and vegetable oil sprays

Gases are found in household or commercial products and used as medical anesthetics:

- Household or commercial products, including butane lighters and propane tanks, whipped cream aerosols or dispensers (whippets), and refrigerant gases

- Medical anesthetics, such as ether, chloroform, halothane, and nitrous oxide ("laughing gas")

Nitrites are used primarily as sexual enhancers:

- Organic nitrites are volatiles that include cyclohexyl, butyl, and amyl nitrites, commonly known as "poppers"; amyl nitrite is still used in certain diagnostic medical procedures (when marketed for illicit use, organic nitrites are often sold in small brown bottles labeled as "video head cleaner," "room odorizer," "leather cleaner," or "liquid aroma")

Chapter 21

Narcotics (Opioids)

Chapter Contents

Section 21.1

Introduction to Narcotics

Excerpted from "Drugs of Abuse," Drug Enforcement Administration, U.S. Department of Justice (www.justice.gov/dea), 2011.

What are narcotics?

Also known as "opioids," the term "narcotic" comes from the Greek word for "stupor" and originally referred to a variety of substances that dulled the senses and relieved pain. Though some people still refer to all drugs as "narcotics," today "narcotic" refers to opium, opium derivatives, and their semi-synthetic substitutes. A more current term for these drugs, with less uncertainty regarding its meaning, is "opioid." Examples include the illicit drug heroin and pharmaceutical drugs like OxyContin, Vicodin, codeine, morphine, methadone, and fentanyl.

What is their origin?

The poppy *Papaver somniferum* is the source for all natural opioids, whereas synthetic opioids are made entirely in a lab and include meperidine, fentanyl, and methadone. Semi-synthetic opioids are synthesized from naturally occurring opium products, such as morphine and codeine, and include heroin, oxycodone, hydrocodone, and hydromorphone. Teens can obtain narcotics from friends, family members, medicine cabinets, pharmacies, nursing homes, hospitals, hospices, doctors, and the internet.

What do they look like?

Narcotics/opioids come in various forms, including tablets, capsules, skin patches, powder, chunks in varying colors (from white to shades of brown and black), liquid form for oral use and injection, syrups, suppositories, and lollipops.

What is their effect on the mind?

Besides their medical use, narcotics/opioids produce a general sense of well-being by reducing tension, anxiety, and aggression. These effects are helpful in a therapeutic setting but contribute to the drugs' abuse. Narcotic/opioid use comes with a variety of unwanted effects, including drowsiness, inability to concentrate, and apathy.

Psychological dependence: Use can create psychological dependence. Long after the physical need for the drug has passed, the addict may continue to think and talk about using drugs and feel overwhelmed coping with daily activities. Relapse is common if there are not changes to the physical environment or the behavioral motivators that prompted the abuse in the first place.

What is their effect on the body?

Narcotics/opioids are prescribed by doctors to treat pain, suppress cough, cure diarrhea, and put people to sleep. Effects depend heavily on the dose, how it's taken, and previous exposure to the drug. Negative effects include slowed physical activity, constriction of the pupils, flushing of the face and neck, constipation, nausea, vomiting, and slowed breathing.

As the dose is increased, both the pain relief and the harmful effects become more pronounced. Some of these preparations are so potent that a single dose can be lethal to an inexperienced user. However, except in cases of extreme intoxication, there is no loss of motor coordination or slurred speech.

Physical dependence and withdrawal: Physical dependence is a consequence of chronic opioid use, and withdrawal takes place when drug use is discontinued. The intensity and character of the physical symptoms experienced during withdrawal are directly related to the particular drug used, the total daily dose, the interval between doses, the duration of use, and the health and personality of the user. These symptoms usually appear shortly before the time of the next scheduled dose.

Early withdrawal symptoms often include watery eyes, runny nose, yawning, and sweating. As the withdrawal worsens, symptoms can include restlessness, irritability, loss of appetite, nausea, tremors, drug craving, severe depression, vomiting, increased heart rate and blood pressure, and chills alternating with flushing and excessive sweating.

However, without intervention, the withdrawal usually runs its course, and most physical symptoms disappear within days or weeks, depending on the particular drug.

What are their overdose effects?

Overdoses of narcotics are not uncommon and can be fatal. Physical signs of narcotics/opioid overdose include constricted (pinpoint) pupils, cold clammy skin, confusion, convulsions, extreme drowsiness, and slowed breathing.

Which drugs cause similar effects?

With the exception of pain relief and cough suppression, most central nervous system depressants (like barbiturates, benzodiazepines, and alcohol) have similar effects, including slowed breathing, tolerance, and dependence.

What is their legal status in the United States?

Narcotics/opioids are controlled substances that vary from schedule I to schedule V, depending on their medical usefulness, abuse potential, safety, and drug dependence profile. Schedule I narcotics, like heroin, have no medical use in the U.S. and are illegal to distribute, purchase, or use outside of medical research.

Section 21.2

Buprenorphine

"Buprenorphine," Drug Enforcement Administration
Office of Diversion Control, U.S. Department of Justice
(www.deadiversion.usdoj.gov), November 2012.

Buprenorphine was first marketed in the United States in 1985 as a schedule V narcotic analgesic. Initially, the only available buprenorphine product in the United States had been a low-dose (0.3 mg/ml) injectable formulation under the brand name Buprenex. Diversion, trafficking, and abuse of other buprenorphine products have occurred in Europe and other areas of the world.

In October 2002, the Food and Drug Administration (FDA) approved two buprenorphine products (Suboxone and Subutex) for the treatment of narcotic addiction. Both products are high dose (two and eight milligram) sublingual (under the tongue) tablets: Subutex is a single entity buprenorphine product and Suboxone is a combination product with buprenorphine and naloxone in a four to one ratio, respectively. After reviewing the available data and receiving a schedule III recommendation from the Department of Health and Human Services (DHHS), the DEA placed buprenorphine and all products containing buprenorphine into schedule III in 2002. Since 2003, diversion, trafficking, and abuse of buprenorphine have become more common in the United States. In June 2010, FDA approved an extended release transdermal film containing buprenorphine (Butrans) for the management of moderate to severe chronic pain in patients requiring a continuous, extended period, around-the-clock opioid analgesic.

Licit Uses

Buprenorphine is intended for the treatment of pain (Buprenex) and opioid addiction (Suboxone and Subutex).In 2001, 2005, and 2006, the Narcotic Addict Treatment Act was amended to allow qualified physicians, under certification of the DHHS, to prescribe schedule III–V narcotic drugs (FDA approved for the indication of narcotic treatment) for narcotic addiction, up to 30 patients per physician at any time, outside the context of clinic-based narcotic treatment programs. This limit was increased to 100 patients per physician, who meet the specified criteria, under the Office of National Drug Control Policy Reauthorization Act, which became effective on December 29, 2006.

Suboxone and Subutex are the only treatment drugs that meet the requirement of this exemption. Currently, there are nearly 15,700 physicians who have been approved by the Substance Abuse and Mental Health Services Administration (SAMHSA) and the DEA for office-based narcotic buprenorphine treatment. Of those physicians, approximately 13,150 were approved to treat up to 30 patients per provider and about 2,500 were approved to treat up to 100 patients. More than 3,000 physicians have submitted their intention to treat up to 100 patients per provider.

IMS Health National Prescription Audit Plus indicates that 7.69 million buprenorphine prescriptions were dispensed in the U.S. in 2011. From January to June 2012, 4.43 million buprenorphine prescriptions were dispensed.

Chemistry/Pharmacology

Buprenorphine has a unique pharmacological profile. It produces the effects typical of both pure mu agonists (e.g., morphine) and partial agonists (e.g., pentazocine) depending on dose, pattern of use, and population taking the drug. It is about 20–30 times more potent than morphine as an analgesic, and like morphine it produces dose-related euphoria, drug liking, papillary constriction, respiratory depression, and sedation. However, acute, high doses of buprenorphine have been shown to have a blunting effect on both physiological and psychological effects due to its partial opioid activity.

Buprenorphine is a long-acting (24–72 hours) opioid that produces less respiratory depression at high doses than other narcotic treatment drugs. However, severe respiratory depression can occur when buprenorphine is combined with other central nervous system depressants, especially benzodiazepines. Deaths have resulted from this combination.

The addition of naloxone in the Suboxone product is intended to block the euphoric high resulting from the injection of this drug by non-buprenorphine maintained narcotic abusers.

User Population

In countries where buprenorphine has gained popularity as a drug of abuse, it is sought by a wide variety of narcotic abusers: young naive individuals, non-addicted opioid abusers, heroin addicts, and buprenorphine treatment clients.

Illicit Uses

Like other opioids commonly abused, buprenorphine is capable of producing significant euphoria. Data from other countries indicate that buprenorphine has been abused by various routes of administration (sublingual, intranasal, and injection) and has gained popularity as a heroin substitute and as a primary drug of abuse. Large percentages of the drug-abusing populations in some areas of France, Ireland, Scotland, India, Nepal, Bangladesh, Pakistan, and New Zealand have reported abusing buprenorphine by injection and in combination with a benzodiazepine.

The National Forensic Laboratory Information System (NFLIS) is a DEA database that collects scientifically verified data on drug items and cases submitted to and analyzed by state and local forensic laboratories. The System to Retrieve Information from Drug Evidence (STRIDE) provides information on drug seizures reported to and analyzed by DEA laboratories. In 2011, federal, state, and local forensic laboratories identified 10,252 drug exhibits as buprenorphine; nearly eight times the number of buprenorphine exhibits (1,291) identified in 2006. In the first six months of 2012, 4,961 buprenorphine exhibits were identified.

According to the Drug Abuse Warning Network (DAWN), an estimated 15,778 emergency department visits were associated with nonmedical use of buprenorphine in 2010, more than three and a half times the 4,440 estimated number of buprenorphine ED visits in 2006. The American Association of Poison Control Centers Annual Report indicates that U.S. poison centers recorded 771 case mentions involving toxic exposure from buprenorphine in 2010.

Control Status

Buprenorphine and all products containing buprenorphine are controlled in schedule III of the Controlled Substances Act.

Section 21.3

Fentanyl

"Fentanyl," National Institute on Drug Abuse
(www.drugabuse.gov), December 2012.

Fentanyl is a powerful synthetic opiate analgesic similar to but more potent than morphine. It is typically used to treat patients with severe pain or to manage pain after surgery. It is also sometimes used to treat people with chronic pain who are physically tolerant to opiates. It is a schedule II prescription drug.

Names

In its prescription form, fentanyl is known as Actiq, Duragesic, and Sublimaze. Street names for the drug include Apache, China girl, China white, dance fever, friend, goodfella, jackpot, murder 8, TNT, as well as Tango and Cash.

Effects

Like heroin, morphine, and other opioid drugs, fentanyl works by binding to the body's opiate receptors, highly concentrated in areas of the brain that control pain and emotions. When opiate drugs bind to these receptors, they can drive up dopamine levels in the brain's reward areas, producing a state of euphoria and relaxation. Medications called opiate receptor antagonists act by blocking the effects of opiate drugs. Naloxone is one such antagonist. Overdoses of fentanyl should be treated immediately with an opiate antagonist.

When prescribed by a physician, fentanyl is often administered via injection, transdermal patch, or in lozenge form. However, the type of fentanyl associated with recent overdoses was produced in clandestine laboratories and mixed with (or substituted for) heroin in a powder form.

Mixing fentanyl with street-sold heroin or cocaine markedly amplifies their potency and potential dangers. Effects include euphoria, drowsiness/respiratory depression and arrest, nausea, confusion, constipation, sedation, unconsciousness, coma, tolerance, and addiction.

Section 21.4

Heroin

Excerpted from "DrugFacts: Heroin," National Institute on
Drug Abuse (www.drugabuse.gov), April 2013.

Heroin is an opiate drug that is synthesized from morphine, a naturally occurring substance extracted from the seed pod of the Asian opium poppy plant. Heroin usually appears as a white or brown powder or as a black sticky substance, known as "black tar heroin."

In 2011, 4.2 million Americans aged 12 or older (or 1.6%) had used heroin at least once in their lives. It is estimated that about 23% of individuals who use heroin become dependent on it.

How is heroin used?

Heroin can be injected, inhaled by snorting or sniffing, or smoked. All three routes of administration deliver the drug to the brain very rapidly, which contributes to its health risks and to its high risk for addiction, which is a chronic relapsing disease caused by changes in the brain and characterized by uncontrollable drug seeking no matter the consequences.

How does heroin affect the brain?

When it enters the brain, heroin is converted back into morphine, which binds to molecules on cells known as opioid receptors. These receptors are located in many areas of the brain (and in the body), especially those involved in the perception of pain and in reward. Opioid receptors are also located in the brain stem, which controls automatic processes critical for life, such as blood pressure, arousal, and respiration. Heroin overdoses frequently involve a suppression of breathing, which can be fatal.

After an intravenous injection of heroin, users report feeling a surge of euphoria ("rush") accompanied by dry mouth, a warm flushing of the skin, heaviness of the extremities, and clouded mental functioning. Following this initial euphoria, the user goes "on the nod," an alternately wakeful and drowsy state. Users who do not inject the drug may not experience the initial rush, but other effects are the same.

Regular heroin use changes the functioning of the brain. One result is tolerance, in which more of the drug is needed to achieve the same intensity of effect. Another result is dependence, characterized by the need to continue use of the drug to avoid withdrawal symptoms.

Can prescription opioid abuse be a first step to heroin use?

Prescription opioid pain medications such as OxyContin and Vicodin can have effects similar to heroin when taken in doses or in ways other than prescribed, and they are currently among the most commonly abused drugs in the United States. Research now suggests that abuse of these drugs may open the door to heroin abuse.

Nearly half of young people who inject heroin surveyed in three recent studies reported abusing prescription opioids before starting to use heroin. Some individuals reported taking up heroin because it is cheaper and easier to obtain than prescription opioids.

Many of these young people also report that crushing prescription opioid pills to snort or inject the powder provided their initiation into these methods of drug administration.

What is the connection between injection drug use and HIV and hepatitis C (HCV) infection?

People who inject drugs are at high risk of contracting HIV and HCV. This is because these diseases are transmitted through contact with blood or other bodily fluids, which can occur when sharing needles or other injection drug use equipment. (HCV is the most common bloodborne infection in the Unites States.) HIV (and less often HCV) can also be contracted during unprotected sex, which drug use makes more likely.

Because of the strong link between drug abuse and the spread of infectious disease, drug abuse treatment can be an effective way to prevent the latter. People in drug abuse treatment, which often includes risk reduction counseling, stop or reduce their drug use and related risk behaviors, including risky injection practices and unsafe sex.

What are the other health effects of heroin?

Heroin abuse is associated with a number of serious health conditions, including fatal overdose, spontaneous abortion, and infectious diseases like hepatitis and HIV. Chronic users may develop collapsed veins, infection of the heart lining and valves, abscesses, constipation and gastrointestinal cramping, and liver or kidney disease. Pulmonary complications, including various types of pneumonia, may result from the poor health of the user as well as from heroin's effects on breathing.

In addition to the effects of the drug itself, street heroin often contains toxic contaminants or additives that can clog blood vessels leading to the lungs, liver, kidneys, or brain, causing permanent damage to vital organs.

Chronic use of heroin leads to physical dependence, a state in which the body has adapted to the presence of the drug. If a dependent user reduces or stops use of the drug abruptly, he or she may experience severe symptoms of withdrawal. These symptoms—which can begin as early as a few hours after the last drug administration—can include restlessness, muscle and bone pain, insomnia, diarrhea and vomiting, cold flashes with goose bumps ("cold turkey"), and kicking movements ("kicking the habit"). Users also experience severe craving for the drug during withdrawal, which can precipitate continued abuse and/ or relapse.

Besides the risk of spontaneous abortion, heroin abuse during pregnancy (together with related factors like poor nutrition and inadequate prenatal care) is also associated with low birth weight, an important risk factor for later delays in development. Additionally, if the mother is regularly abusing the drug, the infant may be born physically dependent on heroin and could suffer from neonatal abstinence syndrome (NAS), a drug withdrawal syndrome in infants that requires hospitalization. According to a recent study, treating opioid-addicted pregnant mothers with buprenorphine (a medication for opioid dependence) can reduce NAS symptoms in babies and shorten their hospital stays.

How is heroin addiction treated?

A range of treatments including behavioral therapies and medications are effective at helping patients stop using heroin and return to stable and productive lives.

Medications include buprenorphine and methadone, both of which work by binding to the same cell receptors as heroin but more weakly, helping a person wean off the drug and reduce craving; and naltrexone, which blocks opioid receptors and prevents the drug from having an effect (patients sometimes have trouble complying with naltrexone treatment, but a new long-acting version given by injection in a doctor's office may increase this treatment's efficacy). Another drug called naloxone is sometimes used as an emergency treatment to counteract the effects of heroin overdose.

Section 21.5

Hydrocodone

"Hydrocodone," Drug Enforcement Administration Office of Diversion Control, U.S. Department of Justice (www.deadiversion.usdoj.gov), April 2013.

Since 2009, hydrocodone has been the second most frequently encountered opioid pharmaceutical in drug evidence submitted to federal, state, and local forensic laboratories as reported by DEA's National Forensic Laboratory Information System and System to Retrieve Information from Drug Evidence.

Licit Uses

Hydrocodone is an antitussive (cough suppressant) and narcotic analgesic agent for the treatment of moderate to moderately severe pain. Studies indicate that hydrocodone is as effective, or more effective, than codeine for cough suppression and nearly equipotent to morphine for pain relief.

Hydrocodone is the most frequently prescribed opiate in the United States with more than 143 million prescriptions for hydrocodone-containing products dispensed in 2012 (IMS Health). There are several hundred brand name and generic hydrocodone products marketed. All are combination products, and the most frequently prescribed combination is hydrocodone and acetaminophen (Vicodin, Lortab).

Chemistry/Pharmacology

Hydrocodone [4,5α-epoxy-3-methoxy-17-methylmorphinan-6-one tartrate (1:1) hydrate (2:5), dihydrocodeinone] is a semi-synthetic opioid most closely related to codeine in structure and morphine in producing opiate-like effects. The first report, that hydrocodone produces euphoria and habituation symptoms, was published in 1923. The first report of hydrocodone dependence and addiction was published in 1961.

242

Illicit Uses

Hydrocodone is abused for its opioid effects. Widespread diversion via bogus call-in prescriptions, altered prescriptions, theft, and illicit purchases from internet sources are made easier by the present controls placed on hydrocodone products. Hydrocodone pills are the most frequently encountered dosage form in illicit traffic. Hydrocodone is generally abused orally, often in combination with alcohol.

Of particular concern is the prevalence of illicit use of hydrocodone among school-aged children. The 2012 Monitoring the Future Survey reports that 1.3%, 3.0% and 3.8% of 8th, 10th, and 12th graders, respectively, used Vicodin nonmedically in the previous year.

The American Association of Poison Control Centers (AAPCC) reports that in 2011, there were 30,792 total exposures and 37 deaths associated with hydrocodone in the U.S. The 2011 National Survey on Drug Use and Health (NSDUH) reports that 23.2 million people of the U.S. population, aged 12 and older, used hydrocodone for nonmedical purposes in their lifetime. In 2011, an estimated 82,480 emergency department visits were associated with nonmedical use of hydrocodone, according to the Drug Abuse Warning Network (DAWN ED). This number of ED visits represents a 107% significant increase from the number of ED visits reported in 2004 (39,846). The Florida Department of Law Enforcement reported 372 deaths as being related to hydrocodone from January to June 2012. Of these 372 deaths, 118 of them were determined to be caused by hydrocodone.

As with most opiates, abuse of hydrocodone is associated with tolerance, dependence, and addiction. The co-formulation with acetaminophen carries an additional risk of liver toxicity when high, acute doses are consumed. Some individuals who abuse very high doses of acetaminophen-containing hydrocodone products may be spared this liver toxicity if they have been chronically taking these products and have escalated their dose slowly over a long period of time.

User Population

Every age group has been affected by the relative ease of hydrocodone availability and the perceived safety of these products by medical prescribers. Sometimes viewed as a "white collar" addiction, hydrocodone abuse has increased among all ethnic and economic groups.

Illicit Distribution

Hydrocodone has been encountered in tablets, capsules, and liquid form in the illicit market. However, hydrocodone tablets with the co-ingredient acetaminophen is the most frequently encountered form. Hydrocodone is not typically found to be clandestinely produced; diverted pharmaceuticals are the primary source of the drug for abuse purposes. Doctor shopping, altered or fraudulent prescriptions, bogus call-in prescriptions, diversion by some physicians and pharmacists, and drug theft are also major sources of the diverted drug.

The NFLIS is a DEA database that collects scientifically verified data on drug items and cases submitted to and analyzed by state and local forensic laboratories. STRIDE provides information on drug seizures reported to and analyzed by DEA laboratories. In 2012, there were 36,816 hydrocodone reports identified in the NFLIS and STRIDE systems, a decrease from 43,463 reports in 2011.

Control Status

The U.S. Congress placed hydrocodone (bulk or single entity products) in schedule II of the Controlled Substances Act (CSA) and its products containing specified doses in combination with specified amounts of isoquinoline alkaloid of opium or one or more nonnarcotic substances in recognized therapeutic amounts as schedule III products when the CSA was enacted.

Section 21.6

Hydromorphone

Excerpted from "Drugs of Abuse," Drug Enforcement Administration,
U.S. Department of Justice (www.justice.gov/dea), 2011.

What is hydromorphone?

Hydromorphone belongs to a class of drugs called "opioids," which includes morphine. It has an analgesic potency of two to eight times that of morphine but has a shorter duration of action and greater sedative properties.

What is its origin?

Hydromorphone is legally manufactured and distributed in the United States. However, abusers can obtain hydromorphone from forged prescriptions, "doctor-shopping," theft from pharmacies, and from friends and acquaintances.

What are the street names?

Common street names include D, Dillies, Dust, Footballs, Juice, and Smack.

What does it look like?

Hydromorphone comes in tablets, rectal suppositories, oral solutions, and injectable formulations.

How is it abused?

Users may abuse hydromorphone tablets by ingesting them. Injectable solutions, as well as tablets that have been crushed and dissolved in a solution, may be injected as a substitute for heroin.

What is its effect on the mind?

When used as a drug of abuse, and not under a doctor's supervision, hydromorphone is taken to produce feelings of euphoria, relaxation, sedation, and reduced anxiety. It may also cause mental clouding, changes in mood, nervousness, and restlessness. It works centrally (in the brain) to reduce pain and suppress cough. Hydromorphone use is associated with both physiological and psychological dependence.

What is its effect on the body?

Hydromorphone may cause constipation, papillary constriction, urinary retention, nausea, vomiting, respiratory depression, dizziness, impaired coordination, loss of appetite, rash, slow or rapid heartbeat, and changes in blood pressure.

What are its overdose effects?

Acute overdose of hydromorphone can produce severe respiratory depression, drowsiness progressing to stupor or coma, lack of skeletal muscle tone, cold and clammy skin, constricted pupils, and reduction in blood pressure and heart rate.

Severe overdose may result in death due to respiratory depression.

Which drugs cause similar effects?

Drugs that have similar effects include heroin, morphine, hydrocodone, fentanyl, and oxycodone.

What is its legal status in the United States?

Hydromorphone is a schedule II drug under the Controlled Substances Act with an accepted medical use as a pain reliever. Hydromorphone has a high potential for abuse, and use may lead to severe psychological or physical dependence.

Section 21.7

Methadone

Excerpted from "Drugs of Abuse," Drug Enforcement Administration,
U.S. Department of Justice (www.justice.gov/dea), 2011.

What is methadone?

Methadone is a synthetic (man-made) narcotic.

What is its origin?

German scientists synthesized methadone during World War II because of a shortage of morphine. Methadone was introduced into the United States in 1947 as an analgesic (Dolophine).

What are common street names?

Common street names include Amidone, Chocolate Chip Cookies, Fizzies, Maria, Pastora, Salvia, Street Methadone, and Wafer.

What does it look like?

Methadone is available as a tablet, disc, oral solution, or injectable liquid. Tablets are available in 5 mg and 10 mg formulations. As of January 1, 2008, manufacturers of methadone hydrochloride tablets 40 mg (dispersible) have voluntarily agreed to restrict distribution of this formulation to only those facilities authorized for detoxification and maintenance treatment of opioid addiction and hospitals. Manufacturers will instruct their wholesale distributors to discontinue supplying this formulation to any facility not meeting this criteria.

How is it abused?

Methadone can be swallowed or injected.

What is its effect on the mind?

Abuse of methadone can lead to psychological dependence.

What is its effect on the body?

When an individual uses methadone, he/she may experience physical symptoms like sweating, itchy skin, or sleepiness. Individuals who abuse methadone risk becoming tolerant of and physically dependent on the drug. When use is stopped, individuals may experience withdrawal symptoms including anxiety, muscle tremors, nausea, diarrhea, vomiting, and abdominal cramps.

The effects of a methadone overdose are slow and shallow breathing, blue fingernails and lips, stomach spasms, clammy skin, convulsions, weak pulse, coma, and possible death.

Which drugs cause similar effects?

Although chemically unlike morphine or heroin, methadone produces many of the same effects.

What is its legal status in the United States?

Methadone is a schedule II drug under the Controlled Substances Act. While it may legally be used under a doctor's supervision, its nonmedical use is illegal.

Section 21.8

Oxycodone

Excerpted from "Drugs of Abuse," Drug Enforcement Administration,
U.S. Department of Justice (www.justice.gov/dea), 2011.

What is oxycodone?

Oxycodone is a semi-synthetic narcotic analgesic and historically has been a popular drug of abuse among the narcotic abusing population.

What is its origin?

Oxycodone is synthesized from thebaine, a constituent of the poppy plant.

What are common street names?

Common street names for oxycodone include Hillbilly Heroin, Kicker, OC, Ox, Roxy, Perc, and Oxy.

What does it look like?

Oxycodone is marketed alone as OxyContin in 10, 20, 40, and 80 mg controlled-release tablets and other immediate-release capsules like 5 mg OxyIR. It is also marketed in combination products with aspirin such as Percodan or acetaminophen such as Roxicet.

How is it abused?

Oxycodone is abused orally or intravenously. The tablets are crushed and sniffed or dissolved in water and injected. Others heat a tablet that has been placed on a piece of foil then inhale the vapors.

What is its effect on the mind?

Euphoria and feelings of relaxation are the most common effects of oxycodone on the brain, which explains its high potential for abuse.

What is its effect on the body?

Physiological effects of oxycodone include pain relief, sedation, respiratory depression, constipation, papillary constriction, and cough suppression. Extended or chronic use of oxycodone containing acetaminophen may cause severe liver damage.

Overdose effects include extreme drowsiness, muscle weakness, confusion, cold and clammy skin, pinpoint pupils, shallow breathing, slow heart rate, fainting, coma, and possible death.

Which drugs cause similar effects?

Drugs that cause similar effects to oxycodone include opium, codeine, heroin, methadone, hydrocodone, fentanyl, and morphine.

What is its legal status in the United States?

Oxycodone products are in schedule II of the federal Controlled Substances Act of 1970.

Chapter 22

Sedatives (Depressants)

Chapter Contents

Section 22.1

Introduction to Depressants

Excerpted from "Drugs of Abuse," Drug Enforcement Administration,
U.S. Department of Justice (www.justice.gov/dea), 2011.

What are depressants?

Depressants will put you to sleep, relieve anxiety and muscle
spasms, and prevent seizures. Barbiturates are older drugs and include
butalbital (Fiorina), phenobarbital, Pentothal, Seconal, and Nembutal.
You can rapidly develop dependence on and tolerance to barbiturates,
meaning you need more and more of them to feel and function normally. This makes them unsafe, increasing the likelihood of coma or death.

Benzodiazepines were developed to replace barbiturates, though
they still share many of the undesirable side effects. Some examples
are Valium, Xanax, Halcion, Ativan, Klonopin, and Restoril. Rohypnol
is a benzodiazepine that is not manufactured or legally marketed in
the United States, but it is used illegally.

Ambien and Sonata are sedative-hypnotic medications approved for
the short-term treatment of insomnia that share many of the properties of benzodiazepines. Other central nervous system (CNS) depressants include meprobamate, methaqualone (Quaalude), and the illicit
drug GHB (gamma hydroxybutyrate).

What is their origin?

Generally, legitimate pharmaceutical products are diverted to
the illicit market. Teens can obtain depressants from the family
medicine cabinet, friends, family members, the internet, doctors,
and hospitals.

What are common street names?

Common street names for depressants include Barbs, Benzos,
Downers, Georgia Home Boy, GHB, Grievous Bodily Harm, Liquid
X, Nerve Pills, Phennies, R2, Reds, Roofies, Rophies, Tranks, and
Yellows.

What do they look like?

Depressants come in the form of pills, syrups, and injectable liquids.

How are they abused?

Individuals abuse depressants to experience euphoria. Depressants are also used with other drugs to add to the other drugs' high or to deal with their side effects. Abusers take higher doses than people taking the drugs under a doctor's supervision for therapeutic purposes. Depressants like GHB and Rohypnol are also misused to facilitate sexual assault.

What is their effect on the mind?

Depressants used therapeutically do what they are prescribed for: put you to sleep, relieve anxiety and muscle spasms, and prevent seizures.

They also cause amnesia, leaving no memory of events that occur while under the influence, reduce your reaction time, impair mental functioning and judgment, and cause confusion.

Long-term use of depressants produces psychological dependence and tolerance.

What is their effect on the body?

Some depressants can relax the muscles. Unwanted physical effects include blurred speech, loss of motor coordination, weakness, headache, lightheadedness, blurred vision, dizziness, nausea, vomiting, low blood pressure, and slowed breathing.

Prolonged use of depressants can lead to physical dependence even at doses recommended for medical treatment. Unlike barbiturates, large doses of benzodiazepines are rarely fatal unless combined with other drugs or alcohol. But unlike the withdrawal syndrome seen with most other drugs of abuse, withdrawal from depressants can be life threatening.

What are their overdose effects?

High doses of depressants or use of them with alcohol or other drugs can slow heart rate and breathing enough to cause death.

Which drugs cause similar effects?

Some antipsychotics, antihistamines, and antidepressants produce sedative effects. Alcohol's effects are similar to those of depressants.

What is their legal status in the United States?

Most depressants are controlled substances that range from schedule I to schedule IV under the Controlled Substances Act, depending on their risk for abuse and whether they currently have an accepted medical use. Many of the depressants have U.S. Food and Drug Administration (FDA)-approved medical uses. Rohypnol is not manufactured or legally marketed in the United States.

Section 22.2

Barbiturates

Excerpted from "Drugs of Abuse," Drug Enforcement Administration, U.S. Department of Justice (www.justice.gov/dea), 2011.

What are barbiturates?

Barbiturates are depressants that produce a wide spectrum of central nervous system depression from mild sedation to coma. They have also been used as sedatives, hypnotics, anesthetics, and anticonvulsants.

Barbiturates are classified as ultrashort, short, intermediate, and long-acting.

What is their origin?

Barbiturates were first introduced for medical use in the 1900s, and today about 12 substances are in medical use.

What are common street names?

Common street names include Barbs, Block Busters, Christmas Trees, Goof Balls, Pinks, Red Devils, Reds & Blues, and Yellow Jackets.

What do they look like?

Barbiturates come in a variety of multicolored pills and tablets. Abusers prefer the short-acting and intermediate barbiturates such as Amytal and Seconal.

How are they abused?

Barbiturates are abused by swallowing a pill or injecting a liquid form. Barbiturates are generally abused to reduce anxiety, decrease inhibitions, and treat unwanted effects of illicit drugs. Barbiturates can be extremely dangerous because overdoses can occur easily and lead to death.

What is their effect on the mind?

Barbiturates cause mild euphoria, lack of inhibition, relief of anxiety, and sleepiness. Higher doses cause impairment of memory, judgment, and coordination; irritability; and paranoid and suicidal ideation.

Tolerance develops quickly and larger doses are then needed to produce the same effect, increasing the danger of an overdose.

What is their effect on the body?

Barbiturates slow down the central nervous system and cause sleepiness.

Effects of overdose include shallow respiration, clammy skin, dilated pupils, weak and rapid pulse, coma, and possible death.

Which drugs cause similar effects?

Drugs with similar effects include alcohol, benzodiazepines like Valium and Xanax, tranquilizers, sleeping pills, Rohypnol, and GHB.

What is their legal status in the United States?

Barbiturates are schedule II, III, and IV depressants under the Controlled Substances Act.

Section 22.3

Benzodiazepines

Excerpted from "Drugs of Abuse," Drug Enforcement Administration,
U.S. Department of Justice (www.justice.gov/dea), 2011.

What are benzodiazepines?

Benzodiazepines are depressants that produce sedation, induce
sleep, relieve anxiety and muscle spasms, and prevent seizures.

What is their origin?

Benzodiazepines are only legally available through prescription.
Many abusers maintain their drug supply by getting prescriptions
from several doctors, forging prescriptions, or buying them illicitly.
Alprazolam and diazepam are the two most frequently encountered
benzodiazepines on the illicit market.

What are common street names?

Common street names include Benzos and Downers.

What do they look like?

The most common benzodiazepines are the prescription drugs Valium, Xanax, Halcion, Ativan, and Klonopin. Tolerance can develop,
although at variable rates and to different degrees. Shorter-acting
benzodiazepines used to manage insomnia include estazolam (Pro-
Som), flurazepam (Dalmane), temazepam (Restoril), and triazolam
(Halcion). Midazolam (Versed), a short-acting benzodiazepine, is utilized for sedation, anxiety, and amnesia in critical care settings and
prior to anesthesia. It is available in the United States as an injectable
preparation and as a syrup (primarily for pediatric patients).

Benzodiazepines with a longer duration of action are utilized to
treat insomnia in patients with daytime anxiety. These benzodiazepines include alprazolam (Xanax), chlordiazepoxide (Librium),
clorazepate (Tranxene), diazepam (Valium), halazepam (Paxipam),

lorazepam (Ativan), oxazepam (Serax), prazepam (Centrax), and quazepam (Doral). Clonazepam (Klonopin), diazepam, and clorazepate are also used as anticonvulsants.

How are they abused?

Abuse is frequently associated with adolescents and young adults who take the drug orally or crush it up and snort it to get high. Abuse is particularly high among heroin and cocaine abusers.

What is their effect on the mind?

Benzodiazepines are associated with amnesia, hostility, irritability, and vivid or disturbing dreams.

What is their effect on the body?

Benzodiazepines slow down the central nervous system and may cause sleepiness. Effects of overdose include shallow respiration, clammy skin, dilated pupils, weak and rapid pulse, coma, and possible death.

Which drugs cause similar effects?

Drugs that cause similar effects include alcohol, barbiturates, sleeping pills, and GHB.

What is their legal status in the United States?

Benzodiazepines are controlled in schedule IV of the Controlled Substance Act.

Section 22.4

Kava

"Kava," Drug Enforcement Administration Office of Diversion Control,
U.S. Department of Justice (www.deadiversion.usdoj.gov), January 2013.

Kava, also known as *Piper methysticum* (intoxicating pepper), is a perennial shrub native to the South Pacific Islands, including Hawaii. It is harvested for its rootstock, which contains the pharmacologically active compounds kavalactones. The term *kava* also refers to the non-fermented, psychoactive beverage prepared from the rootstock. For many centuries, Pacific Island societies have consumed kava beverages for social, ceremonial, and medical purposes. Traditionally, kava beverages are prepared by chewing or pounding the rootstock to produce a cloudy, milky pulp that is then soaked in water before the liquid is filtered to drink.

There is an increasing use of kava for recreational purposes. The reinforcing effects of kava include mild euphoria, muscle relaxation, sedation, and analgesia.

Licit Uses

In the U.S., kava is sold as dietary supplements promoted as natural alternatives to anti-anxiety drugs and sleeping pills. A n analysis of six kava clinical trials found that kava (60–200 mg of kavalactones/day) produced a significant reduction in anxiety compared to placebo. However, the FDA has not made a determination about the ability of dietary supplements containing kava to provide such benefits.

Kava dietary supplements are commonly formulated as tablets and capsules (30%–90% kavalactones; 50–250 mg per capsule). Kava is also available as whole root, powdered root, extracts (powder, paste, and liquid), tea bags, and instant powdered drink mix. Kava is frequently found in products containing a variety of herbs or vitamins, or both.

A number of cases of liver damage (hepatitis and cirrhosis) and liver failure have been associated with commercial extract preparations of kava. In 2002, the FDA issued an advisory alerting consumers and health care providers to the potential risk of liver-related injuries associated with the use of kava dietary supplements.

Chemistry and Pharmacology

The pharmacologically active kavalactones are found in the lipid soluble resin of the kava rootstock. Of the 18 isolated and identified, yangonin, methysticin, dihydromethysticin, dihydrokawain, kawain, and desmethoxyyangonin are the six major kavalactones. Different varieties of kava plants possess varying concentrations of kavalactones.

The pharmacokinetics of the kavalactones has not been extensively studied. Kavalactones are thought to be relatively quickly absorbed in the gut. There may be differences in the bioavailability between each kavalactone.

The limbic structures, amygdala complex, and reticular formation of the brain appear to be the preferential sites of action of kavalactones. However, the exact molecular mechanisms of action are not clear.

Kava has the potential for causing drug interactions through the inhibition of CYP450 enzymes that are responsible for the metabolism of many pharmaceutical agents and other herbal remedies.

Chronic use of kava in large quantities may cause a dry scaly skin or yellow skin discoloration known as kava dermopathy. It may also cause liver toxicity and tremor and abnormal body movement. Individuals may experience a numbing or tingling of the mouth upon drinking kava due to its local anesthetic action. High doses of kavalactones can also produce CNS depressant effects (e.g., sedation and muscle weakness) that appear to be transient.

Illicit Uses

Information on the illicit use of kava in the U.S. is anecdotal. Based on information on the internet, kava is being used recreationally to relax the body and achieve a mild euphoria. It is typically consumed as a beverage made from dried kava root powder, flavored and unflavored powdered extracts, and liquid extract dissolved in pure grain alcohol and vegetable glycerin. Individuals may consume 25 grams of kavalactones, which is about 125 times the daily dose in kava dietary supplements.

Intoxicated individuals typically have sensible thought processes and comprehensive conversations but have difficulty coordinating movement and often fall asleep. Kava users do not exhibit the generalized confusion and delirium that occurs with high levels of alcohol intoxication. While kava alone does not produce the motor and cognitive impairments caused by alcohol, kava does potentiate both the perceived and measured impairment produced by alcohol.

The American Association of Poison Control Centers reported 42 case mentions and 21 single exposures associated with kava in 2010.

User Population

Information on user population in the U.S. is very limited. In the 1980s, kava was introduced to Australian Aboriginal communities where it quickly became a drug of abuse. It has become a serious social problem in regions of Northern Australia.

Distribution

Kava is widely available on the internet. Some websites promoting and selling kava products also sell other uncontrolled psychoactive products such as *Salvia divinorum* and kratom.

Several kava bars and lounges in the U.S. sell kava drinks. The National Forensic Laboratory Information System (NFLIS) and the System to Retrieve Information from Drug Evidence (STRIDE) do not indicate any kava reports.

Control Status

Kava is not a controlled substance in the U.S. Due to concerns of liver toxicity, many countries including Australia, Canada, France, Germany, Malaysia, Singapore, Switzerland, and the United Kingdom have placed regulatory controls on kava. These controls range from warning consumers of the dangers of taking kava to removing kava products from the marketplace.

Chapter 23

Stimulants

Chapter Contents

Section 23.1

Introduction to Stimulants

Excerpted from "Drugs of Abuse," Drug Enforcement Administration,
U.S. Department of Justice (www.justice.gov/dea), 2011.

What are stimulants?

Stimulants speed up the body's systems. This class of drugs includes prescription drugs such as amphetamines (Adderall and Dexedrine), methylphenidate (Concerta and Ritalin), diet aids (such as Didrex, Bontril, Preludin, Fastin, Adipex P, Ionamin, and Meridia), and illicitly produced drugs such as methamphetamine, cocaine, and methcathinone.

What is their origin?

Stimulants are diverted from legitimate channels and clandestinely manufactured exclusively for the illicit market.

What are common street names?

Common street names include Bennies, Black Beauties, Cat, Coke, Crank, Crystal, Flake, Ice, Pellets, R-Ball, Skippy, Snow, Speed, Uppers, and Vitamin R.

What do they look like?

Stimulants come in the form of pills, powder, rocks, and injectable liquids.

How are they abused?

Stimulants can be pills or capsules that are swallowed. Smoking, snorting, or injecting stimulants produces a sudden sensation known as a "rush" or a "flash." Abuse is often associated with a pattern of binge use—sporadically consuming large doses of stimulants over a short period of time. Heavy users may inject themselves every few hours, continuing until they have depleted their drug supply or reached a point of delirium, psychosis, and physical exhaustion. During heavy use, all other interests become secondary to recreating the initial euphoric rush.

What is their effect on the mind?

When used as drugs of abuse and not under a doctor's supervision, stimulants are frequently taken to produce a sense of exhilaration, enhance self-esteem, improve mental and physical performance, increase activity, reduce appetite, extend wakefulness for prolonged period, and "get high."

Chronic, high-dose use is frequently associated with agitation, hostility, panic, aggression, and suicidal or homicidal tendencies. Paranoia, sometimes accompanied by both auditory and visual hallucinations, may also occur.

Tolerance, in which more and more drug is needed to produce the usual effects, can develop rapidly, and psychological dependence occurs. In fact, the strongest psychological dependence observed occurs with the more potent stimulants, such as amphetamine, methylphenidate, methamphetamine, cocaine, and methcathinone.

Abrupt cessation is commonly followed by depression, anxiety, drug craving, and extreme fatigue, known as a "crash."

What is their effect on the body?

Stimulants are sometimes referred to as uppers and reverse the effects of fatigue on both mental and physical tasks. Therapeutic levels of stimulants can produce exhilaration, extended wakefulness, and loss of appetite. These effects are greatly intensified when large doses of stimulants are taken.

Taking too large a dose at one time or taking large doses over an extended period of time may cause such physical side effects as dizziness, tremors, headache, flushed skin, chest pain with palpitations, excessive sweating, vomiting, and abdominal cramps.

In overdose, unless there is medical intervention, high fever, convulsions, and cardiovascular collapse may precede death. Because accidental death is partially due to the effects of stimulants on the body's cardiovascular and temperature-regulating systems, physical exertion increases the hazards of stimulant use.

Which drugs cause similar effects?

Some hallucinogenic substances, such as ecstasy, have a stimulant component to their activity.

What is their legal status in the United States?

Many stimulants have a legitimate medical use for the treatment of conditions such as obesity, narcolepsy, and attention deficit and hyperactivity disorder. Such stimulants vary in their level of control from schedules II to IV, depending on their potential for abuse and dependence.

A number of stimulants have no medical use in the United States but have a high potential for abuse. These stimulants are controlled in schedule I. Some prescription stimulants are not controlled, and some stimulants like tobacco and caffeine don't require a prescription—though society's recognition of their adverse effects has resulted in a proliferation of caffeine-free products and efforts to discourage cigarette smoking.

Stimulant chemicals in over-the-counter products, such as ephedrine and pseudoephedrine, can be found in allergy and cold medicine. As required by the Combat Methamphetamine Epidemic Act of 2005, a retail outlet must store these products out of reach of customers, either behind the counter or in a locked cabinet. Regulated sellers are required to maintain a written or electronic form of a logbook to record sales of these products. In order to purchase these products, customers must now show a photo identification issued by a state or federal government. They are also required to write or enter into the logbook: their name, signature, address, date, and time of sale. In addition, there are daily and monthly sales limits set for customers.

Section 23.2

Amphetamine and Methylphenidate

"DrugFacts: Stimulant ADHA Medications—Methylphenidate
and Amphetamines," National Institute on Drug Abuse
(www.drugabuse.gov), June 2009.

Stimulant medications (e.g., methylphenidate and amphetamines)
are often prescribed to treat individuals diagnosed with attention-
deficit hyperactivity disorder (ADHD). ADHD is characterized by a
persistent pattern of inattention and/or hyperactivity-impulsivity that
is more frequently displayed and more severe than is typically observed
in individuals at a comparable level of development. This pattern of
behavior usually becomes evident in the preschool or early elementary
years, and the median age of onset of ADHD symptoms is seven years.
For many individuals, ADHD symptoms improve during adolescence
or as age increases, but the disorder can persist into adulthood. In the
United States, ADHD is diagnosed in an estimated 8% of children ages
4–17 and in 2.9%–4.4% percent of adults.

How do prescription stimulants affect the brain?

All stimulants work by increasing dopamine levels in the brain—
dopamine is a brain chemical (or neurotransmitter) associated with
pleasure, movement, and attention. The therapeutic effect of stimulants is achieved by slow and steady increases of dopamine, which
are similar to the natural production of the chemical by the brain.
The doses prescribed by physicians start low and increase gradually
until a therapeutic effect is reached. However, when taken in doses
and routes other than those prescribed, stimulants can increase brain
dopamine in a rapid and highly amplified manner—as do most other
drugs of abuse—disrupting normal communication between brain cells,
producing euphoria, and increasing the risk of addiction.

What is the role of stimulants in the treatment of ADHD?

Treatment of ADHD with stimulants, often in conjunction with
psychotherapy, helps to improve the symptoms of ADHD, as well as the

self-esteem, cognition, and social and family interactions of the patient. The most commonly prescribed medications include amphetamines (e.g., Adderall, a mix of amphetamine salts) and methylphenidate (e.g., Ritalin and Concerta—a formulation that releases medication in the body over a period of time). These medications have a paradoxically calming and "focusing" effect on individuals with ADHD. Researchers speculate that because methylphenidate amplifies the release of dopamine, it can improve attention and focus in individuals who have dopamine signals that are weak.

One of the most controversial issues in child psychiatry is whether the use of stimulant medications to treat ADHD increases the risk of substance abuse in adulthood. Research thus far suggests that individuals with ADHD do not become addicted to their stimulant medications when taken in the form and dosage prescribed by their doctors. Furthermore, several studies report that stimulant therapy in childhood does not increase the risk for subsequent drug and alcohol abuse disorders later in life. More research is needed, however, particularly in adolescents treated with stimulant medications.

Why and how are prescription stimulants abused?

Stimulants have been abused for both "performance enhancement" and recreational purposes (i.e., to get high). For the former, they suppress appetite (to facilitate weight loss), increase wakefulness, and increase focus and attention. The euphoric effects of stimulants usually occur when they are crushed and then snorted or injected. Some abusers dissolve the tablets in water and inject the mixture. Complications from this method of use can arise because insoluble fillers in the tablets can block small blood vessels.

What adverse effects does prescription stimulant abuse have on health?

Stimulants can increase blood pressure, heart rate, and body temperature and decrease sleep and appetite, which can lead to malnutrition and its consequences. Repeated use of stimulants can lead to feelings of hostility and paranoia. At high doses, they can lead to serious cardiovascular complications, including stroke.

Addiction to stimulants is also a very real consideration for anyone taking them without medical supervision. This most likely occurs because stimulants, when taken in doses and routes other than those prescribed by a doctor, can induce a rapid rise in dopamine in the brain. Furthermore, if stimulants are used chronically, withdrawal symptoms—including fatigue, depression, and disturbed sleep patterns—can emerge when the drugs are discontinued.

How widespread is prescription stimulant abuse?

Each year, the Monitoring the Future (MTF) survey assesses the extent of drug use among 8th, 10th, and 12th graders nationwide. For amphetamines and methylphenidate, the survey measures only past-year use, which refers to use at least once during the year preceding an individual's response to the survey. Use outside of medical supervision was first measured in the study in 2001; nonmedical use of stimulants has been falling since then, with total declines between 25% and 42% at each grade level surveyed. MTF data for 2008 indicate past-year nonmedical use of Ritalin by 1.6% of 8th graders, 2.9% of 10th graders, and 3.4% of 12th graders.

Since its peak in the mid-1990s, annual prevalence of amphetamine use fell by one-half among 8th graders to 4.5% and by nearly one-half among 10th graders to 6.4% in 2008. Amphetamine use peaked some-what later among 12th graders and has fallen by more than one-third to 6.8% by 2008. Although general nonmedical use of prescription stimulants is declining in this group, when asked, "What amphet-amines have you taken during the last year without a doctor's orders?" 2.8% of all 12th graders surveyed in 2007 reported they had used Ad-derall. Amphetamines rank third among 12th graders for past-year illicit drug use.

Section 23.3

BZP

"N-Benzylpiperazine," Drug Enforcement Administration
Office of Diversion Control, U.S. Department of Justice
(www.deadiversion.usdoj.gov), July 2012.

N-benzylpiperazine (BZP) was first synthesized in 1944 as a potential antiparasitic agent. It was subsequently shown to possess antidepressant activity and amphetamine-like effects, but was not developed for marketing. The amphetamine-like effects of BZP attracted the attention of drug abusers. Since 1996, BZP has been abused by drug abusers; as evidenced by the encounters of this substance by law enforcement officials in various states and the District of Columbia.

The Drug Enforcement Administration (DEA) placed BZP in schedule I of the Controlled Substances Act (CSA) because of its high abuse potential and lack of accepted medical use or safety.

Licit Uses

BZP is used as an intermediate in chemical synthesis. It has no known medical use in the United States.

Chemistry and Pharmacology

BZP is an N-monosubstituted piperazine derivative available as either base or the hydrochloride salt. The base form is a slightly yellowish-green liquid. The hydrochloride salt is a white solid. BZP base is corrosive and causes burns. The salt form of BZP is an irritant to eyes, respiratory system, and skin.

Both animal studies and human clinical studies have demonstrated that the pharmacological effects of BZP are qualitatively similar to those of amphetamine. BZP has been reported to be similar to amphetamine in its effects on chemical transmission in brain. BZP fully mimics discriminative stimulus effects of amphetamine in animals. BZP is self-administered by monkeys indicating reinforcing effects. Subjective effects of BZP were amphetamine-like in drug-naive volunteers and in volunteers with a history of stimulant dependence. BZP acts as a stimulant in humans and produces euphoria and cardiovascular effects, namely increases in heart rate and systolic blood pressure. BZP is about 10 to 20 times less potent than amphetamine in producing these effects. Experimental studies demonstrate that the abuse, dependence potential, pharmacology, and toxicology of BZP are similar to those of amphetamine. Public health risks of BZP are similar to those of amphetamine.

Illicit Uses

BZP is often abused in combination with 1-[3-(trifluoro-methyl) phenyl]piperazine (TFMPP), a noncontrolled substance. This combination has been promoted to the youth population as a substitute for 3,4-methylenedioxymethamphetamine (MDMA) at raves (all-night dance parties). However, there are no clinical studies that directly compared the behavioral effects of BZP to those of MDMA. BZP may also be abused alone for its stimulant effects. BZP is generally administered orally as either powder or tablets and capsules. Other routes of administration included smoking and snorting. In 2001, a report from University in Zurich, Switzerland, described the death of a young female that was attributed to the combined use of BZP and MDMA.

User Population

Youth and young adults are the main abusers of BZP.

Illicit Distribution

According to DEA's System to Retrieve Information from Drug Evidence (STRIDE) and National Forensic Laboratory Information System (NFLIS), the number of reports submitted to federal, state, and local forensic laboratories and identified as BZP increased 149% from 6,088 in 2008 to 15,170 in 2009. In 2010, the number of BZP reports decreased to 8,708 and in 2011, it decreased to 5,288. In the first quarter of 2012, there were 836 reports of BZP.

Illicit distributions occur through smuggling of bulk powder through drug trafficking organizations with connections to overseas sources of supply. The bulk powder is then processed into capsules and tablets. BZP is encountered as pink, white, off-white, purple, orange, tan, and mottled orange-brown tablets. These tablets bear imprints commonly seen on MDMA tablets such as house fly, crown, heart, butterfly, smiley face or bull's head logos and are often sold as "ecstasy." BZP has been found in powder or liquid form which is packaged in small convenience sizes and sold on the internet.

Control Status

BZP was temporarily placed into schedule I of the Controlled Substances Act (CSA) on September 20, 2002 (67 FR 59161). On March 18, 2004, the DEA published a Final Rule in the Federal Register permanently placing BZP in schedule I.

Section 23.4

Cocaine

Excerpted from "DrugFacts: Cocaine,"
National Institute on Drug Abuse (www.drugabuse.gov), April 2013.

Cocaine is a powerfully addictive stimulant drug made from the leaves of the coca plant native to South America. It produces short-term euphoria, energy, and talkativeness in addition to potentially dangerous physical effects like raising heart rate and blood pressure.

How is cocaine used?

The powdered form of cocaine is either inhaled through the nose (snorted), where it is absorbed through the nasal tissue, or dissolved in water and injected into the bloodstream.

Crack is a form of cocaine that has been processed to make a rock crystal (also called "freebase cocaine") that can be smoked. The crystal is heated to produce vapors that are absorbed into the blood-stream through the lungs. (The term "crack" refers to the crackling sound produced by the rock as it is heated.)

The intensity and duration of cocaine's pleasurable effects depend on the way it is administered. Injecting or smoking cocaine delivers the drug rapidly into the bloodstream and brain, producing a quicker and stronger but shorter-lasting high than snorting. The high from snorting cocaine may last 15 to 30 minutes; the high from smoking may last 5 to 10 minutes.

In order to sustain their high, people who use cocaine often use the drug in a binge pattern—taking the drug repeatedly within a relatively short period of time, at increasingly higher doses. This practice can easily lead to addiction, a chronic relapsing disease caused by changes in the brain and characterized by uncontrollable drug seeking no matter the consequences.

How does cocaine affect the brain?

Cocaine is a strong central nervous system stimulant that increases levels of the neurotransmitter dopamine in brain circuits regulating pleasure and movement.

Normally, dopamine is released by neurons in these circuits in response to potential rewards (like the smell of good food) and then recycled back into the cell that released it, thus shutting off the signal between neurons. Cocaine prevents the dopamine from being recycled, causing excessive amounts to build up in the synapse, or junction between neurons. This amplifies the dopamine signal and ultimately disrupts normal brain communication. It is this flood of dopamine that causes cocaine's characteristic high.

With repeated use, cocaine can cause long-term changes in the brain's reward system as well as other brain systems, which may lead to addiction. With repeated use, tolerance to cocaine also often develops; many cocaine abusers report that they seek but fail to achieve as much pleasure as they did from their first exposure. Some users will increase their dose in an attempt to intensify and prolong their high, but this can also increase the risk of adverse psychological or physiological effects.

What are the other health effects of cocaine?

Cocaine affects the body in a variety of ways. It constricts blood vessels, dilates pupils, and increases body temperature, heart rate, and blood pressure. It can also cause headaches and gastrointestinal complications such as abdominal pain and nausea. Because cocaine tends to decrease appetite, chronic users can become malnourished as well.

Most seriously, people who use cocaine can suffer heart attacks or strokes, which may cause sudden death. Cocaine-related deaths are often a result of the heart stopping (cardiac arrest) followed by an arrest of breathing.

People who use cocaine also put themselves at risk for contracting HIV, even if they do not share needles or other drug paraphernalia. This is because cocaine intoxication impairs judgment and can lead to risky sexual behavior.

Some effects of cocaine depend on the method of taking it. Regular snorting of cocaine, for example, can lead to loss of the sense of smell, nosebleeds, problems with swallowing, hoarseness, and a chronically runny nose. Ingesting cocaine by the mouth can cause severe bowel gangrene as a result of reduced blood flow. Injecting cocaine can bring about severe allergic reactions and increased risk for contracting HIV, hepatitis C, and other bloodborne diseases.

Binge-patterned cocaine use may lead to irritability, restlessness, and anxiety. Cocaine abusers can also experience severe paranoia—a temporary state of full-blown paranoid psychosis—in which they lose touch with reality and experience auditory hallucinations.

Cocaine is more dangerous when combined with other drugs or alcohol (polydrug use). For example, the combination of cocaine and heroin (known as a "speedball") carries a particularly high risk of fatal overdose.

Section 23.5

Khat

"DrugFacts: Khat," National Institute on Drug Abuse
(www.drugabuse.gov), April 2013.

Khat (pronounced "cot") is a stimulant drug derived from a shrub (*Catha edulis*) that is native to East Africa and southern Arabia. The khat plant itself is not scheduled under the Controlled Substances Act; however, because one of the mind-altering chemicals found in it, cathinone, is a schedule I drug (a controlled substance with no recognized therapeutic use), the federal government considers khat use illegal.

How is khat used?

Leaves of the khat shrub are typically chewed and held in the cheek, like chewing tobacco, to release their stimulant chemicals.

How does khat affect the brain?

The main psychoactive ingredients in khat are cathinone and cathine. These chemicals are structurally similar to amphetamine and result in similar stimulant effects in the brain and body, although they are less potent. Like other stimulants, cathinone and cathine stimulate the release of the stress hormone and neurotransmitter norepinephrine and raise the level of the neurotransmitter dopamine in brain circuits regulating pleasure and movement.

Who uses khat?

It is estimated that as many as 10 million people worldwide chew khat. It is commonly found in the southwestern part of the Arabian Peninsula and in East Africa, where it has been used for centuries as part of an established cultural tradition. In one large study in Yemen, 82% of men and 43% of women reported at least one lifetime episode of khat use. Its current use among particular migrant communities in the United States and in Europe has caused concern among policy makers and health care professionals. No reliable estimates of prevalence in the United States exist.

Chewing khat leaves is reported to induce a state of euphoria and elation as well as feelings of increased alertness and arousal. The effects begin to subside after about 90 minutes to 3 hours but can last 24 hours. At the end of a khat session, the user may experience a depressed mood, irritability, loss of appetite, and difficulty sleeping.

What are the other health effects of khat?

In addition to its psychological effects, khat users can also experience physiological effects typically produced by stimulants, including an increase in blood pressure and heart rate.

There are a number of adverse physical effects that have been associated with heavy or long-term use of khat, including tooth decay and periodontal disease; gastrointestinal disorders such as constipation, ulcers, inflammation of the stomach, and increased risk of upper gastrointestinal tumors; and cardiovascular disorders such as irregular heartbeat, decreased blood flow, and heart attack.

There is also consistent epidemiologic evidence for a weak association between chronic khat use and mental disorders. Although there is no evidence that khat use causes mental illness, chewing khat leaves may worsen symptoms in patients who have preexisting psychiatric conditions.

It is unclear whether khat causes tolerance, physical dependency, addiction, or withdrawal, but long-term users have reported mild depression, nightmares, and trembling after ceasing to chew khat.

Section 23.6

Kratom

"Kratom (*Mitragyna speciosa korth*)," Drug Enforcement
Administration Office of Diversion Control, U.S. Department of
Justice (www.deadiversion.usdoj.gov), January 2013.

Kratom (*Mitragyna speciosa korth*) is a tropical tree indigenous
to Thailand, Malaysia, Myanmar, and other areas of Southeast Asia.
Kratom is in the same family as the coffee tree (*Rubiaceae*). The tree
reaches heights of 50 feet with a spread of over 15 feet.

Kratom has been used by natives of Thailand and other regions of
Southeast Asia as an herbal drug for decades. Traditionally, kratom
was mostly used as a stimulant by Thai and Malaysian laborers and
farmers to overcome the burdens of hard work. They chewed the
leaves to make them work harder and provide energy and relief from
muscle strains. Kratom was also used in Southeast Asia and by Thai
natives to substitute for opium when opium is not available. It has
also been used to manage opioid withdrawal symptoms by chronic
opioid users.

In 1943, the Thai government passed the Kratom Act 2486 that
made planting of the tree illegal. In 1979, the Thai government enacted
the Narcotics Act B.E. 2522, placing kratom along with marijuana
in Category V of a five category classification of narcotics. Kratom
remains a popular drug in Thailand. It has been reported that young
Thai militants drink a "4x100" kratom formula to make them "more
bold and fearless and easy to control." The two "4x100" kratom formu-
las are described as a mixture of boiled kratom leaves and mosquito
coils and cola or a mixture of boiled cough syrup, kratom leaves, and
cola served with ice. In this report it was also mentioned use of that
the "4x100" formula was gaining popularity among Muslim youngsters
in several districts of Yala (Southern Thailand) and was available in
local coffee and tea shops.

Kratom is promoted as a legal psychoactive product on numerous
websites in the U.S. On those websites, topics range from vendors
listings and preparation of tea and recommended doses, to alleged
medicinal uses and user reports of drug experiences.

Licit Uses

There is no legitimate medical use for kratom in the U.S.

Chemistry and Pharmacology

Over 25 alkaloids have been isolated from kratom; mitragynine is the primary active alkaloid in the plant.

Pharmacology studies show that mitragynine has opioid-like activity in animals. It inhibits electrically stimulated ileum and vas deferens smooth muscle contraction. Through actions on centrally located opioid receptor, it inhibits gastric secretion and reduces pain response.

Kratom has been described as producing both stimulant and sedative effects. At low doses, it produces stimulant effects, with users reporting increased alertness, physical energy, talkativeness, and sociable behavior. At high doses, opiate effects are produced, in addition to sedative and euphoric effects. Effects occur within 5 to 10 minutes after ingestion and last for two to five hours. Acute side effects include nausea, itching, sweating, dry mouth, constipation, increased urination, and loss of appetite.

Kratom consumption can lead to addiction. In a study of Thai kratom addicts, it was observed that some addicts chewed kratom daily for 3 to 30 years (mean of 18.6 years). Long-term use of kratom produced anorexia, weight loss, insomnia, skin darkening, dry mouth, frequent urination, and constipation. A withdrawal syndrome was observed, consisting of symptoms of hostility, aggression, emotional lability, wet nose, achy muscles and bones, and jerky movement of the limbs. Furthermore, several cases of kratom psychosis were observed, where kratom addicts exhibited psychotic symptoms that included hallucinations, delusion, and confusion.

Illicit Uses

Information on the illicit use of kratom in the U.S. is anecdotal. Based on information posted on the internet, kratom is mainly being abused orally as a tea. Chewing kratom leaves is another method of consumption. Doses of 2 to 10 grams are recommended to achieve the desired effects. Users report that the dominant effects are similar to those of psychostimulant drugs.

Other countries are reporting emerging new trends in the use of kratom. In the United Kingdom, kratom is promoted as an "herbal speedball." In Malaysia, kratom (known as ketum) juice preparations are illegally available.

User Population

Information on user population in the U.S. is limited. Kratom abuse is not monitored by any national drug abuse surveys.

Illicit Distribution

STRIDE, a federal database for the seized drugs analyzed by DEA forensic laboratories, and the NFLIS, which collects drug analysis information from state and local forensic laboratories, indicate that there was one drug report of mitragynine, the primary active alkaloid in kratom, in 2010, 44 reports in 2011, and 81 reports in the first six months of 2012.

Kratom is widely available on the internet. There are numerous vendors within and outside of the U.S. selling kratom. Forms of kratom available through the internet include leaves (whole or crushed), powder, extract, encapsulated powder, and extract resin "pies" (40 g pellets made from reduced extract). Seeds and whole trees are also available from some vendors through the internet, suggesting the possibility of domestic cultivation.

Control Status

Kratom is not scheduled under the Controlled Substances Act.

Section 23.7

Methamphetamine

Excerpted from "DrugFacts: Methamphetamine,"
National Institute on Drug Abuse (www.drugabuse.gov), March 2010.

Methamphetamine is a central nervous system stimulant drug that is similar in structure to amphetamine. Due to its high potential for abuse, methamphetamine is classified as a schedule II drug and is available only through a prescription that cannot be refilled. Although methamphetamine can be prescribed by a doctor, its medical uses are limited, and the doses that are prescribed are much lower than those typically abused. Most of the methamphetamine abused in this country comes from foreign or domestic superlabs, although it can also be made in small, illegal laboratories, where its production endangers the people in the labs, neighbors, and the environment.

How is methamphetamine abused?

Methamphetamine is a white, odorless, bitter-tasting crystalline powder that easily dissolves in water or alcohol and is taken orally, intranasally (snorting the powder), by needle injection, or by smoking.

How does methamphetamine affect the brain?

Methamphetamine increases the release and blocks the reuptake of the brain chemical (or neurotransmitter) dopamine, leading to high levels of the chemical in the brain—a common mechanism of action for most drugs of abuse. Dopamine is involved in reward, motivation, the experience of pleasure, and motor function. Methamphetamine's ability to release dopamine rapidly in reward regions of the brain produces the intense euphoria, or "rush," that many users feel after snorting, smoking, or injecting the drug.

Chronic methamphetamine abuse significantly changes how the brain functions. Noninvasive human brain imaging studies have shown alterations in the activity of the dopamine system that are associated with reduced motor skills and impaired verbal learning. Recent studies in chronic methamphetamine abusers have also revealed severe

277

structural and functional changes in areas of the brain associated with emotion and memory, which may account for many of the emotional and cognitive problems observed in chronic methamphetamine abusers.

Repeated methamphetamine abuse can also lead to addiction—a chronic, relapsing disease characterized by compulsive drug seeking and use, which is accompanied by chemical and molecular changes in the brain. Some of these changes persist long after methamphetamine abuse is stopped. Reversal of some of the changes, however, may be observed after sustained periods of abstinence (e.g., more than one year).

What other adverse effects does methamphetamine have on health?

Taking even small amounts of methamphetamine can result in many of the same physical effects as those of other stimulants, such as cocaine or amphetamines, including increased wakefulness, increased physical activity, decreased appetite, increased respiration, rapid heart rate, irregular heartbeat, increased blood pressure, and hyperthermia.

Long-term methamphetamine abuse has many negative health consequences, including extreme weight loss, severe dental problems ("meth mouth"), anxiety, confusion, insomnia, mood disturbances, and violent behavior. Chronic methamphetamine abusers can also display a number of psychotic features, including paranoia, visual and auditory hallucinations, and delusions (for example, the sensation of insects crawling under the skin).

Transmission of HIV and hepatitis B and C can be consequences of methamphetamine abuse. The intoxicating effects of methamphetamine, regardless of how it is taken, can also alter judgment and inhibition and can lead people to engage in unsafe behaviors, including risky sexual behavior. Among abusers who inject the drug, HIV/AIDS and other infectious diseases can be spread through contaminated needles, syringes, and other injection equipment that is used by more than one person. Methamphetamine abuse may also worsen the progression of HIV/AIDS and its consequences. Studies of methamphetamine abusers who are HIV-positive indicate that HIV causes greater neuronal injury and cognitive impairment for individuals in this group compared with HIV-positive people who do not use the drug.

What treatment options exist?

Currently, the most effective treatments for methamphetamine addiction are comprehensive cognitive-behavioral interventions. For example, the Matrix Model—a behavioral treatment approach that combines behavioral therapy, family education, individual counseling, 12-step support, drug testing, and encouragement for nondrug-related activities—has been shown to be effective in reducing methamphetamine abuse. Contingency management interventions, which provide tangible incentives in exchange for engaging in treatment and maintaining abstinence, have also been shown to be effective. There are no medications at this time approved to treat methamphetamine addiction; however, this is an active area of research for NIDA.

How widespread is methamphetamine abuse?

Methamphetamine use among teens appears to have dropped significantly in recent years, according to data revealed by the 2009 Monitoring the Future survey. The number of high-school seniors reporting past-year use is now only at 1.2%, which is the lowest since questions about methamphetamine were added to the survey in 1999; at that time, it was reported at 4.7%. Lifetime use among 8th graders was reported at 1.6% in 2009, down significantly from 2.3% in 2008. In addition, the proportion of 10th graders reporting that crystal methamphetamine was easy to obtain has dropped to 14%, down from 19.5% five years ago.

According to the 2008 National Survey on Drug Use and Health, the number of past-month methamphetamine users age 12 and older decreased by over half between 2006 and 2008. Current (past-month) users were numbered at 731,000 in 2006, 529,000 in 2007, and 314,000 in 2008. Significant declines from 2002 and 2008 also were noted for lifetime and past-year use in this age group.

From 2002 to 2008, past-month use of methamphetamine declined significantly among youths aged 12 to 17, from 0.3% to 0.1%, and young adults aged 18 to 25 also reported significant declines in past-month use, from 0.6% in 2002 to 0.2% in 2008.

Chapter 24

New and Emerging Drugs of Abuse

Chapter Contents

Section 24.1

Law Banning New Synthetic Drugs

"Obama Approves Law to Ban Synthetic Drugs," Get Smart About Drugs, Drug Enforcement Administration (www.getsmartabout drugs.com), July 9, 2012, and excerpts from "Synthetic Drugs Fact Sheet," White House Office of National Drug Control Policy (www .whitehouse.gov/ondcp), February 2012.

Obama Approves Law to Ban Synthetic Drugs

President Barack Obama has signed far-reaching legislation banning chemicals found in dangerous synthetic drugs like 2C-E, "K2," "Spice," and "bath salts." The legislation attacks a U.S. epidemic that was responsible for the death of a Minnesota teenager in 2011. Law enforcement officials in Minnesota and other states have been calling for congressional action to fight the epidemic of designer drugs like 2C-E, which is thought to be the drug responsible for the death of Blaine, Minnesota, 19-year-old Trevor Robinson.

"In Minnesota and across the country, we are seeing more and more tragedies where synthetic drugs are taking lives and tearing apart families," said U.S. senator Amy Klobuchar of Minnesota, a champion of the provisions. Klobuchar cited Robinson's death in advocating for a ban on dangerous chemicals in synthetic drugs like 2C-E, a synthetic hallucinogen. Other chemicals that the new law makes illegal are chemicals found in synthetic marijuana (also called "Spice" or "K2"). Similarly, "bath salts," synthetic drugs that mimic the effects of cocaine and methamphetamine on the body, are also now illegal.

Minnesota and more than 30 other states have already banned a variety of synthetic drug compounds, but new and different compounds are regularly emerging in a market that is spread across the nation via the internet. Congress decided that law enforcement would benefit from response on the national level.

Synthetic Drugs

Synthetic marijuana (often known as "K2" or "Spice") and bath salts products are often sold in legal retail outlets as "herbal incense" and

282

"plant food," respectively, and labeled "not for human consumption" to mask their intended purpose and avoid FDA regulatory oversight of the manufacturing process.

Synthetic marijuana consists of plant material that has been laced with substances (synthetic cannabinoids) that users claim mimics delta-9-tetrahydrocannabinol (THC), the primary psychoactive active ingredient in marijuana, and are marketed toward young people as a "legal" high.

Use of synthetic marijuana is alarmingly high. According to data from the 2011 Monitoring the Future survey of youth drug-use trends, 11.4% of 12th graders used Spice or K2 in the past year, making it the second most commonly used illicit drug among seniors.

Bath salts contain manmade chemicals related to amphetamines that often consist of methylenedioxypyrovalerone (MDPV), mephedrone, and methylone, also known as substituted cathinones.

A Rapidly Emerging Threat

Synthetic cannabinoids in herbal incense products were first detected in the United States in November 2008, by the Drug Enforcement Administration (DEA)'s forensic laboratory. These products were first encountered by U.S. Customs and Border Protection.

According to the American Association of Poison Control Centers, 2,906 calls relating to human exposure to synthetic marijuana were received in 2010. Twice that number (6,959) were received in 2011, and 639 had been received as of January 2012.

According to the American Association of Poison Control Centers, the number of calls related to bath salt exposure received by poison control centers across the country increased by more than 20 times in 2011 alone, up from 304 in 2010 to 6,138.

Sources and Continuing Availability

According to U.S. Customs and Border Protection, a number of synthetic marijuana and bath salts products appear to originate overseas and are manufactured in the absence of quality controls and devoid of governmental regulatory oversight.

Law enforcement personnel have also encountered the manufacture of herbal incense products in such places as residential neighborhoods. These products and associated synthetic cannabinoids are readily accessible via the internet.

The large profits from sales, plus the fact that these chemicals can be easily synthesized to stay one step ahead of control, indicate there is no incentive to discontinue retail distribution of synthetic cannabinoid products under the current statutory and regulatory scheme.

Government Efforts to Ban Synthetic Drug Products

The DEA and state drug control agencies have recognized the need to monitor and, when necessary, control these chemicals. The Comprehensive Crime Control Act of 1984 amends the Controlled Substances Act (CSA) to allow the attorney general to place a substance temporarily in schedule I when it is necessary to avoid an imminent hazard to the public safety (21 U.S.C. §811(h)).

On October 21, 2011, DEA exercised its emergency scheduling authority to control some of the synthetic substances used to manufacture bath salts; these synthetic stimulants are now designated as schedule I substances.

In March 2011, five synthetic cannabinoids were temporarily categorized as schedule I substances under the CSA. Unless permanently controlled, the ban on these five substances is set to expire in March 2012.

At least 38 states have taken action to control one or more of these chemicals. Prior to 2010, synthetic cannabinoids were not controlled by any state or at the federal level.

Section 24.2

"Bath Salts"

"DrugFacts: Synthetic Cathinones ('Bath Salts'),"
National Institute on Drug Abuse (www.drugabuse.gov), November 2012.

The term "bath salts" refers to an emerging family of drugs containing one or more synthetic chemicals related to cathinone, an amphetamine-like stimulant found naturally in the Khat plant.

Reports of severe intoxication and dangerous health effects associated with use of bath salts have made these drugs a serious and growing public health and safety issue. The synthetic cathinones in bath salts can produce euphoria and increased sociability and sex drive, but some users experience paranoia, agitation, and hallucinatory delirium; some even display psychotic and violent behavior, and deaths have been reported in several instances.

The synthetic cathinone products marketed as "bath salts" to evade detection by authorities should not be confused with products such as Epsom salts that are sold to improve the experience of bathing. The latter have no psychoactive (drug-like) properties.

Bath salts typically take the form of a white or brown crystalline powder and are sold in small plastic or foil packages labeled "not for human consumption." Sometimes also marketed as "plant food"—or, more recently, as "jewelry cleaner" or "phone screen cleaner"—they are sold online and in drug paraphernalia stores under a variety of brand names, such as "Ivory Wave," "Bloom," "Cloud Nine," "Lunar Wave," "Vanilla Sky," "White Lightning," and "Scarface."

When bath salts emerged at the end of the last decade, they rapidly gained popularity in the U.S. and Europe as "legal highs." In October 2011, the U.S. Drug Enforcement Administration placed three common synthetic cathinones under emergency ban pending further investigation, and in July 2012, President Barack Obama signed legislation permanently making two of them—mephedrone and MDPV—illegal along with several other synthetic drugs often sold as marijuana substitutes ("Spice").

Although the new law also prohibits chemically similar "analogues" of the named drugs, manufacturers are expected to respond by creating new drugs different enough from the banned substances to evade legal restriction. After mephedrone was banned in the United Kingdom in 2010, for example, a chemical called naphyrone quickly replaced it and is now being sold as "jewelry cleaner" under the brand name "Cosmic Blast."

How are bath salts abused?

Bath salts are typically taken orally, inhaled, or injected, with the worst outcomes being associated with snorting or needle injection.

How do bath salts affect the brain?

Common synthetic cathinones found in bath salts include MDPV, mephedrone ("Drone," "Meph," or "Meow Meow"), and methylone, but there are many others. Much is still unknown about how these substances affect the human brain, and each one may have somewhat different properties. Chemically, they are similar to amphetamines (such as methamphetamine) as well as to MDMA (ecstasy).

The energizing and often agitating effects reported in people who have taken bath salts are consistent with other drugs like amphetamines and cocaine that raise the level of the neurotransmitter dopamine in brain circuits regulating reward and movement. A surge in dopamine in these circuits causes feelings of euphoria and increased activity. A similar surge of the transmitter norepinephrine can raise heart rate and blood pressure. Bath salts have been marketed as cheap (and until recently, legal) substitutes for those stimulants. A recent study found that MDPV—the most common synthetic cathinone found in the blood and urine of patients admitted to emergency departments after bath salts ingestion—raises brain dopamine in the same manner as cocaine but is at least 10 times more potent.

The hallucinatory effects often reported in users of bath salts are consistent with other drugs such as MDMA or LSD that raise levels of another neurotransmitter, serotonin. A recent analysis of the effects in rats of mephedrone and methylone showed that these drugs raised levels of serotonin in a manner similar to MDMA.

What are the other health effects of bath salts?

Bath salts have been linked to an alarming surge in visits to emergency departments and poison control centers across the country. Common reactions reported for people who have needed medical attention after using bath salts include cardiac symptoms (such as racing heart, high blood pressure, and chest pains) and psychiatric symptoms including paranoia, hallucinations, and panic attacks.

Patients with the syndrome known as "excited delirium" from taking bath salts also may have dehydration, breakdown of skeletal muscle tissue, and kidney failure. Intoxication from several synthetic cathinones including MDPV, mephedrone, methedrone, and butylone has proved fatal in several instances.

Early indications are that synthetic cathinones have a high abuse and addiction potential. In a study of the rewarding and reinforcing effects of MDPV, rats showed self-administration patterns and escalation of drug intake nearly identical to methamphetamine. Bath salts users have reported that the drugs trigger intense cravings (or a compulsive urge to use the drug again) and that they are highly addictive. Frequent consumption may induce tolerance, dependence, and strong withdrawal symptoms when not taking the drug.

The dangers of bath salts are compounded by the fact that these products may contain other, unknown ingredients that may have their own harmful effects.

Also, drug users who believe they are purchasing other drugs such as ecstasy may be in danger of receiving synthetic cathinones instead. For example, mephedrone has been found commonly substituted for MDMA in pills sold as ecstasy in the Netherlands.

Section 24.3

Pump-It Powder

First there was K2 (Spice) and the slew of synthetic cannabinoids. Then came bath salts; they were new and they were legal. These drugs were available and sold as over-the-counter products in an international web-based marketplace. Many of them were sold in head shops and medical marijuana clinics in the United States. But now these synthetics are all banned, well, most of them anyway. But into the fray now comes *"Pump-It Powder,"* an "enhanced plant vitamin." It's the latest synthetic drug to be manufactured and sold under the ruse of a substance "not intended for human consumption."

With myriad bath salts and plant food products available in the marketplace, uncertainty already reigns. No one quite knows what is in these synthetics. The Internet is full of supposition, but it is not clear at all what manufacturers are putting into their final products. Nevertheless, a great deal of discussion has centered on the role of geranamine as primary constituent of *Pump-It*. Geranamine is also known as methylhexanamine, an old-time amphetamine-related stimulant and decongestant that is found naturally in the geranium plant, hence its name. Methylhexanamine is a legal substance; it is not scheduled by the DEA. The drug has not been widely studied. It was patented in 1944 and for the most part has been dormant since that time. But in the world of energy drinks and aphrodisiac potions, methylhexanamine has been a prime player. Users of *Pump-It* have flooded Internet message boards with questions and stories about the product. It is the users who we should turn to for expert opinion. From what our MEDTOX DAR [drug abuse recognition] instructor-experts can determine, *Pump-It Powder* indeed performs in a way that is similar to those effects that would be expected with the use of methylhexanamine. But, then again, many users purport the drug to be quite similar to pre-ban bath salts that contained MDPV. Many in fact report that *Pump-It Powder* has become an addictive routine.

We do know that emergency rooms have begun to feel the sting of *Pump-It Powder*. Patients have reported to the emergency rooms having suffered seizures, hallucinations, and paranoia. Users report to physicians that they are experiencing effects that are similar, but more powerful than, cocaine and methamphetamine. The drug appears to have a regional appeal. *Pump-It Powder* is popular in the Midwest and plains states. It does not have a great following on the Pacific Coast, yet. It can be found on the Internet, but more alarming is the fact that it is available as an over-the-counter product in gas stations and novelty stores.

Of great concern is the potential effect that this drug has on teenagers. It is easy to find and it is relatively cheap, $30 for a tin container packed with the powder. The drug can be snorted or "bumped," injected, or smoked. Of additional concern is that the onset of this drug's high is somewhat delayed. This situation then prompts users to "bump" a double or triple dose because the onset of effects is not felt right away. Those actions then lead to absorption of a hyper dose and the experience of grossly exaggerated effects and a likely trip to the hospital.

Like bath salts, a *Pump-It Powder* high will trigger DAR signs and symptoms that are consistent with both central nervous system stimulants and hallucinogens. Heart rate, body temperature, and the internal clock will all be accelerated. The pupils will dilate and may exhibit sluggishness in response to direct light. There may be piloerection (gooseflesh) and user claims of sensory distortions. Users may exhibit behaviors of gross paranoia. The high will last for 4–6 hours, although some users claim that they were held "high" for 12 hours and longer. The symptoms appear to be dose dependent.

Stay tuned to the *MEDTOX Journal* for further news about this drug and others like it. Readers with questions or stories involving *Pump-It Powder* may contact agilberts@medtox.com at the *MEDTOX Journal*.

Section 24.4

Spice/K2

"DrugFacts: Spice (Synthetic Marijuana)," National Institute on Drug Abuse (www.drugabuse.gov), December 2012.

"Spice" refers to a wide variety of herbal mixtures that produce experiences similar to marijuana (cannabis) and that are marketed as "safe," legal alternatives to that drug. Sold under many names, including K2, fake weed, Yucatan Fire, Skunk, Moon Rocks, and others—and labeled "not for human consumption"—these products contain dried, shredded plant material and chemical additives that are responsible for their psychoactive (mind-altering) effects.

Labels on Spice products often claim that they contain "natural" psychoactive material taken from a variety of plants. Spice products do contain dried plant material, but chemical analyses show that their active ingredients are synthetic (or designer) cannabinoid compounds.

For several years, Spice mixtures have been easy to purchase in head shops and gas stations and via the internet. Because the chemicals used in Spice have a high potential for abuse and no medical benefit, the DEA has designated the five active chemicals most frequently found in Spice as schedule I controlled substances, making it illegal to sell, buy, or possess them. Manufacturers of Spice products attempt to evade these legal restrictions by substituting different chemicals in their mixtures, while the DEA continues to monitor the situation and evaluate the need for updating the list of banned cannabinoids.

Spice products are popular among young people; of the illicit drugs most used by high-school seniors, they are second only to marijuana. (They are more popular among boys than girls—in 2012, nearly twice as many male 12th graders reported past-year use of synthetic marijuana as females in the same age group.) Easy access and the misperception that Spice products are "natural" and therefore harmless have likely contributed to their popularity. Another selling point is that the chemicals used in Spice are not easily detected in standard drug tests.

How is spice abused?

Some Spice products are sold as "incense," but they more closely resemble potpourri. Like marijuana, Spice is abused mainly by smoking. Sometimes Spice is mixed with marijuana or is prepared as an herbal infusion for drinking.

How does spice affect the brain?

Spice users report experiences similar to those produced by marijuana—elevated mood, relaxation, and altered perception—and in some cases the effects are even stronger than those of marijuana. Some users report psychotic effects like extreme anxiety, paranoia, and hallucinations.

So far, there have been no scientific studies of Spice's effects on the human brain, but we do know that the cannabinoid compounds found in Spice products act on the same cell receptors as THC, the primary psychoactive component of marijuana. Some of the compounds found in Spice, however, bind more strongly to those receptors, which could lead to a much more powerful and unpredictable effect. Because the chemical composition of many products sold as Spice is unknown, it is likely that some varieties also contain substances that could cause dramatically different effects than the user might expect.

What are the other health effects of spice?

Spice abusers who have been taken to Poison Control Centers report symptoms that include rapid heart rate, vomiting, agitation, confusion, and hallucinations. Spice can also raise blood pressure and cause reduced blood supply to the heart (myocardial ischemia), and in a few cases it has been associated with heart attacks. Regular users may experience withdrawal and addiction symptoms.

We still do not know all the ways Spice may affect human health or how toxic it may be, but one public health concern is that there may be harmful heavy metal residues in Spice mixtures. Without further analyses, it is difficult to determine whether this concern is justified.

Part Four

The Causes and Consequences of Drug Abuse and Addiction

Chapter 25

Understanding Drug Abuse and Addiction

Chapter Contents

Section 25.1

Drug Addiction Is a Chronic Disease

"Drug Abuse and Addiction," National Institute on Drug Abuse
(www.drugabuse.gov), August 2010.

What is drug addiction?

Addiction is defined as a chronic, relapsing brain disease that is
characterized by compulsive drug seeking and use, despite harmful
consequences. It is considered a brain disease because drugs change
the brain—they change its structure and how it works. These brain
changes can be long lasting and can lead to the harmful behaviors seen
in people who abuse drugs.

Why do people take drugs?

In general, people begin taking drugs for a variety of reasons:

- **To feel good:** Most abused drugs produce intense feelings of
  pleasure. This initial sensation of euphoria is followed by other
  effects, which differ with the type of drug used. For example,
  with stimulants such as cocaine, the "high" is followed by feelings of power, self-confidence, and increased energy. In contrast,
  the euphoria caused by opiates such as heroin is followed by feelings of relaxation and satisfaction.

- **To feel better:** Some people who suffer from social anxiety,
  stress-related disorders, and depression begin abusing drugs in
  an attempt to lessen feelings of distress. Stress can play a major
  role in beginning drug use, continuing drug abuse, or relapse in
  patients recovering from addiction.

- **To do better:** The increasing pressure that some individuals
  feel to chemically enhance or improve their athletic or cognitive
  performance can similarly play a role in initial experimentation
  and continued drug abuse.

- **Curiosity and "because others are doing it":** In this respect
  adolescents are particularly vulnerable because of the strong

influence of peer pressure; they are more likely, for example, to engage in "thrilling" and "daring" behaviors.

If taking drugs makes people feel good or better, what's the problem?

At first, people may perceive what seem to be positive effects with drug use. They also may believe that they can control their use; however, drugs can quickly take over their lives. Consider how a social drinker can become intoxicated, put himself behind a wheel, and quickly turn a pleasurable activity into a tragedy for him and others. Over time, if drug use continues, pleasurable activities become less pleasurable, and drug abuse becomes necessary for abusers to simply feel "normal." Drug abusers reach a point where they seek and take drugs, despite the tremendous problems caused for themselves and their loved ones. Some individuals may start to feel the need to take higher or more frequent doses, even in the early stages of their drug use.

Table 25.1. Examples of Risk and Protective Factors

Risk Factors	Domain	Protective Factors
Early aggressive behavior	Individual	Self-control
Poor social skills	Individual	Positive relationships
Lack of parental supervision	Family	Parental monitoring and support
Substance abuse	Peer	Academic competence
Drug availability	School	Anti-drug use policies
Poverty	Community	Strong neighborhood attachment

Is continued drug abuse a voluntary behavior?

The initial decision to take drugs is mostly voluntary. However, when drug abuse takes over, a person's ability to exert self-control can become seriously impaired. Brain imaging studies from drug-addicted individuals show physical changes in areas of the brain that are critical to judgment, decision making, learning and memory, and behavior control. Scientists believe that these changes alter the way the brain works and may help explain the compulsive and destructive behaviors of addiction.

No single factor determines whether a person will become addicted to drugs.

Why do some people become addicted to drugs, while others do not?

As with any other disease, vulnerability to addiction differs from person to person. In general, the more risk factors an individual has, the greater the chance that taking drugs will lead to abuse and addiction. "Protective" factors reduce a person's risk of developing addiction.

What factors determine if a person will become addicted?

No single factor determines whether a person will become addicted to drugs. The overall risk for addiction is affected by the biological makeup of the individual—it can even be influenced by gender or ethnicity, his or her developmental stage, and the surrounding social environment (e.g., conditions at home, at school, and in the neighborhood).

Which biological factors increase risk of addiction?

Scientists estimate that genetic factors account for between 40% and 60% of a person's vulnerability to addiction, including the effects of environment on gene expression and function. Adolescents and individuals with mental disorders are at greater risk of drug abuse and addiction than the general population.

Children's earliest interactions within the family are crucial to their healthy development and risk for drug abuse.

What environmental factors increase the risk of addiction?

Home and family: The influence of the home environment is usually most important in childhood. Parents or older family members who abuse alcohol or drugs, or who engage in criminal behavior, can increase children's risks of developing their own drug problems.

Peer and school: Friends and acquaintances have the greatest influence during adolescence. Drug-abusing peers can sway even those without risk factors to try drugs for the first time. Academic failure or poor social skills can put a child further at risk for drug abuse.

What other factors increase the risk of addiction?

Early use: Although taking drugs at any age can lead to addiction, research shows that the earlier a person begins to use drugs the more likely they are to progress to more serious abuse. This may reflect the harmful effect that drugs can have on the developing brain; it also may result from a constellation of early biological and social vulnerability factors, including genetic susceptibility, mental illness, unstable family relationships, and exposure to physical or sexual abuse. Still, the fact remains that early use is a strong indicator of problems ahead, among them, substance abuse and addiction.

Method of administration: Smoking a drug or injecting it into a vein increases its addictive potential. Both smoked and injected drugs enter the brain within seconds, producing a powerful rush of pleasure. However, this intense "high" can fade within a few minutes, taking the abuser down to lower, more normal levels. It is a starkly felt contrast, and scientists believe that this low feeling drives individuals to repeated drug abuse in an attempt to recapture the high pleasurable state.

Addiction is a developmental disease—it typically begins in childhood or adolescence. The brain continues to develop into adulthood and undergoes dramatic changes during adolescence.

One of the brain areas still maturing during adolescence is the prefrontal cortex—the part of the brain that enables us to assess situations, make sound decisions, and keep our emotions and desires under control. The fact that this critical part of an adolescent's brain is still a work-in-progress puts them at increased risk for poor decisions (such as trying drugs or continued abuse). Also, introducing drugs while the brain is still developing may have profound and long-lasting consequences.

Section 25.2

Common Risk and Protective Factors for Drug Use

"Common Risk and Protective Factors for Alcohol and Drug Use," Substance Abuse and Mental Health Services Administration Center for the Application of Prevention Technologies (captus.samhsa.gov), 2010.

Decades of research have helped to identify several patterns of risk and protective factors contributing to alcohol and drug use in adolescence and in later life. The presence and impact of these factors and their interactions with one another can vary depending on the population for which prevention interventions are planned. Limiting risk factors while strengthening and increasing the availability of protective resources will help to reduce substance abuse and create healthier individuals and communities. The following are some of the most important risk and protective factors identified in the literature:

Age of onset: Alcohol and drug use tends to begin in mid-to-late adolescence, though it is greater among individuals who experience early puberty (O'Connell et al., 2009). The earlier the age at which someone starts drinking the greater the risk that s/he will develop alcohol-related problems later in life. A delay in drinking until 20 to 21 years old reduces the risk of developing alcohol-related problems (Chou et al., 1992).

Youth perception that parents approve of their alcohol or drug use: One of the most consistent risk factors for adolescent drinking is perceived parental approval (Donovan, 2004). Reported maternal care perception has been shown to be significantly lower among those who abuse alcohol and those who use multiple drugs (Gerra et al., 2004).

Peers engaging in problem behavior: Associating with drug- or alcohol-using peers, or being rejected by peers, can create problem behaviors and influence attitudes and norms related to substance use (O'Connell et al., 2009). Exposure to peer problem behavior is correlated with increased alcohol and other substance use in the same month (Dishion et al., 2000). Those who drink in a social setting, or who have peers who do so, are more likely to abuse alcohol later in life (Beck et al., 1996).

Early and persistent problem behaviors, risk taking, and high sensation seeking: Early aggressiveness or antisocial behavior persisting into early adolescence predicts later adolescent aggressiveness, drug abuse, and alcohol problems (Hawkins et al., 1995).

Parental monitoring (or perception of monitoring): Adolescents who report low parental monitoring are significantly more likely to use a variety of substances (Shillington et al., 2005). Positive parental style and close monitoring by parents are proven protective factors for adolescents' use of alcohol and other drugs (Stewart, 2002).

Parent or older sibling drug use (or perception of use): Familial alcohol-using behaviors are strong predictors of adolescent alcohol use (Birckmayer et al., 2004). In a 2003 study, alcohol initiation most often occurred during family gatherings. Moreover, a family history of alcoholism was a significant risk factor for the development of adolescent problem drinking (Warner et al., 2003).

Low perception of harm: Low perception of harm towards alcohol and drug use is a risk factor for use (Henry et al., 2005). Individuals with attitudes or values favorable to alcohol or drugs are more likely to initiate substance use (Hawkins et al., 1992).

Strong parent and adolescent relationship and family cohesion: Adolescents who have a close relationship with their parents are less likely to become alcohol involved (Birckmayer et al., 2004).

Youth access and availability: The majority of alcohol consumed by youth is obtained through social sources, such as parents and friends, at underage parties and at home (Birckmayer et al., 2004). Availability of alcohol or illegal drugs leads to increased use (Hawkins et al., 1995).

Poor school achievement and low school bonding: Adolescents who have a low commitment to school or do poorly are more likely to become alcohol involved (Birckmayer et al., 2004).

References

Beck, K., and Treiman, K.A. (1996). The relationship of social context of drinking, perceived social norms, and parental influence to various drinking patterns of adolescents. *Addictive Behaviors*, 21(5), 633–644.

Birckmayer, J.D., Holder, H.D., Yacoubian, G.S., and Friend, K.B. (2004). A general causal model to guide alcohol, tobacco, and illicit drug prevention: Assessing the research evidence. *Journal of Drug Education*, 34(2), 121–153.

Chou, S. P. and R. P. Pickering. (1992). Early onset of drinking as a risk factor for lifetime alcohol-related problems. *British Journal of Addiction*, 87(8), 1199–1204.

Dishion, T. J. and N. M. Skaggs. (2000). An ecological analysis of monthly "bursts" in early adolescent substance use. *Applied Developmental Science*, 4, 89–97.

Donovan, J.E. (2004). Adolescent alcohol initiation: A review of psychosocial risk factors. *Journal of Adolescent Health*, 35(6), 529.

Gerra, G., L. Angioni, et al. (2004). Substance use among high-school students: Relationships with temperament, personality traits, and parental care perception. *Substance Use & Misuse*, 39(2), 345–367.

Hawkins, J. D., M. W. Arthur, et al. (1995). Preventing substance abuse. From *Building a Safer Society: Strategic Approaches to Crime Prevention*, Volume 19, P 343–427, 1995, Michael Tonry & David P Farrington, eds. United States.

Hawkins, D. J., Catalano, R. F., and Miller, J. Y. (1992). Risk and protective factors for alcohol and other substance problems in adolescence and early adulthood: Implications for substance abuse prevention. *Psychological Bulletin*, 112(1), 64–105.

Henry, K. L., M. D. Slater, et al. (2005). Alcohol use in early adolescence: The effect of changes in risk taking, perceived harm and friends' alcohol use. *Journal of Studies on Alcohol*, 66(2), 275–283.

O'Connell, M. E., Boat, T., and Warner, K. E., eds. (2009). Preventing mental, emotional, and behavioral disorders among young people: Progress and possibilities. Committee on the Prevention of Mental Disorders and Substance Abuse Among Children, Youth and Young Adults, Institute of Medicine. Washington, DC: National Academies Press.

Shillington, A. M., S. Lehman, et al. (2005). Parental monitoring: Can it continue to be protective among high-risk adolescents? *Journal of Child & Adolescent Substance Abuse*, 15(1), 1–15.

Stewart, C. (2002). Family factors of low-income African-American youth associated with substance use: An exploratory analysis. *Journal of Ethnicity in Substance Abuse*, 1(1), 97–111.

Warner, L. A., and H. R. White. (2003). Longitudinal effects of age at onset and first drinking situations on problem drinking. *Substance Use & Misuse*, 38(14), 1983–2016.

Section 25.3

How Drugs Affect the Brain

"Drugs and the Brain," National Institute on Drug Abuse
(www.drugabuse.gov), August 2010.

The human brain is the most complex organ in the body. This three-pound mass of gray and white matter sits at the center of all human activity—you need it to drive a car, to enjoy a meal, to breathe, to create an artistic masterpiece, and to enjoy everyday activities. In brief, the brain regulates your basic body functions; enables you to interpret and respond to everything you experience; and shapes your thoughts, emotions, and behavior.

The brain is made up of many parts that all work together as a team. Different parts of the brain are responsible for coordinating and performing specific functions. Drugs can alter important brain areas that are necessary for life-sustaining functions and can drive the compulsive drug abuse that marks addiction. Brain areas affected by drug abuse are the following:

- The brain stem controls basic functions critical to life, such as heart rate, breathing, and sleeping.

- The limbic system contains the brain's reward circuit—it links together a number of brain structures that control and regulate our ability to feel pleasure. Feeling pleasure motivates us to repeat behaviors such as eating—actions that are critical to our existence. The limbic system is activated when we perform these activities—and also by drugs of abuse. In addition, the limbic system is responsible for our perception of other emotions, both positive and negative, which explains the mood-altering properties of many drugs.

- The cerebral cortex is divided into areas that control specific functions. Different areas process information from our senses, enabling us to see, feel, hear, and taste. The front part of the cortex, the frontal cortex or forebrain, is the thinking center of the brain; it powers our ability to think, plan, solve problems, and make decisions.

How does the brain communicate?

The brain is a communications center consisting of billions of neurons, or nerve cells. Networks of neurons pass messages back and forth to different structures within the brain, the spinal column, and the peripheral nervous system. These nerve networks coordinate and regulate everything we feel, think, and do.

- **Neuron to neuron:** Each nerve cell in the brain sends and receives messages in the form of electrical impulses. Once a cell receives and processes a message, it sends it on to other neurons.

- **Neurotransmitters (the brain's chemical messengers):** The messages are carried between neurons by chemicals called neurotransmitters. (They transmit messages between neurons.)

- **Receptors (the brain's chemical receivers):** The neurotransmitter attaches to a specialized site on the receiving cell called a receptor. A neurotransmitter and its receptor operate like a "key and lock," an exquisitely specific mechanism that ensures that each receptor will forward the appropriate message only after interacting with the right kind of neurotransmitter.

- **Transporters (the brain's chemical recyclers):** Located on the cell that releases the neurotransmitter, transporters recycle these neurotransmitters (i.e., bringing them back into the cell that released them), thereby shutting off the signal between neurons.

How do drugs work in the brain?

Drugs are chemicals. They work in the brain by tapping into the brain's communication system and interfering with the way nerve cells normally send, receive, and process information. Some drugs, such as marijuana and heroin, can activate neurons because their chemical structure mimics that of a natural neurotransmitter. This similarity in structure "fools" receptors and allows the drugs to lock onto and activate the nerve cells. Although these drugs mimic brain chemicals, they don't activate nerve cells in the same way as a natural neurotransmitter, and they lead to abnormal messages being transmitted through the network.

Other drugs, such as amphetamine or cocaine, can cause the nerve cells to release abnormally large amounts of natural neurotransmitters or prevent the normal recycling of these brain chemicals. This disruption produces a greatly amplified message, ultimately disrupting communication channels. The difference in effect can be described as the difference between someone whispering into your ear and someone shouting into a microphone.

How do drugs work in the brain to produce pleasure?

Most drugs of abuse directly or indirectly target the brain's reward system by flooding the circuit with dopamine. Dopamine is a neurotransmitter present in regions of the brain that regulate movement, emotion, cognition, motivation, and feelings of pleasure. The overstimulation of this system, which rewards our natural behaviors, produces the euphoric effects sought by people who abuse drugs and teaches them to repeat the behavior.

How does stimulation of the brain's pleasure circuit teach us to keep taking drugs?

Our brains are wired to ensure that we will repeat life-sustaining activities by associating those activities with pleasure or reward. Whenever this reward circuit is activated, the brain notes that something important is happening that needs to be remembered and teaches us to do it again and again, without thinking about it. Because drugs of abuse stimulate the same circuit, we learn to abuse drugs in the same way.

Why are drugs more addictive than natural rewards?

When some drugs of abuse are taken, they can release 2 to 10 times the amount of dopamine that natural rewards do. In some cases, this occurs almost immediately (as when drugs are smoked or injected), and the effects can last much longer than those produced by natural rewards. The resulting effects on the brain's pleasure circuit dwarfs those produced by naturally rewarding behaviors such as eating and sex. The effect of such a powerful reward strongly motivates people to take drugs again and again. This is why scientists sometimes say that drug abuse is something we learn to do very, very well.

What happens to your brain if you keep taking drugs?

Just as we turn down the volume on a radio that is too loud, the brain adjusts to the overwhelming surges in dopamine (and other neurotransmitters) by producing less dopamine or by reducing the number of receptors that can receive signals. As a result, dopamine's impact on the reward circuit of a drug abuser's brain can become abnormally low, and the ability to experience any pleasure is reduced. This is why the abuser eventually feels flat, lifeless, and depressed and is unable to enjoy things that previously brought them pleasure. Now, they need to take drugs just to try and bring their dopamine function back up to normal. And, they must take larger amounts of the drug than they first did to create the dopamine high—an effect known as tolerance.

How does long-term drug taking affect brain circuits?

We know that the same sort of mechanisms involved in the development of tolerance can eventually lead to profound changes in neurons and brain circuits, with the potential to severely compromise the long-term health of the brain. For example, glutamate is another neurotransmitter that influences the reward circuit and the ability to learn. When the optimal concentration of glutamate is altered by drug abuse, the brain attempts to compensate for this change, which can cause impairment in cognitive function. Similarly, long-term drug abuse can trigger adaptations in habit or nonconscious memory systems. Conditioning is one example of this type of learning, whereby environmental cues become associated with the drug experience and can trigger uncontrollable cravings if the individual is later exposed to these cues, even without the drug itself being available. This learned "reflex" is extremely robust and can emerge even after many years of abstinence.

What other brain changes occur with abuse?

Chronic exposure to drugs of abuse disrupts the way critical brain structures interact to control and inhibit behaviors related to drug abuse. Just as continued abuse may lead to tolerance or the need for higher drug dosages to produce an effect, it may also lead to addiction, which can drive an abuser to seek out and take drugs compulsively. Drug addiction erodes a person's self-control and ability to make sound decisions, while sending intense impulses to take drugs.

Section 25.4

The Spectrum of Substance Use Disorders

Excerpted from "Protecting Children in Families Affected by Substance Use Disorders. Chapter 2, The Nature of Substance Use Disorders," Child Welfare Information Gateway, U.S. Department of Health and Human Services (www .childwelfare.gov), 2009, and "Substance Use Disorders in People with Physical and Sensory Disabilities," Substance Abuse and Mental Health Services Administration (www.samhsa.gov), August 2011.

Protecting Children in Families Affected by Substance Use Disorders: The Nature of Substance Abuse Disorders

The Continuum of Alcohol and Drug Use

Substance use, like many human behaviors, occurs along a broad continuum from no use to extremely heavy use. The likelihood of an individual experiencing problems stemming from substance use typically increases as the rate of use increases. The continuum for the use of substances includes substance use, substance abuse, and substance dependence or addiction.

Substance use is the consumption of low or infrequent doses of alcohol or drugs, such that damaging consequences are rare or minor. In reference to alcohol, this means drinking in a way that does not impair functioning or lead to negative consequences, such as violence. In reference to prescription drugs, use involves taking medications as prescribed by a physician. Regarding over-the-counter medications, use is defined as taking the substance as recommended for alleviating symptoms. Some people who choose to use substances may use them periodically, never use them to an extreme, or never experience life consequences because of their use.

Substance abuse is a pattern of substance use that leads to significant impairment or distress, reflected by one or more of the following:

- Failure to fulfill major role obligations at work, school, or home (e.g., substance-related absences from work, suspension from school, neglect of a child's need for regular meals)

307

- Continued use in spite of physical hazards (e.g., driving under the influence)

- Trouble with the law (e.g., arrests for substance-related disorderly conduct)

- Interpersonal or social problems

Additionally, use of a medication in a manner different from how it is prescribed or recommended and use of an intravenous drug that is not medically required are considered substance abuse.

Individuals may abuse one or more substances for a certain period of time and then modify their behaviors because of internal or external pressures. Abuse is characterized by periodic events of abusive use of substances, which may be accompanied by life consequences directly related to its use. With proper intervention, an individual with substance abuse problems can avert progression to addiction. At this level of progression, the abusers often are not aware or, if they are, they may not be honest with themselves that the negative consequences they experience are linked to their substance use. With proper intervention, these individuals are able to choose to limit or to cease substance use because of the recognition of the connection between use and consequences. Other people, however, may continue abusing substances until they become addicted.

Substance dependence or addiction is the progressive need for alcohol or drugs that results from the use of that substance. This need creates both psychological and physical changes that make it difficult for the users to control when they will use the substance or how much they will use. Psychological dependence occurs when a user needs the substance to feel normal or to engage in typical daily activities. Physical dependence occurs when the body adapts to the substance and needs increasing amounts to ward off the effects of withdrawal and to maintain physiological functioning. Dependence can result in the following:

- **The continued use of a substance despite negative consequences:** The individual continues drug or alcohol use despite incidents, such as accidents, arrests, or a lack of money to pay for food because it was spent on drugs.

- **An increase in tolerance to the substance:** The individual requires more of the alcohol or drug to obtain the same effect.

- **Withdrawal symptoms:** The individual needs to consume the substance in order not to experience unpleasant withdrawal effects, such as uncontrollable shaking and tremors or intense nausea.

- **Behavioral changes:** The individual who is dependent shows these characteristics:

  - Uses more than intended

  - Spends a majority of the time either obtaining, using, or withdrawing from the use of the substance

  - Cannot stop using until the substance is gone or the individual passes out

Criteria for diagnosing substance dependence and substance abuse as a substance abuse disorder (SUD) have been defined in the *Diagnostic and Statistical Manual of Mental Disorders, 4th Edition, Text Revision* (DSM-IV-TR), the American Psychiatric Association's classification index for mental disorders.

In Brief: Substance Use Disorders

Numerous signs may suggest the presence of an active SUD. These include, but are not limited to, the following:

- Dilated or constricted pupils

- Slurred speech

- Inability to focus, visually or cognitively

- Unsteady gait

- Blackouts

- Insomnia

- Irritability or agitation

- Depression, anxiety, low self-esteem, resentment

- Odor of alcohol on breath

- Excessive use of aftershave or mouthwash (to mask the odor of alcohol)

- Mild tremor

- Nasal irritation (suggestive of cocaine insufflation)

- Eye irritation (suggestive of exposure to marijuana smoke)

- Odor of marijuana on clothing

- Abuse of drugs or alcohol by family members

- Many missed appointments with vocational rehabilitation counselors, job interviews, and the like

- Difficulty learning new tasks

- Attention deficits

- Lack of initiative

Some manifestations of certain disabilities may be difficult to distinguish from these signs of SUDs. For example, people with multiple sclerosis may have an unsteady gait, slurred speech, and memory impairment. Other signs, such as depression or anxiety, may indicate a different, distinct behavioral health condition.

Screening for SUDs

Screening is not the same as diagnosing; it simply indicates whether further evaluation by an SUD professional is indicated. Drug abuse screening tests can be found at the following:

- **Project Cork:** www.projectcork.org/clinical_tools/html/DAST.html

- **National Institute on Drug Abuse (NIDA):** www.drugabuse .gov/nmassist

Types of SUD Services

SUD services include the following:

- **Prevention education:** Information in various formats that helps people understand the risks of substance use

- **In-depth assessment:** An evaluation by a treatment provider to determine whether an SUD is present and, if so, what level of care is needed and what treatment options are available

- **Outpatient or inpatient detoxification:** Medically supervised withdrawal from alcohol or drugs

- **Outpatient treatment:** Psychosocial interventions and individual and group counseling on substance use

- **Medication-assisted treatment and counseling:** Methadone, buprenorphine, and other medications for opioid dependence or acamprosate, disulfiram, and naltrexone for alcohol use disorders; medication-assisted treatment works best if combined with psychosocial counseling interventions

- **Residential programs:** Short- and long-term structured living to help people reenter their community

In addition, people in recovery often attend mutual-help groups, such as Alcoholics Anonymous (AA), Narcotics Anonymous (NA), and SMART (Self Management and Recovery Training) Recovery to share experiences and support one another's recovery efforts.

Chapter 26

Polydrug Use and Coexisting Drug and Alcohol Dependence

Chapter Contents

Section 26.1

Polydrug Use

From Kedia, S., Sell, M., and Relyea, G. Mono- versus polydrug abuse patterns among publicly funded clients. *Substance Abuse Treatment, Prevention, and Policy.* 2007, 2:33. © 2007 Kedia et al; licensee BioMed Central Ltd. The original work has been modified: the text has been excerpted. This is an Open Access article distributed under the terms of the Creative Commons Attribution License (http://creativecommons.org/licenses/by/3.0). Reviewed by David A. Cooke, MD, FACP, July 2013.

Background

Alcohol and illicit drug abuse continues to be a major public health concern in the United States. According to the U.S. Department of Health and Human Services (DHHS)'s 2005 National Survey on Drug Use and Health, 6.6% (16 million) of Americans age 12 or older reported heavy drinking, 22.7% (55 million) reported binge drinking, and 8.1% (19.7 million) reported using illicit drugs within the month prior to the survey. A DHHS survey in 2002 found that 56% of all admissions to publicly funded treatment facilities were for multiple substances; among these admissions, 76% abused alcohol, 55% abused marijuana, 48% abused cocaine, 27% abused opiates, and 26% abused other drugs. Despite the high rates of polydrug abuse, the literature on this issue is limited. In addition, there are few studies reporting the probability of mono- versus polydrug abuse across various demographic characteristics. Drawing upon seven years (1998–2004) of admission data, this study examines the patterns of mono- versus polydrug abuse among admissions to publicly funded alcohol and drug abuse treatment programs in Tennessee.

The World Health Organization defines polydrug abuse as the concurrent (taken at the same time) or sequential (one drug taken followed by another) abuse of more than one drug or type of drug, with dependence upon at least one. Such abuse has been increasingly reported in emergency room admissions and has been linked to drug-related deaths as well as nonfatal overdoses. The abuse of multiple substances has a long recorded history in the United States, dating to the early 20th century when combination drug abuse was found among 11.9%

of narcotic addicts in New York and 1% of patients in Louisiana. During the 1960s, polydrug abuse increased drastically; for example, barbiturate abuse was noted among 29% of heroin addicts and 32.4% of narcotic addicts in Lexington, Kentucky, as well as among the urban heroin addicts who would alternate alcohol with illicit drug abuse, at times as a detoxification method.

Alcohol abusers often report abuse of other substances. In a study of 248 alcoholics seeking substance abuse treatment, 68% reported using additional drugs in the 90 days prior to admission. Another recent study found that over 80% of the alcoholics in treatment were dependent on at least one other substance, most often marijuana or cocaine. Conversely, alcohol abuse was noted among admissions who were primarily in treatment for dependence on illicit drugs—84% for cocaine, 71% for barbiturates, 67% for opiates, and 64% for hallucinogens.

Other studies have revealed a prevalence for polydrug abuse as well. Darke and Hall ["Levels and correlates of polydrug use among heroin users and regular amphetamine users," *Drug Alcohol Depend* 1995, 39:231–235] found that monodrug abuse was rare among 329 heroin abusers and 301 amphetamine abusers during a six-month study period. Leri et al. ["Understanding polydrug use: Review of heroin and cocaine co-use," *Addiction* 2003, 98:7–22] surveyed 1,111 injection drug abusers regarding their combination of cocaine and heroin abuse and found that approximately 15% not being treated in methadone maintenance programs were co-abusers of the drugs. This study also found that the individuals who abused both drugs tended to abuse them sequentially as opposed to simultaneously. Additionally, researchers have noted that polydrug abusers who combine cocaine and heroin do so to achieve specific effects not attainable with just one substance; this practice can transform primary abuse of one drug into a pattern of polydrug abuse.

While there has been some research examining predictive variables associated with polydrug abuse, these studies have focused on psychological aspects of the abusers, including high scores on various psychometric scales or a range of psychosocial factors such as depression, psychological distress, family support/bonding, and social conformity as a proxy for traditional values. The study presented here statistically examines demographic characteristics and drug abuse patterns of a large statewide dataset of publicly funded admissions to substance abuse treatment programs over a seven-year period (1998–2004) in Tennessee. The goals of this study include: 1) determining patterns of mono- or polydrug abuse; 2) identifying the most prevalent combinations of polydrug abuse; and 3) examining the probability of mono- versus polydrug abuse by demographic variables.

Discussion

This study revealed that for both mono- and polydrug abusers, alcohol was the predominant substance of choice, followed by cocaine and marijuana, findings consistent with those reported by other national surveys. These three substances were also the most common in two- and three-substance combinations reported by this study sample—at least one of these substances was part of 13 of the top 14 substance pairings and at least two were found in 11 of the top 15 triads. This strongly concurs with earlier studies in which the most frequent polydrug combinations included alcohol, specifically marijuana with alcohol, followed by alcohol with other illicit drugs, and marijuana with other illicit drugs. Whereas some other researchers used the general category of "illicit drugs," this study explicitly identified cocaine as the illicit substance. In terms of total overall abuse, cocaine abuse was second only to alcohol and was reported in the most frequently abused two- and three-substance combinations.

Despite these similarities, in many ways the results of this research are quite different from those reported in previous studies. We found slightly lower polydrug abuse rates than the national trends reported by the Treatment Episode Data Set (TEDS; see wwwdasis.samhsa .gov/teds05/tedsad2k5web.pdf). In a report of longitudinal trends of substance abuse from 1994–2005, only 44.2% of all admissions in 2005 reported no substance abuse in addition to the primary substance. The TEDS data also indicated that roughly half of adolescents between the ages of 12 and 17 who were admitted for substance abuse treatment were being treated for a combination of both alcohol and marijuana, although that proportion has been steadily decreasing since 1999 to about 43% of admissions in 2005. While the majority (55.1%) of admissions for treatment of alcohol did not report abuse of other substances, admissions with other substances as the primary substance of abuse reported roughly 24.7% to 41.7% being treated for a single substance. So far, TEDS has not reported polydrug data by state, preventing a direct comparison with the results of this research in Tennessee.

Examinations of demographic characteristics of polydrug abusers, such as age, gender, and ethnicity, in order to identify trends have found that, in general, polydrug abuse was lowest for those over 40 years old and highest among those under 20. For example, Chen and Kandel ["The natural history of drug use from adolescence to the mid-thirties in a general population sample," *Am J Public Health* 1995, 85:41–47] found a tendency for polydrug abusers to be young, with initiation of illicit polydrug abuse being extremely rare after age 20. The DHHS found that 65% of admissions under 20 reported polydrug abuse, whereas only 41%

of admissions over 45 did so. Examining polydrug abuse by age group among national admissions to publicly funded substance abuse treatment, Henderson [*Age differences in multiple drug use: National admissions to publicly funded substance abuse treatment*, chap. 4, http://www.oas.samhsa.gov/aging/chap4.htm] found peak polydrug abuse among those younger than 40. Earleywine and Newcomb ["Concurrent versus simultaneous polydrug use," *Exp Clin Psychopharmacol* 1997, 5:353–364] found that a majority of polydrug abuse took place among those age 28–32, who constituted 31% of the combination abusers of marijuana and alcohol, 28% of alcohol and illicit drugs other than marijuana, and 22% of marijuana with other illicit drugs. Collins et al. ["Simultaneous polydrug use among teens," *J Subst Abuse* 1998, 10:233–253] found polydrug abuse in 29% of 12th graders studied. The American Academy of Family Physicians reported the abuse of multiple drugs by more than two thirds of patients age 20–30 and among more than four fifths of those under 20. Several other studies found high levels of polydrug abuse among adolescents. At the same time, research has suggested that the incidence of polydrug abuse may decline with age. For example, Raveis and Kandel ["Changes in drug behavior from the middle to the late twenties," *Am J Public Health* 1987, 77:607–611] determined that 85%–95% of abusers, other than those who were marijuana and alcohol dependent, had ceased multiple drug abuse by age 28–29, and Darke and Hall (Ibid.) noted that among heroin and amphetamine abusers the number of drugs used tended to decrease with age. In contrast to these previous studies, this research found that while polydrug abuse was higher among clients between the ages of 18 and 44, monodrug abuse prevailed among minors and adults over 55.

Earlier research also found that males exhibited more polydrug abuse than females. In this study, however, males and females were equally likely to be polydrug abusers. With regard to ethnicity, our research differed from previous studies as well. Asians have been shown to be less likely than African Americans, Hispanics, or Caucasians to be polydrug abusers, and African Americans have been found to be less likely to be polydrug abusers than Hispanics or Caucasians. Our findings indicated that Caucasians were more likely to be monodrug abusers and African Americans were more likely to be polydrug abusers, in direct contrast to prior reports of lower rates of polydrug abuse among African Americans than Caucasians. Additionally, although there is little in the substance abuse literature regarding rural versus urban polydrug abuse in the United States, this study found that admissions in urban areas were more likely to be for polydrug abuse, while rural admissions were more likely to be for monodrug abuse.

The variation in study results discussed here suggests that accounting for regional differences in substance abuse patterns may be very important, if not determinant, in the implementation of public health policy at the state level. National estimates, even the state breakdowns provided in the Substance Abuse and Mental Health Services Administration (SAMHSA)'s National Survey on Drug Use and Health, may be less reliable than comprehensive, multiyear research derived from local treatment providers, such as the findings presented here.

Section 26.2

Drug and Alcohol Dependence

Excerpted from "Alcohol Alert: Alcohol and Other Drugs," National Institute on Alcohol Abuse and Alcoholism (niaaa.nih.gov), July 2008. Reviewed by David A. Cooke, MD, FACP, July 2013.

Drug and alcohol dependence often go hand in hand. Research shows that people who are dependent on alcohol are much more likely than the general population to use drugs, and people with drug dependence are much more likely to drink alcohol. For example, certain researchers found that, of 248 alcoholics seeking treatment, 64% met the criteria for a drug use disorder at some point in their lifetime.

Patients with co-occurring alcohol and other drug use disorders also are likely to have more severe dependence-related problems than those without combined disorders—that is, they meet a higher number of diagnostic criteria for each disorder (three out of seven criteria are required to meet the diagnosis of dependence). People with co-occurring alcohol and other drug use disorders are more likely to have psychiatric disorders such as personality, mood, and anxiety disorders; they are more likely to attempt suicide and to suffer health problems. People who use both alcohol and drugs also are at risk for dangerous interactions between these substances. For example, a person who uses alcohol with benzodiazepines, whether these drugs are prescribed or taken illegally, is at increased risk of fatal poisoning.

Epidemiology: How Common Is Alcohol and Other Drug Addiction?

How common is alcohol and other drug use, and how often do alcohol and drug use disorders co-occur? To answer these questions, the National Institute on Alcohol Abuse and Alcoholism (NIAAA) conducted the National Epidemiologic Survey on Alcohol and Related Conditions (NESARC), one of the largest surveys of its kind ever performed. It examined the prevalence of alcohol and other drug use and abuse in the United States. According to NESARC, 8.5% of adults in the United States met the criteria for an alcohol use disorder, whereas 2% met the criteria for a drug use disorder and 1.1% met the criteria for both. People who are dependent on drugs are more likely to have an alcohol use disorder than people with alcoholism are to have a drug use disorder. Young people ages 18–24 had the highest rates of co-occurring alcohol and other drug use disorders. Men were more likely than women to have problems with alcohol, drugs, or the two substances combined.

Because many people suffer from both alcohol and drug dependence, scientists speculate that these disorders may have some common causes and risk factors.

The Genetics of Alcohol and Other Drug Use Disorders—Shared Risk Factors?

Research has established that some of the risk for addiction to both drugs and alcohol is inherited. Children of alcoholics are 50% to 60% more likely to develop alcohol use disorders than people in the general population. Similarly, children of parents who abuse illicit drugs may be 45% to 79% more likely to do so themselves than the general public. This suggests that some of the risk factors for alcohol and other drug use are rooted in genetics, though studies of specific families have not proven a genetic contribution.

Researchers believe that some of the same genes that increase a person's risk for problems with alcohol also might put him or her at greater risk for drug dependence. Moreover, those same genes might increase the risk for other psychiatric problems, such as conduct disorder and adult antisocial behavior (i.e., externalizing behaviors).

Much of the most compelling evidence for this apparent genetic link is based on twin and adoption studies. Adoption studies compare the risk of alcoholism in biological relatives with the risk in adoptive relatives of alcoholics (e.g., an adopted-away child of an alcoholic parent). Twin studies compare the risk of alcoholism in pairs of twins reared in the same environment, examining both identical twins (i.e., twins who share 100% of their genes) and fraternal twins (i.e., twins who share, on average, only 50% of their genes).

For example, in 2003, researchers analyzed data from the Virginia Twin Registry. They compared rates of alcohol, drug, and other externalizing disorders in identical and fraternal twins. They found that, in identical twins, when one twin was dependent on alcohol or on drugs, the second twin was much more likely (than a second fraternal twin) to have a problem with drugs or alcohol or to have an externalizing disorder. The study suggested that certain genes put people at risk for both alcohol and other drug use disorders, as well as externalizing disorders, whereas other genes put people at risk for specific types of disorders. These disorder-specific genes often are linked to how the body breaks down (or metabolizes) specific drugs and alcohol.

Diagnosing Substance Use Disorders: Barriers and Challenges

An accurate diagnosis is the first step toward treatment and recovery. However, diagnosing people with drug and alcohol disorders can be complicated, especially when these disorders occur concurrently. There are barriers to diagnosis: For example, patients may be unwilling to talk about their addiction, and clinicians may be unaware of the signs and symptoms of abuse and dependence.

Clinicians should screen patients for alcohol and other drug use disorders in a systematic, step-by-step fashion. Despite careful screening, however, some substance use disorders go undetected. Patients often misreport their substance use because of the stigma associated with an alcohol or other drug use disorder diagnosis, or they may fear legal reprisals. To address these fears, clinicians should make sure patients know the scope of confidentiality required by law. Clinicians also should make an effort to be empathic, accepting, and nonjudgmental; to ask questions in a direct and straightforward manner; and to deal with their own discomfort regarding drug use so as not to communicate their anxiety to their patients.

Although not as common, some patients overreport their substance use. For example, a patient suffering from untreated or inadequately treated pain may exaggerate his or her use of opiates in order to obtain methadone or buprenorphine (drugs used to treat opioid addiction) to alleviate that pain. Such patients would benefit from treatment by a pain specialist.

Additionally, clinicians may fail to recognize substance use disorders because they do not routinely screen for substance use, especially in patients who do not look like "typical substance users." According to

NESARC data, there is no typical substance user; problem alcohol and drug use occurs in people across genders, age groups, and ethnic backgrounds. It is important that clinicians evaluate all patients for substance use disorders.

Treatment

Behavioral therapies: For most patients, the most effective treatment approaches combine behavioral treatments (i.e., motivation enhancement therapy [MET] and cognitive-behavioral therapy [CBT]) and pharmacological treatments. MET seeks to motivate patients who are resistant to treatment, and CBT gives people the skills to reduce their drinking or to abstain from drinking. Contingency management interventions are another tool. These interventions center on rewarding positive behavior. Behavioral therapy also is an important tool for helping patients comply with medication regimens.

Pharmacotherapies: In addition to behavioral therapy, pharmacotherapies can help patients to curb their use of alcohol and other drugs. The following are traditional and new medications available to treat alcohol and drug dependence:

- **Disulfiram:** Disulfiram interferes with the breakdown of alcohol. When a person taking disulfiram drinks alcohol, it causes a buildup of acetaldehyde—a toxic byproduct of alcohol—in the body. This causes a variety of unpleasant effects, including reddening or flushing of the face and neck, nausea, and nervousness. The U.S. Food and Drug Administration (FDA) approved disulfiram in 1949 for the treatment of alcohol use disorders. In a study of 600 male veterans, overall, disulfiram had no effect on long-term abstinence. Among individuals who drank, however, the active dosage of the medication (250 mg/day) reduced the number of days the subjects spent drinking. Disulfiram can cause potentially serious effects when combined with alcohol, so the patient's goal must be abstinence. Patients who respond well to disulfiram tend to be older, with greater social stability and motivation for recovery; they tend to have a longer drinking history, attend Alcoholics Anonymous meetings, and be free of alcohol-related dementia and other cognitive problems.

  Disulfiram may be useful in treating cocaine addiction, both by producing an adverse reaction similar to that produced with alcohol and by reducing the euphoria associated with the drug. Successful treatment with disulfiram requires strict adherence to the medication regimen—patients who take disulfiram must be highly motivated to continue treatment.

- **Naltrexone:** Naltrexone blocks the activity of a class of molecules (i.e., opiate receptors). These molecules are involved in relaying chemical messages in the brain that are involved in addiction. In addition to an oral form, the FDA has approved a long-acting, injectable form of naltrexone for the treatment of alcohol dependence. Research shows that naltrexone reduces the risk of relapse in heavy drinkers; however, there is less evidence that it reduces the number of drinking days or that it helps patients to maintain total abstinence.

  Studies also have shown that naltrexone may be useful in treating drug use disorders, including opioid and cocaine dependence. Naltrexone has been approved by the FDA for the treatment of opioid dependence; however, because it can cause acute withdrawal from opiates (potentially making the patient feel very ill), patients should be drug-free for at least seven days before beginning treatment. Additionally, patients should be warned that if they return to using opiates heavily, they run the risk of death because naltrexone will reduce their tolerance to opiates and put them at risk for overdose.

- **Acamprosate:** Acamprosate also affects certain chemical messengers (i.e., neurotransmitters) in the brain. Although the FDA approved acamprosate for the treatment of alcohol dependence, research with this medication has produced mixed results. European studies have shown that acamprosate not only reduces the risk of heavy drinking, but nearly doubles the likelihood that patients will achieve abstinence. These studies suggest that acamprosate is most useful in patients who develop alcohol dependence later in life, who do not have a family history of alcohol dependence, and who display physical dependence and higher than usual levels of anxiety. It is important to note that other studies show that acamprosate is no more effective than placebo.

- **Anticonvulsant medications:** Topirimate has been shown to be an effective treatment for alcohol dependence and may be beneficial for cocaine dependence treatment. Other anticonvulsants, including carbamazepine and valproate, also have shown some effectiveness in treating alcohol use disorders, and they may be especially useful in patients with co-occurring alcohol dependence and bipolar disorder.

- **Serotonergic and other medications:** Although studies are scarce, some research has shown that medications which target other mechanisms in the brain (selective serotonin reuptake inhibitors [SSRIs], atypical antipsychotic medications, or lithium) may be useful in treating substance use disorders. The medications appear to be particularly useful for treating certain subgroups of alcohol-dependent patients, based on the age of onset of problem drinking.

Conclusion

Addictive disorders represent a major health issue both in the United States and worldwide. Because alcohol and drug dependence are likely to co-occur, exploring how alcohol addiction may relate to and interact with other addictions is important. Current research is exploring the underlying causes of addiction, and why alcohol and other drug use disorders co-occur so frequently, as well as how behavioral and drug therapies can best treat these disorders. There is no "magic bullet" for treating addiction—no treatment will work for everyone in every situation. More research is needed to identify effective treatments for different populations, especially youth, older people, and patients with co-occurring psychiatric disorders. Such research is vital to better understand the mechanisms and course of addiction as well as its diagnosis and treatment.

Chapter 27

Prescription and Over-the-Counter Drug Abuse

Chapter Contents

Section 27.1

Causes and Prevalence of Prescription Drug Abuse

"Topics in Brief: Prescription Drug Abuse," December 2011, and excerpts from "Prescription Drugs: Abuse and Addiction: How Many People Suffer Adverse Health Consequences from Abusing Prescription Drugs?" October 2011, National Institute on Drug Abuse (www.drugabuse.gov).

Prescription Drug Abuse

Prescription drug abuse is the intentional use of a medication without a prescription, in a way other than as prescribed, or for the experience or feeling it causes. It is not a new problem, but one that deserves renewed attention. For although prescription drugs can be powerful allies, they also pose serious health risks related to their abuse.

Prescription drug abuse remains a significant problem in the United States.

- In 2010, approximately 7.0 million persons were current users of psychotherapeutic drugs taken nonmedically (2.7% of the U.S. population), an estimate similar to that in 2009. This class of drugs is broadly described as those targeting the central nervous system, including drugs used to treat psychiatric disorders (National Survey on Drug Use and Health, NSDUH, 2010). The medications most commonly abused are the following:

  - **Pain relievers:** 5.1 million

  - **Tranquilizers:** 2.2 million

  - **Stimulants:** 1.1 million

  - **Sedatives:** 0.4 million

- Among adolescents, prescription and over-the-counter medications account for most of the commonly abused illicit drugs by high school seniors.

  - Nearly 1 in 12 high school seniors reported nonmedical use of Vicodin; 1 in 20 reported abuse of OxyContin.

- When asked how prescription narcotics were obtained for nonmedical use, 70% of 12th graders said they were given to them by a friend or relative (Monitoring the Future, MTF, 2011). The number obtaining them over the internet was negligible.

- Among those who abuse prescription drugs, high rates of other risky behaviors, including abuse of other drugs and alcohol, have also been reported.

What is driving this high prevalence?

Multiple factors are likely at work:

- **Misperceptions about their safety:** Because these medications are prescribed by doctors, many assume that they are safe to take under any circumstances. This is not the case. Prescription drugs act directly or indirectly on the same brain systems affected by illicit drugs. Using a medication other than as prescribed can potentially lead to a variety of adverse health effects, including overdose and addiction.

- **Increasing environmental availability:** Between 1991 and 2010, prescriptions for stimulants increased from 5 million to nearly 45 million and for opioid analgesics from about 75.5 million to 209.5 million.

- **Varied motivations for their abuse:** Underlying reasons include to get high; to counter anxiety, pain, or sleep problems; or to enhance cognition. Whatever the motivation, prescription drug abuse comes with serious risks.

What are the risks of commonly abused prescription drugs?

Opioids are used to treat pain.

- **Addiction:** Prescription opioids act on the same receptors as heroin and can be highly addictive. People who abuse them sometimes alter the route of administration (e.g., snorting or injecting) to intensify the effect; some even report moving from prescription opioids to heroin. NSDUH estimates about 1.9 million people in the U.S. meet abuse or dependence criteria for prescription opioids.

- **Overdose:** Abuse of opioids, alone or with alcohol or other drugs, can depress respiration and lead to death. Unintentional overdose deaths involving prescription opioids have quadrupled since 1999 and now outnumber those from heroin and cocaine combined.

- **Heightened HIV risk:** Injecting opioids increases the risk of HIV and other infectious diseases through use of unsterile or shared equipment. Noninjection drug use can also increase these risks through drug-altered judgment and decision making.

Central nervous system (CNS) depressants are used to treat anxiety and sleep problems.

- **Addiction and dangerous withdrawal symptoms:** These drugs are addictive, and, in chronic users or abusers, discontinuing them absent a physician's guidance can bring about severe withdrawal symptoms, including seizures that can be life-threatening.

- **Overdose:** High doses can cause severe respiratory depression. This risk increases when CNS depressants are combined with other medications or alcohol.

Stimulants are used to treat ADHD and narcolepsy.

- **Addiction and other health consequences:** These include psychosis, seizures, and cardiovascular complications.

What treatments are available for prescription drug abuse?

Available options for effectively treating addiction to prescription drugs depend on the medication being abused. Approaches to treating pain reliever addiction are drawn from research on treating heroin addiction and include medications combined with behavioral counseling. A recent large-scale clinical trial supported by the National Institute on Drug Abuse (NIDA) showed that Suboxone (buprenorphine + naloxone), prescribed in primary care settings, helped about half of participants reduce their pain reliever abuse during extended Suboxone treatment. Another promising approach includes long-acting formulations of medications, such as Vivitrol, a depot formulation of the opioid receptor blocker naltrexone, recently approved by the U.S. Food and Drug Administration (FDA) to treat opioid addiction. With effects that last for weeks instead of hours or days, long-acting formulations stand to aid in treatment retention and abstinence.

Although no medications yet exist to treat addiction to CNS depressants or to prescription stimulants, behavioral therapies proven effective in treating other drug addictions may be used. NIDA is also supporting multiple studies to identify promising medications for stimulant addiction.

What research on prescription drug abuse does NIDA support?

NIDA-supported researchers are conducting large-scale epidemiological studies investigating the patterns and sources of nonmedical use of prescription medications in high school and college students. Results suggest that prevention efforts should include a focus on the motivations behind the abuse, which often have an age and gender bias.

NIDA is also leading efforts to develop pain medications with diminished abuse potential, such as those that bypass the reward system of the brain. This is particularly important in light of returning veteran and growing elderly populations. To that end, NIDA is supporting research to better understand how to effectively treat people with chronic pain, which may predispose someone to become addicted to prescription pain relievers, and what can be done to prevent it among those at risk.

How Many People Suffer Adverse Health Consequences from Abusing Prescription Drugs?

The Drug Abuse Warning Network (DAWN), which monitors emergency department (ED) visits in selected areas across the nation, reported that approximately 1 million ED visits in 2009 could be attributed to prescription drug abuse. Roughly 343,000 involved prescription opioid pain relievers, a rate more than double that of five years prior. ED visits also more than doubled for CNS stimulants, involved in nearly 22,000 visits in 2009, as well as CNS depressants (anxiolytics, sedatives, and hypnotics), involved in 363,000 visits. Of the latter, benzodiazepines (e.g., Xanax) comprised the vast majority. Rates for a popular prescribed nonbenzodiazepine sleep aid, zolpidem (Ambien), rose from roughly 13,000 in 2004 to 29,000 in 2009. More than half of ED visits for prescription drug abuse involved multiple drugs.

Section 27.2

Boys More Likely than
Girls to Abuse Over-the-Counter Drugs

As crackdowns get tougher on alcohol, tobacco sales, and illicit drugs, there's a growing trend among youth to turn to another source to get high: their parents' medicine cabinet. A new University of Cincinnati [UC] study suggests adolescent males are at a higher risk of reporting longtime use of over-the-counter drugs, compared with their female peers.

Early results of the study by Rebecca Vidourek, a UC assistant professor of health promotion, and Keith King, a University of Cincinnati professor of health promotion, will be presented on Oct. 29, at the 140th annual meeting of the American Public Health Association in San Francisco.

The study examined over-the-counter (OTC) drug use among 7th- to 12th-grade students in 133 schools across Greater Cincinnati. The data was collected by the Coalition for a Drug Free Greater Cincinnati as part of the 2009–2010 Pride Survey on adolescent drug use in America. The survey was distributed to more than 54,000 students.

Early analysis found that 10% of the students reported abusing over-the-counter drugs. "Findings from this study highlight and underscore OTC drugs as an increasing and significant health issue affecting young people," says Vidourek, who adds that commonly abused OTC medications include cough syrup containing Dextromethorphan (DXM) and decongestants. The researchers say that high rates of OTC use were also found among male and female junior high school students.

Vidourek says that OTC abuse can result in unintentional poisoning, seizures, and physical and psychological addictions.

The researchers say that youth who reported involvement in positive activities, such as school clubs, sports, community and church organizations, were less likely to report abusing OTC medications. Teens more likely to report taking OTC drugs were also more likely to report that they had attended parties with the drugs or had friends who abused OTC drugs.

Section 27.3

Misuse of Over-the-Counter Cough and Cold Medicines

"Cough and Cold Medicine Abuse," February 2013, reprinted with permission from www.kidshealth.org. This information was provided by KidsHealth®, one of the largest resources online for medically reviewed health information written for parents, kids, and teens. For more articles like this, visit www.KidsHealth.org, or www.TeensHealth.org. Copyright © 1995–2013 The Nemours Foundation. All rights reserved.

Chugging cough medicine for an instant high isn't a new practice for teens, who have raided the medicine cabinet for a quick, cheap, and legal high for decades. And unfortunately, this dangerous, potentially deadly practice still goes on.

So it's important for parents to understand the risks and know how to prevent their kids from intentionally overdosing on cough and cold medicine.

Why Do Kids Abuse Cough and Cold Remedies?

Before the FDA replaced the narcotic codeine with dextromethorphan as an over-the-counter (OTC) cough suppressant in the 1970s, teens were simply guzzling down cough syrup for a quick buzz.

Over the years, teens discovered that they still could get high by taking large doses of any OTC medicine containing dextromethorphan (also called DXM).

Dextromethorphan-containing products—tablets, capsules, gel caps, lozenges, and syrups—are labeled DM, cough suppressant, or Tuss (or contain "tuss" in the title).

Medicines containing dextromethorphan are easy to find, affordable for cash-strapped teens, and perfectly legal. Getting access to the dangerous drug is often as easy as walking into the local drugstore with a few dollars or raiding the family medicine cabinet. And because it's found in over-the-counter medicines, many teens naively assume that DXM can't be dangerous.

Then and Now

DXM abuse is common, according to recent studies, and easy access to OTC medications in stores and over the internet probably contributes to this.

The major difference between current abuse of cough and cold medicines and that in years past is that teens now use the internet to not only buy DXM in pure powder form, but to learn how to abuse it. Because drinking large volumes of cough syrup causes vomiting, the drug is being extracted from cough syrups and sold on the internet in a tablet that can be swallowed or a powder that can be snorted. Online dosing calculators even teach abusers how much they'll need to take for their weight to get high.

One way teens get their DXM fixes is by taking "Triple-C"— Coricidin HBP Cough and Cold—which contains 30 mg of DXM in little red tablets. Users taking large volumes of Triple-C run additional health risks because it contains an antihistamine as well.

The list of other ingredients—decongestants, expectorants, and pain relievers—contained in other Coricidin products and OTC cough and cold preparations compound the risks associated with DXM and could lead to a serious drug overdose.

Besides Triple-C, other street names for DXM include: Candy, C-C-C, Dex, DM, Drex, Red Devils, Robo, Rojo, Skittles, Tussin, Velvet, and Vitamin D. Users are sometimes called "syrup heads" and the act of abusing DXM is often called "dexing," "robotripping," or "robodosing" (because users chug Robitussin or another cough syrup to achieve their desired high).

What Happens When Teens Abuse DXM?

Although DXM can be safely taken in 15- to 30-milligram doses to suppress a cough, abusers tend to consume as much as 360 milligrams or more. Taking mass quantities of products containing DXM can cause hallucinations, loss of motor control, and "out-of-body" (dissociative) sensations.

Other possible side effects of DXM abuse include: confusion, impaired judgment, blurred vision, dizziness, paranoia, excessive sweating, slurred speech, nausea, vomiting, abdominal pain, irregular heartbeat, high blood pressure, headache, lethargy, numbness of fingers and toes, facial redness, dry and itchy skin, loss of consciousness, seizures, brain damage, and even death.

When consumed in large quantities, DXM can also cause hyperthermia, or high fever. This is a real concern for teens who take DXM while in a hot environment or while exerting themselves at a rave or dance club, where DXM is often sold and passed off as similar-looking drugs like PCP [phencyclidine]. And the situation becomes even more dangerous if these substances are used with alcohol or another drug.

Being on the Lookout

You can help prevent your teen from abusing over-the-counter medicines. Here's how:

- Lock your medicine cabinet or keep those OTC medicines that could potentially be abused in a less accessible place.

- Avoid stockpiling OTC medicines. Having too many at your teen's disposal could make abusing them more tempting.

- Keep track of how much is in each bottle or container in your medicine cabinet.

- Keep an eye out not only for traditional-looking cough and cold remedies in your teen's room, but also strange-looking tablets (DXM is often sold on the internet and on the street in its pure form in various shapes and colors).

- Watch out for the possible warning signs of DXM abuse.

- Monitor your teen's internet use. Be on the lookout for suspicious websites and emails that seem to be promoting the abuse of DXM or other drugs, both legal and illegal.

Above all, talk to your kids about drug abuse and explain that even though taking lots of a cough or cold medicine seems harmless, it's not. Even when it comes from the family medicine cabinet or the corner drugstore, when taken in large amounts DXM is a drug that can be just as deadly as any sold on a seedy street corner. And even if you don't think your teens are doing it, chances are they know others who are.

Section 27.4

Alcohol Abuse Makes Prescription Drug Abuse More Likely

"Alcohol Abuse Makes Prescription Drug Abuse More Likely," National Institute on Drug Abuse (www.drugabuse.gov), March 1, 2008. Reviewed by David A. Cooke, MD, FACP, July 2013.

Men and women with alcohol use disorders (AUDs) are 18 times more likely to report nonmedical use of prescription drugs than people who don't drink at all, according to researchers at the University of Michigan. Dr. Sean Esteban McCabe and colleagues documented this link in two NIDA-funded studies; they also discovered that young adults were most at risk for concurrent or simultaneous abuse of both alcohol and prescription drugs.

"The message of these studies is that clinicians should conduct thorough drug use histories, particularly when working with young adults," says Dr. McCabe. "Clinicians should ask patients with alcohol use disorders about nonmedical use of prescription drugs [NMUPD] and in turn ask nonmedical users of prescription medications about their drinking behaviors." The authors also recommend that college staff educate students about the adverse health outcomes associated with using alcohol and prescription medications at the same time.

Two Studies

The authors' first study looked at the prevalence of AUDs and NMUPD in 43,093 individuals 18 and older who participated in the National Epidemiologic Survey on Alcohol and Related Conditions (NESARC) between 2001 and 2005. Participants lived across the United States in a broad spectrum of household arrangements and represented white, African American, Asian, Hispanic, and Native American populations. Although people with AUDs constituted only 9% of NESARC's total sample, they accounted for more than a third of those who reported NMUPD.

Since the largest group of alcohol/prescription drug abusers were between the ages of 18 and 24, the team's second study focused entirely on this population and involved 4,580 young adults at a large, public, Midwestern university. The participants completed a self-administered web survey, which revealed that 12% of them had used both alcohol and prescription drugs nonmedically within the last year but at different times (concurrent use), and 7% had taken them at the same time (simultaneous use).

When alcohol and prescription drugs are used simultaneously, severe medical problems can result, including alcohol poisoning, unconsciousness, respiratory depression, and sometimes death. In addition, college students who drank and took prescription drugs simultaneously were more likely than those who did not to black out, vomit, and engage in other risky behaviors such as drunk driving and unplanned sex.

Who, What, and When

The prescription drugs that were combined with alcohol in order of prevalence included prescription opiates (e.g., Vicodin, OxyContin, Tylenol 3 with codeine, Percocet), stimulant medication (e.g., Ritalin, Adderall, Concerta), sedative/anxiety medication (e.g., Ativan, Xanax, Valium), and sleeping medication (e.g., Ambien, Halcion, Restoril). The college study asked about the respondent's use of medications prescribed for other people while the NESARC explored both use of someone else's prescription medications as well as the use of one's own prescription medications in a manner not intended by the prescribing clinician (e.g., to get high).

The researchers found that the more alcohol a person drank and the younger he or she started drinking, the more likely he or she was to report NMUPD. Compared with people who did not drink at all, drinkers who did not binge were almost twice as likely to engage in NMUPD; binge drinkers with no AUDs were three times as likely; people who abused alcohol but were not dependent on alcohol were nearly seven times as likely; and people who were dependent on alcohol were 18 times as likely to report NMUPD.

While the majority of the respondents in both studies were white (71% in NESARC and 65% in the college group), an even higher percentage of the simultaneous polydrug users in the college study were white males who had started drinking in their early teens. The NESARC study also found that whites in general were two to five times more likely than African Americans to report NMUPD during the past year. Native Americans were at increased risk for NMUPD, and the authors indicated that this subpopulation should receive greater research attention in the future.

Dr. McCabe emphasizes that many people who simultaneously drink alcohol and use prescription medications have no idea how dangerous the interactions between these substances can be. "Passing out is a protective mechanism that stops people from drinking when they are approaching potentially dangerous blood alcohol concentrations," he explains. "But if you take stimulants when you drink, you can potentially override this mechanism and this could lead to life-threatening consequences."

Dr. James Colliver, formerly of NIDA's Division of Epidemiology, Services and Prevention Research, offers perspective on these studies. "Prescription sedatives, tranquilizers, painkillers, and stimulants are generally safe and effective medications for patients who take them as prescribed by a clinician," Dr. Colliver states. "They are used to treat acute and chronic pain, attention deficit hyperactivity disorder, anxiety disorders, and sleep disorders.

"The problem is that many people think that, because prescription drugs have been tested and approved by the Food and Drug Administration, they are always safe to use; but they are safe only when used under the direction of a physician for the purpose for which they are prescribed."

Chapter 28

Legal, Financial, and Social Consequences of Drug Abuse

Chapter Contents

Section 28.1

Consequences of Drug Abuse

Excerpted from "Consequences of Drug Abuse," Get Smart About Drugs, Drug Enforcement Administration (getsmartaboutdrugs.com), 2009. Despite its older publication date, the material in this section is considered accurate and relevant.

Drug abuse is not an issue to be taken lightly—as you know, there are serious consequences for all ages, and for all members of your family. It's important to fully understand the variety of consequences someone may experience if he or she gets caught up in drug abuse.

Legal Consequences of Drug Use

Having a criminal record: Criminal convictions are recorded for some offenses, and these records may exist forever. This can affect your or your child's life in many ways.

Career: Certain types of work can be closed to someone with a criminal record. For example, some types of jobs require certifications or registrations with a professional association when your academic training is finished, and that association can refuse to accept a person with a criminal record.

Employment: Some employers will check applicants for a criminal record. A person may not be able to get a job in the armed or police services, in security or public services, or in business or industry if he or she has a conviction. A person who is convicted of an offense while employed could be fired.

Licenses: Having a criminal record can prevent a person from getting many sorts of licenses; for example, licenses for driving a taxi, running a liquor store, or owning a gun.

Travel: Many countries require that people traveling there get a visa. These countries can refuse to give a visa to a person who has a criminal record.

Social status: Many individuals and groups of people discriminate against someone with a criminal record. A criminal record can affect your standing in the community, the attitudes of your co-workers and neighbors, and your relationships with your family and friends.

The Impact of Drugs on Physical Health

Physical health: Drug abuse can adversely affect every major system in the human body.

Another way that drugs can affect your or your child's physical health—as well as potentially that of others—is if one drives while under the influence of drugs. Drugged driving is a major concern because it impairs a driver's motor function, concentration, and perception—all of which increase the likelihood of road accidents. Marijuana, for example, can impair a driver's abilities for up to three hours after use and can remain in a person's system for up to 24 hours. Approximately one in six (15%) teens reported driving under the influence of marijuana. Combine teens drug use with their inexperience on the road, and you have a recipe for disaster.

Teens who abuse drugs may also engage in behavior that places them at risk of contracting HIV/AIDS or other sexually transmitted diseases. This may happen because they are injecting drugs and sharing used needles, or because of poor judgment and impulse control while experiencing the effects of mood-altering drugs, making them more likely to engage in risky sexual behaviors.

Mental health: Mental health problems such as depression, developmental lags, apathy, withdrawal, and other psychosocial dysfunctions frequently are linked to substance abuse among adolescents. Substance-abusing youth are at higher risk than nonusers for mental health problems, including depression, conduct problems, personality disorders, suicidal thoughts, attempted suicide, and suicide. Marijuana use, which is prevalent among youth, has been shown to interfere with short-term memory, learning, and psychomotor skills.

Addiction: No one thinks that they will ever become addicted to drugs when they start using them—but addiction can and often does happen. Addiction is a compulsive need for and use of habit-forming substances such as drugs. Someone who is addicted loses control and judgment and, when use of the drug is stopped, may suffer severe psychological or physical symptoms, such as anxiety, irritability, unhappiness, and stress. Withdrawal from certain drugs can also result in severe physical discomfort, such as tremors, flu-like symptoms, diarrhea, bone pain, and even seizures. Long-term users of certain drugs may experience pervasive changes in brain function. For example, prolonged exposure to ecstasy can lead to deficits in memory, increased depression, anxiety, and sleep problems.

Social Consequences of Drug Use and Drug Abuse

Drugs alter the brain, so it stands to reason that they would also change the way that humans interact with one another. And drug abuse can radically affect the way you or your child interacts with family, friends, and others.

Families: Substance abuse affects the emotional, financial, and psychological well-being of the entire family. Teens who use drugs withdraw from their family members and family activities, as well as set bad examples for any younger siblings. Because their judgment and decision-making ability become greatly impaired, they may become more hostile toward family members and even steal from them to get money for drugs.

Academics: Teens who abuse drugs have declining grades, a higher rate of absenteeism from school and other activities, as well as an increased potential for dropping out of school. Research has shown that a low level of commitment to education and higher truancy rates appear to be related to substance abuse among adolescents. Cognitive and behavioral problems may also interfere with the academic performance of youth who use alcohol and drugs.

Peers: Teens who abuse drugs are often alienated from and stigmatized by their peers, and they may disengage from school and community activities. For teens who don't use drugs—the best advice is to stay away from kids who do. Experts agree that association with drug-abusing peers is often the most immediate risk for exposing adolescents to drug abuse and delinquent behavior.

Delinquency: Substance abuse and delinquent behavior often go hand in hand. For many youth who abuse drugs, arrest, adjudication, and intervention by the juvenile justice system are eventual consequences they face. While it cannot be claimed that substance abuse causes delinquent behavior—or that delinquency causes alcohol and other drug use—there is an undeniable link between the two behaviors. Substance abuse and delinquency are strongly correlated and often result in involvement with negative peer groups, as well problems in school and at home.

Financial Consequences

Drug use costs society and governments financially in various ways that are well-known:

- Costs to employers for their drug-using employees' absenteeism and reduced productivity, theft, and higher workman's compensation claims due to accidents and injuries

- Costs to the law enforcement and criminal justice systems to arrest, prosecute and incarcerate drug users who commit crimes while under the influence or to obtain money for buying drugs, as well as those who traffic in drugs

- Costs of legitimate businesses closing because they can't compete with businesses using drug money to subsidize their operations

- Costs of artificially inflated financial markets that have been infused with drug money abruptly crashing when governments intervene

- Costs associated with corruption of public and business leaders

- Political costs with financial ramifications, such as the national security costs incurred when the democracies and rule of law of our allies and neighboring countries are threatened by drug cartels

- Costs of putting power and influence in criminals' hands

- Costs to the health care system of caring for drug users and those whom they injure

- Costs to institutions, such as schools, that have to devote policies and processes and personnel to dealing with drug-using students

- Costs to families who break up due to one or both parents' addictions, or who have a drug-using child who needs intervention and treatment

Less often do you find information about the financial cost to users of their own use, costs such as lost aptitudes and abilities and opportunities and, along with those, lost potential financial and other gain. The RAND Corporation is a nonprofit think tank that seeks to improve policy and decision making through research and analysis, and substance abuse is one of their research areas. They have studied groups of drug-using and non-using teenagers well into their adulthood and have posted on their site (www.rand.org/pubs) a number of studies that include information on the costs to users of their own use. Some of those findings include the following:

Impact on jobs: "Adolescent drug use is linked with poorer occupational and job quality outcomes as much as 10 years after high school.

Interestingly, which job-related outcomes are affected by early hard drug use varies by gender. Females who use hard drugs as adolescents end up in lower skill, lower status jobs, while males who use hard drugs as adolescents are more likely to end up in jobs with fewer benefits (e.g., health, retirement)." (From "High School Drug Use Predicts Job-Related Outcomes at Age 29," by Jeanne S. Ringel, Phyllis L. Ellickson and Rebecca L. Collins, published in *Addictive Behaviors*, volume 32, number 3, March 2007, p. [576]–589; RAND's summary of the study is accessible at www.rand.org/pubs/library_reprints/LRP20070301.)

Impact on life satisfaction, including socioeconomic opportunities: "The present study investigated whether adolescent cigarette, alcohol, marijuana, and hard drug use predicts life satisfaction in young adulthood. Survey data were used from a longitudinal cohort of 2,376 adolescents at ages 18 and 29, originally recruited from California and Oregon middle schools at age 13. Results ... indicated that use of cigarettes and hard drugs at age 18 was associated with lower life satisfaction at age 29, controlling for adolescent environmental, social, and behavioral factors related to lower life satisfaction. ... Results suggest that some forms of adolescent substance use limit socio-economic opportunities, and have a lasting effect on health, consequently decreasing life-satisfaction." (From "Are Adolescent Substance Users Less Satisfied With Life as Young Adults and If So, Why?" by Laura M. Bogart, Rebecca L. Collins, Phyllis L. Ellickson, and David J. Klein, published in *Social Indicators Research*, volume 81, number 1, March 2007, p. [149]–169; RAND's summary of the study is accessible at www.rand.org/pubs/library_reprints/LRP20070304/.)

Impact on life adjustment and functioning: A 1990 report by Jonathan Shedler and Jack Block ("Adolescent Drug Use and Psychological Health: A Longitudinal Inquiry," published in *American Psychologist*, volume 45 number 5, pp. 612–630) raised the possibility that "adolescents who experimented with marijuana were better adjusted emotionally and socially than their counterparts who avoided all drugs," a report that generated much discussion among professionals in the field of drug abuse prevention. Because Shedler and Block's study followed only 100 young people, all from the San Francisco Bay Area, RAND decided to revisit the question, "using a wealth of data on youthful substance abuse accumulated since 1985 by the RAND Adolescent/Young Adult Panel Study,... [containing] responses from ... more than 3,000 individuals who were originally recruited from 30 California and Oregon schools ... represent[ing] a wide range of community types, socioeconomic status, and racial/ethnic composition."

These young people were surveyed in grades 7, 8, 9, 10, and 12 and again at ages 23 and 29.

The RAND study found that "Youth who stayed away from marijuana through their senior year of high school functioned better overall than did seniors who experimented with the drug. Compared with experimenters, abstainers had more parental support, devoted more time to homework, spent more time in extracurricular school activities, earned better grades, got into less trouble and were emotionally better off. ... By the time they turn 23, those who had avoided marijuana in high school functioned better overall as young adults than those who had experimented with it in their youth. Compared with experimenters, abstainers were better educated, were happier with their friends, and were less involved in deviant behavior (stealing and drug selling). ... Youth who experiment with marijuana are worse off in many respects than those who abstain throughout their teen years." (From the study by J. S. Tucker, P. L. Ellickson, R. L. Collins, and D. J. Klein, "Are Drug Experimenters Better Adjusted Than Abstainers and Users?: A Longitudinal Study of Adolescent Marijuana Use," published in the *Journal of Adolescent Health*, volume 39, number 4, 2006, pp.488–494, as described in a research brief that can be accessed via www.rand.org/pubs/research_briefs/RB9265.)

Impact on school attendance and its implications for long-term social and economic outcomes: Another study presented by RAND states that "Substance use initiation and frequency are associated with reduced educational attainments among adolescents." The researchers studied 1,084 American adolescents who had been in treatment for drug use and found that "reductions in the frequency of alcohol, stimulants and other drug use and the elimination of marijuana use were each associated independently with increased likelihoods of school attendance." They noted that "... Because years of completed schooling is highly correlated with long-term social and economic outcomes, the possibility that reductions in substance use may improve school attendance" should be taken into account when considering the cost-effectiveness of substance abuse treatment and other interventions. (From "Reducing Substance Use Improves Adolescents' School Attendance," by John Engberg and Andrew R. Morral, published in *Addiction*, volume 101, number 12, December 2006, p. [1741]–1751, which may be accessed via www.rand.org/pubs/library_reprints/LRP20070301.)

Impact on the overall welfare of young adults: RAND studied nearly 6,000 young people from age 13 to 29 for behavioral, socioeconomic, and health outcomes at age 29. The young people were divided into five groups, including abstainers and four groups of marijuana users, grouped according to how old they were when they began using and how much they used. Researchers found that abstainers consistently had the most favorable outcomes, and the young people who used a lot of marijuana when they were young (13) had the worst outcomes despite the fact that they reduced their use as they got older. Their outcomes were worse even than those of the young people who steadily increased the amount of marijuana they used as they aged. (From "Marijuana Use From Adolescence to Young Adulthood: Multiple Developmental Trajectories and Their Associated Outcomes," by Phyllis L. Ellickson, Steven Martino, and Rebecca L. Collins, published in *Health Psychology*, volume 23, number 2, May 2004, pp. 299–307; accessible via www.rand.org/pubs/reprints/RP1192.)

Section 28.2

Drugged Driving

"DrugFacts: Drugged Driving," National Institute on Drug Abuse (www.drugabuse.gov), December 2010.

What is drugged driving?

"Have one [drink] for the road" was once a commonly used phrase in American culture. It has only been within the past 25 years that, as a nation, we have begun to recognize the dangers associated with drunk driving. And through a multipronged and concerted effort involving many stakeholders—including educators, media, legislators, law enforcement, and community organizations such as Mothers Against Drunk Driving—the nation has seen a decline in the numbers of people killed or injured as a result of drunk driving. But it is now time that we recognize and address the similar dangers that can occur with drugged driving.

The principal concern regarding drugged driving is that driving under the influence of any drug that acts on the brain could impair one's motor skills, reaction time, and judgment. Drugged driving is a public health concern because it puts not only the driver at risk but also passengers and others who share the road.

However, despite the knowledge about a drug's potentially lethal effects on driving performance and other concerns that have been acknowledged by some public health officials, policy officials, and constituent groups, drugged driving laws have lagged behind alcohol-related driving legislation, in part because of limitations in the current technology for determining drug levels and resulting impairment. For alcohol, detection of its blood concentration (BAC) is relatively simple, and concentrations greater than 0.08% have been shown to impair driving performance; thus, 0.08% is the legal limit in this country. But for illicit drugs, there is no agreed-upon limit for which impairment has been reliably demonstrated. Furthermore, determining current drug levels can be difficult, since some drugs linger in the body for a period of days or weeks after initial ingestion.

Some states (Arizona, Delaware, Georgia, Indiana, Illinois, Iowa, Michigan, Minnesota, Nevada, North Carolina, Ohio, Pennsylvania, Rhode Island, South Dakota, Utah, Virginia, and Wisconsin) have passed "per se" laws, in which it is illegal to operate a motor vehicle if there is any detectable level of a prohibited drug, or its metabolites, in the driver's blood. Other state laws define "drugged driving" as driving when a drug "renders the driver incapable of driving safely" or "causes the driver to be impaired."

In addition, 44 states and the District of Columbia have implemented Drug Evaluation and Classification Programs, designed to train police officers as drug recognition experts. Officers learn to detect characteristics in a person's behavior and appearance that may be associated with drug intoxication. If the officer suspects drug intoxication, a blood or urine sample is submitted to a laboratory for confirmation.

How many people take drugs and drive?

According to the National Highway Traffic Safety Administration (NHTSA)'s 2007 National Roadside Survey, more than 16% of weekend, nighttime drivers tested positive for illegal, prescription, or over-the-counter medications. More than 11% tested positive for illicit drugs. Another NHTSA study found that in 2009, among fatally injured drivers, 18% tested positive for at least one drug (e.g., illicit, prescription, or over-the-counter), an increase from 13% in 2005. Together, these indicators are a sign that continued substance abuse education, prevention, and law enforcement efforts are critical to public health and safety.

According to the 2009 National Survey on Drug Use and Health (NSDUH), an estimated 10.5 million people aged 12 or older reported driving under the influence of illicit drugs during the year prior to being surveyed. This corresponds to 4.2% of the population aged 12 or older, similar to the rate in 2008 (4%) and not significantly different from the rate in 2002 (4.7%). In 2009, the rate was highest among young adults aged 18 to 25 (12.8%). In addition, NSDUH reported the following:

- In 2009, an estimated 12% of persons aged 12 or older (30.2 million persons) drove under the influence of alcohol at least once in the past year. This percentage has dropped since 2002, when it was 14.2%.

- Driving under the influence of an illicit drug or alcohol was associated with age. In 2009, an estimated 6.3% of youth aged 16 or 17 drove under the influence. This percentage steadily increased with age to reach a peak of 24.8% among young adults aged 21 to 25. Beyond the age of 25, these rates showed a general decline with increasing age.

- Also in 2009, among persons aged 12 or older, males were more likely than females (16.9% versus 9.2%, respectively) to drive under the influence of an illicit drug or alcohol in the past year.

In recent years, more attention has been given to drugs other than alcohol that have increasingly been recognized as hazards to road traffic safety. Some of this research has been done in other countries or in specific regions within the United States, and the prevalence rates for different drugs used vary accordingly. Overall, marijuana is the most prevalent illegal drug detected in impaired drivers, fatally injured drivers, and motor vehicle crash victims. Other drugs also implicated include benzodiazepines, cocaine, opiates, and amphetamines.

A number of studies have examined illicit drug use in drivers involved in motor vehicle crashes, reckless driving, or fatal accidents.

- One study found that about 34% of motor vehicle crash victims admitted to a Maryland trauma center tested positive for "drugs only"; about 16% tested positive for "alcohol only." Approximately 9.9% (or 1 in 10) tested positive for alcohol and drugs, and within this group, 50% were younger than age 18. Although it is interesting that more people in this study tested positive for "drugs only" compared with "alcohol only," it should be noted that this represents one geographic location, so findings cannot be generalized. In fact, the majority of studies among similar populations have found higher prevalence rates of alcohol use compared with drug use.

- Studies conducted in several localities have found that approximately 4% to 14% of drivers who sustained injury or died in traffic accidents tested positive for delta-9-tetrahydrocannabinol (THC), the active ingredient in marijuana.

- In a large study of almost 3,400 fatally injured drivers from three Australian states (Victoria, New South Wales, and Western Australia) between 1990 and 1999, drugs other than alcohol were present in 26.7% of the cases. These included cannabis (13.5%), opioids (4.9%), stimulants (4.1%), benzodiazepines (4.1%), and other psychotropic drugs (2.7%). Almost 10% of the cases involved both alcohol and other drugs.

What about teens and drugged driving?

According to the Centers for Disease Control and Prevention, vehicle accidents are the leading cause of death among young people aged 16 to 19. It is generally accepted that because teens are the least experienced drivers as a group, they have a higher risk of being involved in an accident compared with more experienced drivers. When this lack of experience is combined with the use of marijuana or other substances that impact cognitive and motor abilities, the results can be tragic.

Results from the National Institute on Drug Abuse (NIDA)'s Monitoring the Future survey indicate that in 2007, more than 12% of high school seniors admitted to driving under the influence of marijuana in the two weeks prior to the survey.

The 2007 State of Maryland Adolescent Survey indicates that 11.1% of the state's licensed adolescent drivers reported driving under the influence of marijuana on three or more occasions, and 10% reported driving while using a drug other than marijuana (not including alcohol).

Why is drugged driving hazardous?

Drugs acting on the brain can alter perception, cognition, attention, balance, coordination, reaction time, and other faculties required for safe driving. The effects of specific drugs of abuse differ depending on their mechanisms of action, the amount consumed, the history of the user, and other factors.

Marijuana: THC affects areas of the brain that control the body's movements, balance, coordination, memory, and judgment, as well as sensations. Because these effects are multifaceted, more research is required to understand marijuana's impact on the ability of drivers to react to complex and unpredictable situations. However, we do know the following:

- A meta-analysis of approximately 60 experimental studies—including laboratory, driving simulator, and on-road experiments—found that behavioral and cognitive skills related to driving performance were impaired in a dose-dependent fashion with increasing THC blood levels.

- Evidence from both real and simulated driving studies indicates that marijuana can negatively affect a driver's attentiveness, perception of time and speed, and ability to draw on information obtained from past experiences.

- A study of over 3,000 fatally injured drivers in Australia showed that when marijuana was present in the blood of the driver, he or she was much more likely to be at fault for the accident. Additionally, the higher the THC concentration, the more likely the driver was to be culpable.

- Research shows that impairment increases significantly when marijuana use is combined with alcohol. Studies have found that many drivers who test positive for alcohol also test positive for THC, making it clear that drinking and drugged driving are often linked behaviors.

Prescription drugs: Many medications (e.g., benzodiazepines and opiate analgesics) act on systems in the brain that could impair driving ability. In fact, many prescription drugs come with warnings against the operation of machinery—including motor vehicles—for a specified period of time after use. When prescription drugs are taken without medical supervision (i.e., when abused), impaired driving and other harmful reactions can also result. In short, drugged driving is a dangerous activity that puts us all at risk.

Section 28.3

Drug Use and Crime

This section contains excerpts from "Breaking the Cycle of Drug Use and Crime," November 3, 2011, "Study: More Than Half of Adult Male Arrestees Test Positive for at Least One Drug," May 18, 2012, and "The Arrestee Drug Abuse Monitoring (ADAM II) 2011 Annual Report Highlights," 2011, Office of National Drug Control Policy (www.whitehouse.gov).

Breaking the Cycle of Drug Use and Crime

In 2009, nearly seven million individuals were under supervision of the state and federal criminal justice systems. Nearly two million of these individuals were incarcerated for their crimes, while the remaining five million were on probation or parole. While both the federal and state correctional systems must address this challenge, states generally bear the costs related to this population, and correctional spending has increased accordingly. Between 1988 and 2009, state corrections spending increased from $12 billion to $52 billion per year.

Despite these significant expenditures, far too many offenders return to drug use and crime upon their reentry into society. Part of the reason for this phenomenon is that many offenders are dealing with chronic substance abuse—a disease for which too many are inadequately treated.

Among state prisoners with a substance use disorder, 53% had at least three prior sentences to probation or incarceration, compared to 32% of other inmates. Drug dependent or abusing state prisoners (48%) were also more likely than other inmates (37%) to have been on probation or parole supervision at the time of their arrest. The revolving door of the nation's criminal justice systems is one of the most significant challenges in reducing the devastating consequences of drug use. This cycle deprives too many Americans of their chance to lead healthy, safe, and productive lives.

The administration's strategy promotes a variety of evidence-based alternatives to incarceration for drug-involved offenders. These include Drug Market Interventions (DMI) to disrupt open-air drug markets; Drug and Veterans Treatment Courts designed to effectively treat the substance abuse and mental health disorders of adults, young people, and veterans in the system; smart probation strategies, like Hawaii's Opportunity Probation with Enforcement (HOPE), to use existing community supervision mechanisms to address probationers' underlying substance abuse issues; improved service delivery behind the walls of jail and prison; and reentry support to ensure that offenders don't return to drug use and crime once released.

States are taking steps to improve how their justice systems address substance-abusing offenders and are reexamining and reforming sentencing structures to better align with evidence-based approaches.

More Than Half of Adult Male Arrestees Test Positive for at Least One Drug

Drug use and related crime strain the resources of this country. The latest evidence comes from the 2011 Arrestee Drug Abuse Monitoring Annual Report (ADAM II), released May 18, 2012, which tests for drugs in adult males arrested for a wide variety of crimes in 10 sites across the country. This study found a majority of adult males arrested for crimes tested positive for an illegal drug at the time of their arrest. In fact, positive drug tests among arrestees ranged from 64% in Atlanta, Georgia, to 81% in Sacramento, California.

These data were obtained from individuals booked for all types of crimes, from misdemeanors to felonies, and not just those arrested on drug charges. The ADAM program tests only for drugs marijuana, cocaine, opiates (including heroin and prescription pain relievers), amphetamines/methamphetamine, Darvon, PCP (phencyclidine), benzodiazepines, methadone, and barbiturates—not alcohol.

Although today's data show a high rate of arrestees testing positive for illicit drugs, over the long term, we are actually seeing declines in drug use rates among the general population. Over the past 30 years, the overall rate of current drug use in America has dropped by roughly one-third. And more recently, the rates of current cocaine and meth use have dropped by 40% and 52%, respectively, and the number of cocaine overdoses has dropped by 42%.

The 2011 ADAM II findings are clear evidence of the link between drugs and crime. Too often, underlying substance use disorders are the driving force behind criminal activity. It is imperative, then, that we address our nation's drug problem not just as a criminal justice issue but as a public health issue. We cannot arrest our way out of the drug problem. What we need are evidence-based reforms that break the cycle of drug use and crime, reduce recidivism, and make our communities healthier and safer.

The Arrestee Drug Abuse Monitoring (ADAM II) 2011 Annual Report Highlights

- Drug use among the arrestee population is much higher than in the general U.S. population.

- At the 10 sites participating in the ADAM II study, over 60% of booked arrestees tested positive for at least one illicit drug at the time of their arrest. In 5 of the sites (Chicago, Minneapolis, New York, Portland, and Sacramento), 70% or more tested positive.

- The proportion of arrestees in each site testing positive for any drug ranged from 64% (Atlanta) to 81% (Sacramento).

- Cocaine positives have declined significantly in all ADAM II sites since 2007. In New York and Chicago, cocaine positives dropped from 50% or more in 2000 to half that in 2011.

- The most commonly detected drug in all sites was marijuana (from 36% in Atlanta to 56% in Sacramento).

- Cocaine in powder or crack form was the second most commonly detected substance in 8 of the 10 sites in 2011. In 6 sites, 20% or more of arrestees tested positive for cocaine in 2011.

- The proportion of arrestees in each site who tested positive for multiple drugs in their system ranged from 13% (Charlotte) to 38% (Sacramento).

- The proportion of arrestees testing positive for opiates (heroin and prescription pain relievers) has increased significantly in 5 of 10 sites since 2000 and 2001, more than doubling since 2000 in Denver (to 10%) and more than tripling in Indianapolis (to 10%) in 2011.

- Of those who admitted to drug use in the prior 12 months, less than 16% had been in any outpatient or inpatient treatment in the prior year.
  - Only 2% (Atlanta) to 15% (Portland) reported receiving outpatient drug or alcohol treatment in the past year.
  - 3% (Atlanta) to 16% (Portland) reported receiving inpatient or residential substance abuse treatment in the past year.
  - 2% (Atlanta) to 4% (Portland) reported receiving inpatient mental health or psychiatric treatment.

- Methamphetamine rates remain highest in the two Western sites, with 43% (Sacramento County, California) and 23% (Multnomah County, Oregon) of arrestees testing positive for the drug.

Chapter 29

Health Consequences of Drug Addiction

Chapter Contents

Section 29.1

Poor Health Outcomes of Commonly Abused Drugs

Excerpted from "Health Effects," National Institute on Drug Abuse (www.drugabuse.gov), 2012.

Cannabis (Marijuana) Health Effects

Acute: Heightened sensory perception; euphoria, followed by drowsiness/relaxation; impaired short-term memory, attention, judgment, coordination and balance; increased heart rate; increased appetite

Long-term: Addiction in about 9% of users, about one in six of those who started using in their teens, and 25% to 50% of daily users; mental disorders may be a causal factor in schizophreniform disorders (in those with a preexisting vulnerability); associated with depression and anxiety; smoking-related complications of chronic cough and bronchitis; lung and upper airway cancers undetermined

In combination with alcohol: Magnified tachycardia and effect on blood pressure; amplified impairment of cognitive, psychomotor, and driving performance

Withdrawal symptoms: Irritability, difficulty sleeping, strange nightmares, craving, and anxiety

Cocaine Health Effects

Acute: Dilated pupils; increased body temperature, heart rate, and blood pressure; nausea; increased energy, alertness; euphoria; decreased appetite and sleep

High doses: Erratic and violent behavior, panic attacks

Long-term: Addiction, restlessness, anxiety, irritability, paranoia, panic attacks, mood disturbances; insomnia; nasal damage and difficulty swallowing from snorting; GI problems; HIV

In combination with alcohol: When combined, a greater risk of overdose and sudden death than either substance alone

Withdrawal symptoms: Depression, fatigue, increased appetite, insomnia or hypersomnia, vivid unpleasant dreams, psychomotor retardation or agitation

Pregnancy: Premature delivery, low birth weights, and smaller for gestational age

Prescription Stimulants (Abuse) Health Effects

Amphetamine (Dexedrine, Adderall), Methylphenidate (Ritalin, Concerta)

Acute: Increased alertness, attention, energy; irregular heartbeat, dangerously high body temperature, potential for cardiovascular failure or seizures

Long-term: High doses especially, or alternate routes of administration (e.g., snorting, injecting), can lead to anxiety, hostility, paranoia, psychosis; addiction

In combination with alcohol: Masks the depressant action of alcohol, increasing risk of alcohol overdose; may increase blood pressure; jitters

Withdrawal symptoms: Depression, fatigue, increased appetite, insomnia or hypersomnia, vivid unpleasant dreams, psychomotor retardation or agitation

Mixing with antidepressants or over-the-counter (OTC) cold medicines: May enhance adverse effects, cause blood pressure to become dangerously high, or lead to irregular heart rhythms

Methamphetamine Health Effects

Acute: Enhanced mood; increased heart rate, blood pressure, body temperature, energy and activity; decreased appetite; dry mouth; increased sexuality; jaw clenching

Long-term: Addiction, memory loss; weight loss; impaired cognition; insomnia, anxiety, irritability, confusion, paranoia, aggression, mood disturbances, hallucinations, violent behavior; liver, kidney, lung damage; severe dental problems; cardiac and neurological damage; HIV, hepatitis

Withdrawal symptoms: Depression, anxiety, fatigue, and intense craving for the drug

Pregnancy: Increased risk of premature birth, placental abruption, fetal growth retardation, and heart and brain abnormalities

Inhalants Health Effects

Volatile Solvents, Aerosols, Gases, Nitrites (Poppers)

Acute: Confusion; nausea; slurred speech; lack of coordination; euphoria; dizziness; drowsiness; disinhibition, lightheadedness, hallucinations/delusions; headaches; suffocation; convulsions/seizures; hypoxia; heart failure; coma; sudden sniffing death (butane, propane, and other chemicals in aerosols)

- **Nitrites:** Systemic vasodilation; increased heart rate; brief sensation of heat and excitement; dizziness; headache

Long-term: Myelin break down leading to muscle spasms, tremors, and possible permanent motor impairment; liver/kidney damage; a minority inhale on a regular basis, but among those, some report symptoms of addiction

- **Nitrites:** HIV/AIDS and hepatitis; lipoid pneumonia

- **Nitrites in combination with alcohol:** Increased risk of adverse cardiovascular effects; alcohol may increase the blood-vessel relaxant effect of organic nitrates (such as amyl nitrite) and result in dangerously low blood pressure

Withdrawal symptoms: A mild withdrawal syndrome (e.g., irritability, restlessness, insomnia, headaches, poor concentration) with long-term inhalant abuse

Pregnancy: Although rigorous studies have not been conducted, data from occupational exposure to abused solvents like toluene suggest increased spontaneous abortion and fetal malformations

Prescription Sedatives, Sleeping Pills*, or Anxiolytics (Abuse) Health Effects

Acute: Drowsiness, relaxation; overdose

Long-term: Tolerance, physical dependence, addiction

In combination with alcohol: Slows both heart rate and respiration, which can be fatal

Withdrawal symptoms: Discontinuing prolonged use absent a physician's guidance can lead to serious withdrawal symptoms, including seizures; for barbiturates, abrupt cessation can be life threatening

*Although newer (non-benzodiazepine) sleep medications are thought to have less abuse/addiction liability, ER visits associated with their nonmedical use have been increasing, so these may also present a risk for patients taking them other than as prescribed.

Hallucinogens Health Effects

LSD

Acute: Elation, depression, arousal, paranoia or panic; impulsive behavior, rapid shifts in emotions; distortions in perception; increased body temperature, heart rate, blood pressure; nausea; loss of appetite; sweating; dry mouth; jaw clenching; numbness; sleeplessness; dizziness, weakness, tremors

High doses: Panic, paranoia, feelings of despair, fear of insanity and death

Long-term: Frightening flashbacks, hallucinogen persisting perception disorder (HPPD); low addictive potential—however, tolerance does develop

Psilocybin

Acute: In low doses, relaxation; altered sensory perception; increased energy, heart rate; decreased appetite; in high doses, effects similar to LSD, including visual hallucinations, altered perceptions; nervousness, confusion, panic, paranoia

Long-term: Low addictive potential; however, may produce tolerance

Salvia

Acute: Short-lived, but intense hallucinations, altered visual perception, mood, body sensations; emotional swings, feelings of detachment from one's body; highly modified perception of external reality and self; sweating

Long-term: Unknown addictive potential

PCP (Phencyclidine)

Acute: In low doses, shallow, rapid breathing, increase in heart rate and blood pressure; nausea, blurred vision, dizziness; numbness; slurred speech; confusion; loss of coordination; muscle contractions; analgesia; altered perceptions; feelings of being separated from one's body; in high doses, feelings of invulnerability and exaggerated strength; seizures, coma, hyperthermia

Ketamine

Acute: Anxiety; agitation; insomnia; euphoria; excitement; slurred speech; blurred vision; irregular heartbeat; in low doses, nausea, elevated blood pressure, sedation, analgesia; impaired attention, memory, and motor function; in higher doses, immobility, distortions of auditory and visual perceptions, feelings of being separated from one's body and environment, hallucinations, memory problems

Long-term: Cognitive impairment, including verbal and short-term memory; blurred vision; loss of coordination

In combination with alcohol: Increased risk of adverse effects

MDMA (Ecstasy) Health Effects

Acute: Euphoria; increased energy, alertness, tactile sensitivity, empathy; decreased fear, anxiety; increased/irregular heartbeat; dehydration; chills; sweating; impaired cognition and motor function; reduced appetite; muscle cramping; teeth grinding/clenching; in rare cases—hyperthermia, rhabdomyolysis, and death

Long-term: Impulsiveness; irritability; sleep disturbances; anxiety; addiction

Street Opioids (Heroin, Opium) Health Effects

Acute: Euphoria; warm flushing of skin; dry mouth; heavy feeling in extremities; clouded thinking; alternate wakeful and drowsy states; itching; nausea; depressed respiration

Long-term: Addiction; physical dependence; collapsed veins; abscesses; infection of heart lining and valves; arthritis/other rheumatologic problems; HIV; hepatitis C

In combination with alcohol: Dangerous slowdown of heart rate and respiration, coma, or death

Withdrawal symptoms: Restlessness, muscle and bone pain, insomnia, diarrhea, vomiting, cold flashes with goose bumps ("cold turkey"), and leg movements

Pregnancy: Spontaneous abortions; low birth weight

Prescription Opioids (Abuse) Health Effects

Hydrocodone, Oxycodone, Codeine

Acute: Pain relief, drowsiness, nausea, constipation, euphoria—in some; when taken by routes other than as prescribed (e.g., snorted, injected), increased risk of depressed respiration, leading to coma, death

Long-term: Tolerance, addiction

In combination with alcohol: Dangerous slowing of heart rate and respiration, coma, or death

Withdrawal symptoms: Restlessness, muscle and bone pain, insomnia, diarrhea, vomiting, cold flashes with goose bumps ("cold turkey"), and leg movements

Pregnancy: Spontaneous abortions; low birth weight

Older adults: The higher prevalence of pain in this population renders a greater number of prescriptions written for opioid medications; unintentional misuse or abuse could have more serious health consequences for elderly patients because of comorbid illnesses (and multiple prescriptions), potential for drug interactions, and age-related changes in drug metabolism

Androgenic Anabolic Steroids (Abuse) Health Effects

Acute: Headaches, acne; fluid retention (especially in the extremities), gastrointestinal irritation, diarrhea, stomach pains, and oily skin, jaundice, and hypertension; infections at the injection site

Long-term: Liver damage; cardiovascular disease; high blood pressure; increases in LDL (low-density lipoprotein, "bad" cholesterol) and decreases in HDL (high-density lipoprotein, "good" cholesterol); cardiac hypertrophy, atherosclerosis; addiction potential different from other drugs since abuse is not driven by euphoric effects—nevertheless, individuals often continue abuse despite adverse physical/social consequences

In combination with alcohol: May be synergistic in precipitating impulsive violent behavior (more research is needed)

359

Withdrawal symptoms: Mood swings, fatigue, restlessness, loss of appetite, insomnia, reduced sex drive, steroid cravings, and depression— sometimes leads to suicide attempts

Males: Shrunken testicles, reduced sperm count, infertility, baldness, development of breasts, increased risk for prostate cancer and striae distensae (a skin condition) when injected

Females: Facial hair, male-pattern baldness, changes in or cessation of the menstrual cycle, enlargement of the clitoris, deepened voice, circumscribed hypertrichosis (excessive body hair growth)

Adolescents: Stunted growth due to premature skeletal maturation and accelerated puberty changes

Section 29.2

Substance Abuse and Medical Complications

Excerpted from "Medical Consequences of Drug Abuse," National Institute on Drug Abuse (www.drugabuse.gov), December 2012.

Drug addiction is a brain disease. Although initial drug use might be voluntary, drugs of abuse have been shown to alter gene expression and brain circuitry, which in turn affect human behavior. Once addiction develops, these brain changes interfere with an individual's ability to make voluntary decisions, leading to compulsive drug craving, seeking, and use.

The impact of addiction can be far reaching. Cardiovascular disease, stroke, cancer, HIV/AIDS, hepatitis, and lung disease can all be affected by drug abuse. Some of these effects occur when drugs are used at high doses or after prolonged use; however, some may occur after just one use.

HIV, hepatitis, and other infectious diseases: Drug abuse not only weakens the immune system but is also linked to risky behaviors like needle sharing and unsafe sex. The combination greatly increases the likelihood of acquiring HIV/AIDS, hepatitis, and many other infectious diseases.

Cardiovascular effects: Researchers have found a connection between the abuse of most drugs and adverse cardiovascular effects, ranging from abnormal heart rate to heart attacks. Injection drug use can also lead to cardiovascular problems such as collapsed veins and bacterial infections of the blood vessels and heart valves.

Respiratory effects: Drug abuse can lead to a variety of respiratory problems. Smoking cigarettes, for example, has been shown to cause bronchitis, emphysema, and lung cancer. Marijuana smoke may also cause respiratory problems. The use of some drugs may also cause breathing to slow, block air from entering the lungs, or exacerbate asthma symptoms.

Gastrointestinal effects: Among other adverse effects, many drugs of abuse have been known to cause nausea and vomiting soon after use. Cocaine use can also cause abdominal pain.

Musculoskeletal effects: Steroid use during childhood or adolescence, resulting in artificially high sex hormone levels, can signal the bones to stop growing earlier than they normally would have, leading to short stature. Other drugs may also cause severe muscle cramping and overall muscle weakness.

Kidney damage: Some drugs may cause kidney damage or failure, either directly or indirectly from dangerous increases in body temperature and muscle breakdown.

Liver damage: Chronic use of some drugs, such as heroin, inhalants, and steroids, may lead to significant damage to the liver.

Neurological effects: All drugs of abuse act in the brain to produce their euphoric effects; however, some of them also have severe negative consequences in the brain such as seizures, stroke, and widespread brain damage that can affect all aspects of daily life. Drug use can also cause brain changes that lead to problems with memory, attention, and decision making.

Mental health effects: Chronic use of some drugs of abuse can cause long-lasting changes in the brain, which may lead to paranoia, depression, aggression, and hallucinations.

Hormonal effects: Steroid abuse disrupts the normal production of hormones in the body, causing both reversible and irreversible changes. These changes include infertility and testicle shrinkage in men as well as masculinization in women.

Cancer: Cigarette smoking is the most preventable cause of cancer in the U.S. Smoking cigarettes has been linked to cancer of the mouth, neck, stomach, and lung, among others.

Prenatal effects: The full extent of the effects of prenatal drug exposure on a child is not known; however, studies show that various drugs of abuse may result in premature birth, miscarriage, low birth weight, and a variety of behavioral and cognitive problems.

Other health effects: In addition to the effects various drugs of abuse may have on specific organs of the body, many drugs produce global body changes such as dramatic changes in appetite and increases in body temperature, which may affect a variety of health conditions. Withdrawal from drug use also may lead to numerous adverse health effects, including restlessness, mood swings, fatigue, changes in appetite, muscle and bone pain, insomnia, cold flashes, diarrhea, and vomiting.

Mortality: Drug-related deaths have more than doubled since the early 1980s. There are more deaths, illness, and disabilities from substance abuse than from any other preventable health condition. Today, one in four deaths is attributable to alcohol, tobacco, and illicit drug use.

Section 29.3

Long-Term Marijuana Use Linked to Lower IQ

"NIH-Funded Study Links Long-Term Marijuana Use, Especially When Started During Adolescence, with Decreased IQ and Impaired Cognitive Function," National Institute on Drug Abuse (www.drugabuse.gov), September 10, 2012.

NIH-funded research shows that long-term marijuana use is associated with impaired intellectual functioning, especially if usage starts during the teen years. Over 1,000 study participants were given neuropsychological tests in early adolescence, prior to initiation of marijuana use, and then re-tested in mid adulthood. Study members with more persistent marijuana dependence showed greater IQ decline and greater impairment across five different cognitive domains, especially executive function and processing speed. This is the first long-term prospective study to test young people before their first use of marijuana and again after 20-plus years of use. The study was thus able to rule out preexisting differences in IQ between heavy marijuana users and others; it is also significant for including degree of cannabis exposure and age of onset as factors. Those who started use during the teen years showed greater IQ decline than those who began use as adults. These latter results are especially troubling, given recent data showing increased marijuana use among teens over the last five years, along with declines in perceived risk of harm associated with use. The results of this study are consistent with the notion that cannabis may actually cause some of the neuropsychological deficits seen in regular cannabis users.

The study was funded in part by the National Institute on Drug Abuse, the National Institute on Aging, and the National Institute of Mental Health. For a copy of the study, go to www.pnas.org/content/early/2012/08/22/1206820109.abstract?sid=aaccd18b-26ef-4497-8da0-fa55c5ad15fe.

Chapter 30

Preventing Disease in Drug-Abusing Populations

Chapter Contents

Section 30.1

Drug Abuse and Infectious Diseases

"Integrated Prevention Services for HIV Infection, Viral Hepatitis, Sexually Transmitted Diseases, and Tuberculosis for Persons Who Use Drugs Illicitly: Summary Guidance from CDC and the U.S. Department of Health and Human Services," Centers for Disease Control and Prevention, *Morbidity and Mortality Weekly Report* (www.cdc.gov/mmwr), November 9, 2012.

Illicit Use of Drugs and Infectious Diseases

Rates of HIV infection, viral hepatitis, sexually transmitted diseases (STDs), and tuberculosis (TB) are substantially higher among persons who use drugs illicitly than among persons who do not use drugs illicitly. The term "illicit use of drugs" encompasses all levels of use, abuse, and dependence because each level is associated with behaviors that increase the risk for contracting or transmitting infectious diseases. Persons who use drugs illicitly are defined as those who use, without prescription, prescription drugs (e.g., oxycodone), or as those who use illicit drugs such as opiates (e.g., heroin), stimulants (e.g., powder cocaine, crack cocaine, and methamphetamine), or other so-called "club drugs" (e.g., gamma hydroxybutyrate [GHB], ketamine, flunitrazepam, and ecstasy). Marijuana use and nonmedical use of prescription drugs also are associated with risk for contracting or transmitting infectious diseases.

In general, the risk for acquiring and transmitting infectious disease in a population is a reflection of the prevalence of a given infection in the population, the efficiency of transmission of the organism, and the burden of infectious diseases and patterns of the risk behaviors in which that population engages. The high rates of HIV infection, viral hepatitis, STDs, and TB among persons who use drugs illicitly reflect behavioral, social, cultural, environmental, and structural factors that facilitate disease transmission. Behavioral factors include the use and sharing of contaminated injection equipment (i.e., needles and syringes) and drug preparation equipment (e.g., water, cotton, and a cooker). Bloodborne infections such as HIV infection and viral hepatitis are transmitted efficiently through sharing of contaminated needles. The transmission also can occur through unprotected sex. Illicit use of alcohol by youth, alcohol intoxication, and illicit use of drugs are associated with unsafe sexual behaviors, which are risk factors for HIV infection, viral hepatitis, and STDs. Such social and cultural factors as marginalization, stigma, and lack of social support can contribute to disease transmission; these factors often affect persons who are members of a sexual minority (i.e., lesbian, gay, bisexual, and transgender), persons who use drugs illicitly, or persons who have a mental disorder. Environmental factors common among persons who use drugs illicitly include unstable living conditions and limited availability of sterile injection and drug preparation equipment. Lack of access to and under-enrollment in substance abuse treatment programs are other structural factors contributing to infectious disease transmission. In addition, fear of arrest by law enforcement officers and fear of discrimination by health care providers can discourage persons who use drugs illicitly from using health care services adequately. Persons who use drugs illicitly often have other complex health and social needs, including treatment for substance abuse and for preexisting or concurrent mental disorders.

HIV Infection, Viral Hepatitis, STDs, and TB among Persons Who Use Drugs Illicitly

In the United States, approximately 9%–12% of new HIV cases, 50% of new hepatitis C cases, and 2% of hepatitis A cases are associated with illicit injection of drugs. Among persons who are at risk for infectious diseases, men who have sex with men (MSM) are affected disproportionately by HIV. For example, the Centers for Disease Control and Prevention (CDC) estimates that the rate of new HIV diagnoses among MSM is between 44 and 86 times that among other men, and between 40 and 77 times that among women. A 2008 survey of MSM from cities with high AIDS prevalence indicated that 5% of MSM had ever injected drugs, compared with 1.5% among the general population. The number of new HIV infections is highest among MSM, particularly young MSM, and next highest among persons infected through heterosexual contact, followed by persons who inject drugs.

The epidemiology of HIV infection differs by groups and is influenced by demographic factors affecting use of health care services. For example, persistent racial and ethnic disparities in infectious diseases among persons who use illicit drugs remain a challenge. Data indicate racial and ethnic disparities in use of health care services, including entry and retention in substance abuse treatment programs and other programs. Data also exist on the limited number of gender-sensitive interventions that meet the sex-specific needs of women who use drugs

367

(e.g., negotiation and empowerment for adoption of safer behaviors and providing for needs of children).

A large body of research has demonstrated that illicit drug use, regardless of the route of absorption of the drug, puts users at risk for acquiring HIV infection and STDs. For example, illicit injection of drugs can impair judgment, increasing the likelihood of engaging in risky sexual behaviors. Illicit noninjection drug use also puts users at risk for infectious diseases. Fortunately, prevention efforts aimed at reducing drug injection risk can be successful. For example, in recent years, a convergence in HIV prevalence and incidence among those who engage illicitly in injection or noninjection drug use suggests that a decrease has occurred in HIV transmission; the decrease is associated with safer use of syringes. There has also been a corresponding increase in HIV transmission associated with risky sexual behaviors. Illicit noninjection drug use, particularly use of stimulants, "club drugs," and, to some extent, poppers (e.g., amylnitrite or butylnitrite), and erectile enhancement drugs, plays a substantial role in transmission of infectious diseases although patterns of substance abuse and preferences vary by age group, race, and ethnicity. Many studies highlight the role of methamphetamine and other drugs in risky sexual behavior among MSM as well as the effect of crack cocaine use on exchange of sex for illicit drugs, all of which have implications for infection with HIV and STDs.

The prevalence of STDs among persons who use drugs illicitly varies (range: 1%–6% for syphilis, 1%–5% for Chlamydia, 1%–3% for gonorrhea, and 38%–61% for herpes simplex virus-2 [HSV-2] infection). The moderately high prevalence of bacterial STDs among persons who inject drugs illicitly is not much different from the prevalence among youth at high risk. The high prevalence of HSV-2 among persons who use drugs illicitly contrasts with the 17% prevalence reported for the general population of persons aged 14–49 years. In the United States, approximately one in five patients with active TB either uses a drug illicitly or drinks alcohol in excess, or both. Among U.S.-born TB patients, one in three patients with TB reports substance abuse. In 2008, illicit noninjection drug use was reported in 7.3% of U.S. TB patients, and illicit injection drug use was reported in 1.8%.

Interventions to Reduce Risk Behaviors

Risk-Reduction Programs and Messages

Much of the research on HIV prevention programs for persons who inject drugs illicitly has focused on injection-related risk. In recent years, however, multiple studies have concluded that persons who use drugs illicitly, through injection or noninjection routes, are at increased risk for sexual transmission of HIV, HBV, and other STDs, regardless of the means of introducing the drug into the body. Most persons who use drugs illicitly, through injecting or other means (e.g., inhaling, sniffing, or snorting), are sexually active. Levels of sexual risk are influenced both by the drugs that are used illicitly and by their route of administration. Sexual transmission of HIV among persons who use drugs illicitly is associated with several factors, including a history of other STDs, recent initiation of illicit drug injection, and exchange of sex for money or for illicit drugs. Male-to-male sex as well as illicit use of drugs through noninjection means, including the use of such stimulants as crack cocaine and methamphetamine, is associated with increased risky sexual behaviors; these drugs increase the libido or reduce inhibitions.

Although persons who inject drugs illicitly have reduced their injection risk behaviors in response to behavior-change health interventions, reducing their risky sexual behaviors remains a challenge, similar to the challenge that faces persons who do not use drugs illicitly. Results of two meta-analyses of studies of HIV prevention interventions for persons who use drugs illicitly indicate that multisession psychosocial behavioral interventions that address sexual risk behaviors have a modest added effect compared with the effect of shorter educational interventions and a larger added effect compared with minimal interventions (e.g., waitlist or provision of a self-help booklet). Those results indicate that such interventions should be implemented on a wider scale to reach all persons who use drugs illicitly with messages about safer sex behaviors. However, participants with modest reductions in sexual risk might return to pre-intervention sexual risk (e.g., no condom use or a higher number of sex partners) more rapidly than they would return to pre-intervention injection risk (e.g., use of contaminated needles and sharing of needles).

Persons who use drugs illicitly should be provided with or referred to interventions that include some or all of the following prevention components:

- Information on prevention and transmission of infectious diseases and on safer sex and injection practices

- Assessment of personal risk

- Training in how to use condoms correctly and the importance of using condoms consistently

369

- Counseling to address emotional or practical issues in practicing safe sex

- Training in safer sex negotiation

- HIV testing

- STD screening and treatment

- Referral to substance abuse treatment and social services (e.g., housing)

- Psychosocial support

- Referrals to relevant mental health and family planning services

- Training in overdose prevention and provision of naloxone

Treatment of Substance Use and Mental Disorders to Prevent Infectious Diseases

In general, a short detoxification program from opioids has limited success in leading persons who use drugs illicitly to abstain from such use. For persons who use drugs illicitly, a longer program for substance abuse treatment that includes medication-assisted therapy (e.g., methadone or buprenorphine) and behavioral interventions is helpful for treating illicit drug use as well as for preventing HIV infection, viral hepatitis, STDs, and TB. Reducing or eliminating illicit drug use through substance abuse treatment promotes an overall healthy lifestyle and reduces other negative consequences of illicit drug use, including overdose.

For persons who use drugs illicitly, both lack of motivation to enter substance abuse treatment and the moderately long waiting periods that face them can be barriers to enrollment. Other factors affecting access to substance abuse treatment programs include poverty, lack of health insurance, and fear of being stigmatized as persons who use drugs illicitly.

Substance abuse treatment can reduce such risk behaviors as needle-sharing and exchange of sex for money or for illicit drugs. In addition, substance abuse treatment can serve as an entry point to medical care, and it can improve adherence to medical treatment regimens for infectious diseases. Substance abuse treatment includes nonpharmacologic, psychosocial approaches as well as pharmacologic therapies. Often, a combination of the two approaches is employed. For example, cognitive and behavioral therapies are effective treatments for abuse of amphetamine-type stimulants; the use of such therapies has demonstrated reductions in illicit drug use and in high-risk behaviors. Nonpharmacologic psychotherapies (i.e., behavioral interventions) are valuable when medications are not available or allowable. Adherence interventions might greatly enhance the effects of nonpharmacologic psychotherapies and medications and reduce high-risk behaviors associated with acquisition or transmission of infectious diseases.

An extensive body of evidence demonstrates that therapy with methadone or buprenorphine reduces the frequency of heroin injection, increases rates of retention in substance abuse treatment programs, and markedly decreases criminal activity. For example, methadone maintenance therapy has been associated with reductions in the frequency of illicit injection and sharing of injection equipment. It also has been associated with reductions in the number of sex partners and in the exchange of sex for money or for illicit drugs.

Increased condom use and increased safer sexual behaviors have been reported by persons who have reduced their illicit use of drugs. Substance abuse treatment improves HIV treatment adherence, resulting in lower viral loads and lower likelihood of HIV transmission. Substance abuse treatment also facilitates the prevention of TB among persons who use drugs illicitly. Treatment of TB infection and of TB disease among persons who use drugs illicitly is more successful when integrated with substance abuse treatment, incentives (e.g., food coupons), facilitators (e.g., tokens for transportation), and other services.

Access to Sterile Injection and Drug Preparation Equipment

Evidence suggests that access to sterile injection equipment can reduce transmission of bloodborne pathogens among persons who inject drugs illicitly. However, access to sterile needles and syringes generally is controlled by federal and state-specific laws and regulations that control their sale, distribution, and possession. In December 2011, the U.S. Congress reinstated a ban on the use of federal funds for carrying out any program that distributes sterile needles or syringes for hypodermic injection of illegal drugs.

Distribution policies for sterile injection equipment (e.g., secondary exchange or conditions and numbers of syringes provided) can allow syringe services programs to overcome operational barriers (e.g., limited locations or hours of operation) and can increase access to sterile equipment for persons who inject drugs illicitly.

Although most states do not require a prescription to buy syringes, many states and pharmacies require customers to present personal identification or to sign for the purchase of sterile needles and syringes

371

Participation in no-cost syringe exchange programs leads to a decrease in the frequency of needle-sharing without causing an increase in the frequency of illicit use of drugs.

Existing evidence indicates that syringe exchange programs are effective in reducing the incidence of HIV infection. Syringe exchange programs reduce the risk for infection with HCV, which is the most common bloodborne pathogen among persons who inject drugs illicitly.

In addition to providing sterile syringes, most syringe exchange programs provide other health-related supplies and services to their clients. In 2008, more than 90% of syringe exchange programs provided male condoms, alcohol pads, and education on safer injection practices and on prevention of HIV infection, viral hepatitis, STDs, and abscesses; 87% provided HIV counseling and testing; 65% provided testing and counseling for HCV; 55% provided STD screening; 49% provided vaccination for hepatitis B; 47% provided vaccination for hepatitis A; 24% provided counseling and testing for hepatitis B; 31% provided TB screening; and 18% provided counseling and testing for hepatitis A.

Syringe exchange programs also often provide referrals to substance abuse treatment and social services. Syringe exchange programs also can serve as sites for TB screening and for testing for TB infection, and they can serve as gateways to treatment for HIV or HCV infection.

Interventions to Increase Condom Availability

Increasing the availability of condoms is associated with substantial reductions in HIV risk. Limited condom availability attributable to high cost, a low concentration of sale outlets in a given area, or limits on free distribution of condoms are often cited as barriers to condom use. Distributing condoms free of charge at clinics, substance abuse treatment centers, jails and prisons, businesses, or other community locations (e.g., outreach and syringe services programs) can serve as a public health intervention or a supplement to existing campaigns and interventions, because prices as low as 25 cents per condom have been demonstrated to deter their use. In addition, condom use can reduce risk for oral and vaginal transmission of HIV, viral hepatitis, and bacterial and viral STDs among persons who use drugs illicitly. Because gonorrhea, Chlamydia, syphilis, HSV-2, and HIV can be transmitted by oral sex, condom use also can reduce transmission of these infections through oral sex.

Partner Services and Contact Follow-up

Partner services begin when persons who have an infection are interviewed to obtain information about their partners in a voluntary and confidential manner. Following this step, partners are notified confidentially of their possible exposure to infection. Services that can be offered to infected persons and to their partners include risk-reduction counseling, testing (including partner or couple testing), hepatitis A and B vaccination, treatment or referral to medical care, and referral to other services (e.g., substance abuse treatment, social support, housing assistance, and mental health services). Partner notification services for persons at risk for infections transmitted through illicit injection of drugs (e.g., HIV and HCV) are as effective in reducing transmission of these infections as are the partner notification services for infections transmitted through risky sexual behaviors (e.g., bacterial STDs).

Referrals and Linkage to Care

Persons who use drugs illicitly and who are identified to be infected with HIV, viral hepatitis, STDs, or TB should be referred and linked actively to medical care. Medical care includes treatment for these infections as well as treatment for other health conditions that affect the lives and well-being of persons who use drugs illicitly. Referral to and linkage with mental health services provide a supportive role for persons receiving treatment for infectious diseases and substance use disorders, including persons who are receiving treatment for hepatitis C infection, because HCV treatment regimens are associated with increased levels of depression.

Three approaches to referrals and linkage to care are used commonly. First, persons who use drugs illicitly are referred, following a needs assessment process, for medical treatment, care, and supportive services. Assistance with follow-up can facilitate initial contact with and linkage to appropriate service providers. A second approach is the "strengths-based case management approach," which calls on clients to identify internal strengths and abilities and to develop a personal plan that includes meetings with case managers to acquire needed resources. A third approach is active linking, which can include health care visits accompanied by a linkage coordinator or case manager to ensure that clients obtain appropriate medical care. Such accompaniment is especially important for the first appointment. Linkage-to-care approaches are effective in improving health care outcomes; on the other hand, referral alone has not been effective in enhancing linkage and adherence to care.

Supportive strategies or incentives can be helpful in increasing adherence and linkage to care, e.g., co-location of services, deployment of outreach workers, peer navigators, monetary incentives, and motivational enhancements. Persons interacting with the criminal justice system or leaving correctional facilities (jails or prisons) can benefit particularly from active linkage to HIV medical care, TB linkage interventions, HCV medical care, STD services, substance abuse treatment, and overdose prevention programs.

Medical Treatment for Infectious Diseases

Persons who use drugs illicitly need to receive appropriate treatment for infectious diseases and relevant health education messages from trained personnel. An infected person who receives a diagnosis of HIV infection, viral hepatitis, STDs, or TB should be referred to care providers and receive primary medical care and evaluation for progression of infection to disease, as well as treatment. In addition, infected persons need to be provided with counseling and guidance on how to stay healthy and prevent disease progression. They also should be instructed about how to reduce the risk for transmitting their infections to others, receive encouragement to seek further medical evaluation, and, if necessary, be given information about the importance of adhering to medical treatment regimens. Most persons who use drugs illicitly are capable of adhering actively to complex medical regimens. Therefore, past or current illicit use of drugs should not be considered a contraindication to successful treatment for infectious diseases. Treatment of infectious diseases reduces and potentially prevents transmission of infectious diseases in the communities where persons who use drugs illicitly reside. Sex partners and drug-using partners and contacts of infected persons should be identified and provided with prevention information, in addition to referral for medical evaluation and for treatment, if necessary.

Adherence to treatment of infectious diseases among persons who use drugs illicitly can be enhanced by addressing different comorbid conditions, including mental disorders and such other factors as poverty-related issues, including homelessness and limited access to transportation.

There is a potential for harmful medication interactions or toxic effects in the treatment of persons with multiple infections who inject drugs illicitly. Adverse effects of medications can include the effects of HIV antiretroviral medications on liver, kidney, and neurologic functions. For example, rifampin, a first-line medication for treating TB, interacts both with methadone (for treating addiction to heroin) and with efavirenz and nevirapine (for treating HIV infection).

Before 2002, the National Institutes of Health (NIH) considered illicit use of drugs a contraindication for HCV treatment, meaning that persons who used drugs illicitly were routinely denied medical treatment for HCV infection. In 2002, NIH issued a consensus statement that HCV treatment for persons who use drugs illicitly should be considered on a case-by-case basis. Since then, according to some studies, illicit use of drugs during HCV therapy has been associated with lower rates of adherence and with increased risk for reinfection, although this association has not been demonstrated consistently. Other studies have indicated that HCV treatment adherence among persons who use drugs illicitly was increased by use of integrated service models that included mental health and substance abuse treatment, peer-based support groups, and a specific version of DOT for HCV treatment.

Delivery of Integrated Prevention Services

Persons who use drugs illicitly can benefit from comprehensive (or at least combination) services that meet their individual clinical needs or community needs. They can be expected to benefit from synergy among services that are delivered jointly at the service delivery level as integrated services.

Section 30.2

The Connection between HIV/AIDS and Drug Abuse

"DrugFacts: HIV/AIDS and Drug Abuse:
Intertwined Epidemics," National Institute on Drug Abuse
(www.drugabuse.gov), May 2012.

Drug abuse and addiction have been inextricably linked with HIV/AIDS since the beginning of the epidemic. The link has to do with heightened risk—both of contracting and transmitting HIV and of worsening its consequences.

No vaccine yet exists to protect a person from getting HIV, and there is no cure. However, HIV can be prevented and its transmission curtailed. Drug abuse treatment fosters both of these goals. HIV medications also help prevent HIV transmission and the progression of HIV to AIDS, greatly prolonging lives.

What exactly is HIV/AIDS?

HIV stands for human immunodeficiency virus. This virus severely damages the immune system and causes acquired immune deficiency syndrome, or AIDS, a condition that defeats the body's ability to protect itself against disease.

HIV inflicts this damage by infecting immune cells in our bodies called CD4 positive (CD4+) T cells—essential for fighting infections. HIV converts the CD4+ T cells into "factories" that produce more of the HIV virus to infect other healthy cells, eventually destroying the CD4+ T cells.

As CD4+ T cells are lost and the immune system weakens, a person becomes more prone to illnesses and common infections. AIDS is diagnosed when a person has one or more of these infections and a CD4+ cell count of less than 200.

More than 16,000 people died from AIDS in 2008.

How is HIV spread?

HIV is transmitted by contact with the blood or other body fluids of an infected person. This can occur during unprotected sex or through sharing injecting drug-use equipment. In addition, untreated infected women can pass HIV to their infants during pregnancy, delivery, and breastfeeding.

How do drugs affect HIV?

Most people know that intravenous drug use and needle-sharing can transmit HIV; less known is the role that drug abuse in general plays. A person under the influence of certain drugs is more likely to engage in risky behaviors such as having unsafe sex with an infected partner. Indeed, the most common (but not only) way of contracting HIV is through unsafe sex. This includes "transactional" sex—trading sex for drugs or money.

Drug abuse and addiction can also worsen HIV symptoms, causing greater neuronal injury and cognitive impairment, for example.

Because of the strong link between drug abuse and the spread of HIV, drug abuse treatment can be an effective way to prevent the latter. People in drug abuse treatment, which often includes HIV risk reduction counseling, stop or reduce their drug use and related risk behaviors, including risky injection practices and unsafe sex.

Can anyone get HIV/AIDS?

Yes, anyone is vulnerable to contracting HIV. Although injecting and other drug users are at elevated risk, anyone who has unprotected sex could be exposed to the infection. In 2010, nearly 47,000 people were diagnosed with HIV. Among those newly diagnosed, nearly two-thirds occurred in men who have sex with men (MSM). One-half of all people living with HIV in 2008 were MSM.

HIV infection is also disproportionately represented in the African American community. Over one-half of all newly diagnosed cases in the United States are in African Americans, followed by the white and Hispanic populations.

How is HIV treated?

From the beginning of the HIV/AIDS epidemic in the early 1980s until the mid-1990s, HIV infection was almost guaranteed to result in death from AIDS. The number of deaths declined after 1996, when effective treatments were introduced.

HAART—highly active antiretroviral therapy—is a customized combination of different classes of medications that a physician prescribes to treat HIV. Although it cannot rid the body of the virus, HAART can control the amount of virus in the bloodstream (viral load), helping to delay the onset of symptoms and progression to AIDS, prolonging survival in people with HIV.

Why is HIV testing so important?

A person infected with HIV may look and feel fine for many years and may not even be aware of the infection. In fact, the Centers for Disease Control and Prevention estimates that 1.2 million people are infected with HIV in the United States and that one in five people infected are unaware of it. HIV testing is critical and can help prevent spread of the infection—among those most at risk (e.g., people who abuse drugs) and in general. Getting tested is not complicated. Some tests can even provide results in 20 minutes, although testing is not accurate until about six to eight weeks after exposure to HIV. That time is needed for HIV antibodies to form in amounts detectable by a standard HIV test.

Research shows that seeking out and testing high-risk populations and starting treatment for those who test positive prevents HIV transmission by decreasing viral load, infectivity (the ability to infect others), and subsequent illness—to the benefit of all.

Section 30.3

Hepatitis Infection and Drug Use

Excerpted from "Substance Abuse/Use," Aids.gov, U.S. Department of Health and Human Services (www.aids.gov), June 20, 2011, and "Hepatitis C FAQs for the Public," Centers for Disease Control and Prevention (www.cdc.gov), October 22, 2012.

Substance Abuse/Use

In 2008 alone an estimated 4,444 Americans were infected with HIV by injecting drugs. Sharing drug equipment (or "works") can expose you to HIV-infected blood. If you share works with someone who is HIV-positive, that person's blood can stay on needles or spread to the drug solution. In that case, you can inject HIV directly into your body.

You can get HIV-infected blood into drug solutions by preparing drugs with the following:

- A used syringe

- Used bottle caps, spoons, or other containers ("cookers")

- Used pieces of filtering cotton or cigarette filters ("cottons")

- Water that was already used to dissolve drugs or clean syringes

If you are an injection drug user (IDU), you can also pass HIV to your sex partners.

Drug Use and HIV Infection

According to the most recent CDC data (2008):

- Injection drug users represent 12% of annual new HIV infections in the United States.

- Injection drug users represent 19% of those living with HIV in the United States.

- Among males, 9% of diagnosed HIV infections were attributed to injection drug use and another 4% were attributed to male-to-male sexual contact and injection drug use.

- Among females, 15% of diagnosed HIV infections were attributed to injection drug use.

Injecting Drug Users Are Also At-Risk of Hepatitis Infection

HIV infection isn't the only risk: Injecting drugs is also the main way of becoming infected with the hepatitis C virus (HCV). In fact, 50%–90% of HIV-infected injection drug users are also infected with hepatitis C, a liver disease caused by HCV.

HCV infection sometimes results in an acute illness, but most often becomes a chronic condition that can lead to cirrhosis of the liver and liver cancer. HCV infection is more serious in HIV-infected persons. It leads to liver damage more quickly. Co-infection with HCV may also affect the treatment of HIV infection. Therefore, it's important for people who inject drugs to know whether they are also infected with HCV and, if they aren't, to take steps to prevent infection. To find out if you are infected, your doctor or other health care provider will have to test your blood to check for the virus. Hepatitis C can be treated successfully, even in HIV-infected persons.

Hepatitis C

Hepatitis C is a contagious liver disease that ranges in severity from a mild illness lasting a few weeks to a serious, lifelong illness that attacks the liver. It results from infection with the hepatitis C virus, which is spread primarily through contact with the blood of an infected person. Hepatitis C can be either "acute" or "chronic."

- Acute hepatitis C virus infection is a short-term illness that occurs within the first six months after someone is exposed to the hepatitis C virus. For most people, acute infection leads to chronic infection.

- Chronic hepatitis C virus infection is a long-term illness that occurs when HCV remains in a person's body. Hepatitis C virus infection can last a lifetime and lead to serious liver problems, including cirrhosis (scarring of the liver) or liver cancer.

How common is hepatitis C in the United States?

In 2009, there were an estimated 16,000 acute hepatitis C virus infections reported in the United States. An estimated 3.2 million persons in the United States have chronic hepatitis C virus infection. Most people do not know they are infected because they don't look or feel sick. Approximately 75%–85% of people who become infected with hepatitis C virus develop chronic infection.

How is hepatitis C spread?

Hepatitis C is usually spread when blood from a person infected with the hepatitis C virus enters the body of someone who is not infected. Today, most people become infected with the hepatitis C virus by sharing needles or other equipment to inject drugs. People can become infected with the Hepatitis C virus during such activities as the following:

- Sharing needles, syringes, or other equipment to inject drugs
- Needlestick injuries in health care settings
- Being born to a mother who has hepatitis C

Less commonly, a person can also get hepatitis C virus infection through the following:

- Sharing personal care items that may have come in contact with another person's blood, such as razors or toothbrushes
- Having sexual contact with a person infected with the hepatitis C virus

What are the symptoms of acute hepatitis C?

Approximately 70%–80% of people with acute hepatitis C do not have any symptoms. Some people, however, can have mild to severe symptoms soon after being infected, including the following:

- Fever
- Fatigue
- Loss of appetite
- Nausea
- Vomiting
- Abdominal pain
- Dark urine
- Clay-colored bowel movements
- Joint pain
- Jaundice (yellow color in the skin or eyes)

Many people who are infected with the Hepatitis C virus do not know they are infected because they do not look or feel sick.

How soon after exposure to hepatitis C do symptoms appear?

If symptoms occur, the average time is six to seven weeks after exposure, but this can range from two weeks to six months. However, many people infected with the hepatitis C virus do not develop symptoms.

What are the symptoms of chronic hepatitis C?

Most people with chronic hepatitis C do not have any symptoms. However, if a person has been infected for many years, his or her liver may be damaged. In many cases, there are no symptoms of the disease until liver problems have developed. In persons without symptoms, hepatitis C is often detected during routine blood tests to measure liver function and liver enzyme (protein produced by the liver) level.

How serious is chronic hepatitis C?

Chronic hepatitis C is a serious disease that can result in long-term health problems, including liver damage, liver failure, liver cancer, or even death. It is the leading cause of cirrhosis and liver cancer and the most common reason for liver transplantation in the United States. Approximately 15,000 people die every year from hepatitis C–related liver disease.

What are the long-term effects of hepatitis C?

The following occur out of every 100 people infected with the hepatitis C virus:

- About 75–85 people will develop chronic hepatitis C virus infection.
- Of those, 60–70 people will go on to develop chronic liver disease.
- 5–20 people will go on to develop cirrhosis over a period of 20–30 years.
- 1–5 people will die from cirrhosis or liver cancer.

How is hepatitis C treated?

There is no medication available to treat acute hepatitis C infection. Doctors usually recommend rest, adequate nutrition, and fluids.

Patients with chronic hepatitis should discuss treatment options with a doctor who specializes in treating hepatitis. They should be monitored regularly for signs of liver disease and evaluated for treatment. The treatment most often used for hepatitis C is a combination of two medicines, interferon and ribavirin. However, not every person with chronic hepatitis C needs or will benefit from treatment. In addition, the drugs may cause serious side effects in some patients.

Is it possible to get over hepatitis C?

Yes, approximately 15%–25% of people who get hepatitis C will clear the virus from their bodies without treatment and will not develop chronic infection. Experts do not fully understand why this happens for some people.

What can people with chronic hepatitis C do to take care of their liver?

People with chronic hepatitis C should be monitored regularly by an experienced doctor. They should avoid alcohol because it can cause additional liver damage. They also should check with a health professional before taking any prescription pills, supplements, or over-the-counter medications, as these can potentially damage the liver. If liver damage is present, a person should check with his or her doctor about getting vaccinated against hepatitis A and hepatitis B.

Section 30.4

Sterile Syringe Programs

Introduction

Injection drug use is associated with a high risk of infection by blood-borne diseases such as HIV and hepatitis C. Sterile syringe access programs help lower these risks by limiting syringe sharing and providing safe disposal options. These programs also provide people who inject drugs with referrals to treatment, detoxification, social services, and primary health care.

Increasing access to sterile syringes through syringe exchange programs and non-prescription pharmacy sales is essential to reducing syringe sharing among people who inject drugs. Throughout the world, research has consistently shown that syringe access programs decrease rates of HIV/AIDS and hepatitis C transmission. Syringe access programs have also been shown to increase the safe disposal of used syringes, protecting police officers and the public from accidental exposure to blood-borne diseases.

Despite the benefits of these life-saving programs, legal and bureaucratic barriers still prevent people who use drugs from accessing clean syringes. Repressive drug law enforcement strategies—and the fear of arrest—lead to more risky injecting practices. Often people share syringes because they cannot access sterile ones through pharmacies without a prescription or because carrying sterile syringes is still illegal in their state.

Other times people lack access because syringe access programs are limited by lack of funding. The U.S. Congress recently reinstated the federal ban on funding sterile syringe programs, after finally lifting the two-decade-long ban just two years ago. The federal ban is estimated to have cost thousands of lives and hundreds of millions of dollars.

The Drug Policy Alliance [DPA] is working to ensure wider access to sterile syringes throughout the country. We support removing syringes from the criminal code by ending policies that criminalize syringe possession and limit sterile syringe distribution. DPA was instrumental in eliminating the federal ban on syringe access funding, and we are fighting to make sure the ban gets lifted again. We have led successful efforts to launch syringe access programs and facilities in several states, most recently in New Jersey.

DPA supports the non-prescription, over-the-counter sale of syringes, which is now permitted in all but one state (Delaware). We support state efforts to exempt syringes from paraphernalia laws and broaden the legal definition of medical necessity as it relates to syringe access. We also favor allowing doctors to prescribe syringes to their patients, a practice few states currently permit.

Drug Injection and HIV/AIDS

Globally, injection drug use accounts for approximately one in three new cases of HIV outside of sub-Saharan Africa. In the U.S., estimated HIV prevalence among people who inject drugs is roughly 16%, or one in six. Rates in countries that have comprehensively and consistently funded syringe access programs are far lower—in some cases, close to zero.

Sharing syringes not only puts people who use drugs at risk, but also their sexual partners. Although rates of HIV infection among people who inject drugs have declined in the U.S. over the past decade, unsafe injecting practices continue to transmit the disease.

According to the Centers for Disease Control and Prevention (CDC), people who inject drugs represented 9% (4,500) of all estimated new HIV infections in 2009—an annual figure that has not changed significantly since 2006. CDC estimates that "[s]ince the epidemic began, injection drug use has directly and indirectly accounted for more than one-third (36%) of AIDS cases in the United States," which amounts to more than 350,000 people.

Obstacles to sterile syringe access perpetuate the escalating racial disparities in HIV infection rates. Among people who inject drugs in the U.S., blacks and Latinos have considerably higher rates of HIV compared to whites. Black men and women accounted for the greatest number of new of HIV infections among injection-drug using people in 2009—almost half (48%). Age-adjusted death rates due to HIV/AIDS have been highest among blacks and second-highest among Latinos. Between 2004 and 2007, 152,917 people were diagnosed with HIV in 34 states, including 19,687 people who inject drugs (roughly 13%); however, blacks accounted for more than 57% of these new infections.

Injection drug-related HIV/AIDS also affects women disproportionately. Since the beginning of the epidemic, "57 percent of all AIDS cases among women have been attributed to injection drug use or sex with partners who inject drugs, compared with 31 percent of cases among men" [Steffanie A. Strathdee & Jamila K. Stockman, "Epidemiology of HIV Among Injecting and Non-injecting Drug Users: Current Trends and Implications for Interventions," *Current HIV/AIDS Rep* (2010) 7:99–106 (citing CDC, HIV infection among injection-drug users—34 states, 2004–2007. *Morbidity & Mortality Weekly Report* 2009, 58:1291–1295)].

Syringe Access Saves Lives

More than 200 studies from the U.S. and abroad have reached the same incontrovertible conclusions: syringe access programs are a cost-effective means to reduce the spread of HIV and viral hepatitis, and that these programs do not contribute to increased drug use, drug injection, crime, or unsafe discarding of syringes. A CDC-funded study published in the *Journal of the American Medical Association* credits syringe access with reducing HIV incidence among people who inject drugs by 80% in the past decade.

In some U.S. cities and states, advocates have overcome drug war hostility to implement syringe access programs that have saved thousands of lives with no negative impacts to their communities. For example, New York City experienced one of the largest HIV epidemics among people who inject drugs in the world, but after implementing syringe access programs in 1990, both HIV incidence and HIV prevalence decreased by 75% or more.

According to a global survey, HIV prevalence rates increased in cities without syringe access programs by roughly 6% each year, while prevalence rates decreased by approximately 6% annually in cities with syringe access services. Confirming these findings, another study drawing on data from 99 cities around the world found that HIV prevalence decreased by 18% in cities with syringe access programs, and increased by over 8% in cities without these life-saving programs.

Metropolitan areas that have banned over-the-counter sales of sterile syringes have been shown to have considerably higher rates of HIV prevalence than those that have not, prompting researchers to conclude, "Laws restricting syringe access are associated with HIV transmission and should be repealed" [S Friedman et al., *American Journal of Public Health* 91 (2001): 353].

Most programs not only provide disease prevention education and materials, but also provide referral to drug treatment and other vital health services, including screenings for HIV, hepatitis, and sexually transmitted infections.

"Needle exchange programs have been proven to reduce the transmission of blood-borne diseases ... [and] do not increase drug use."

—Gil Kerlikowske, director of the White House Office of National Drug Control Policy and former Seattle police chief, April 2009

Syringe Access Is Cost Effective

Restricting access to sterile syringes is not only bad public health policy—it's also bad economic policy. Research has consistently shown that not only does syringe access save lives—it saves money.

A sterile syringe costs roughly $0.97, yet in 2006 the lifetime cost of treating someone with AIDS was $618,000, and the lifetime cost of treating someone with hepatitis C is estimated to cost between $100,000 and $300,000. The U.S. can save billions of dollars on medical costs by increasing access to sterile syringes to prevent injection-related HIV and viral hepatitis infections.

Chapter 31

Mental Illness and Addiction

Chapter Contents

Section 31.1

Addiction and Mental Health Disorders

"DrugFacts: Comorbidity: Addiction and Other Mental Disorders,"
National Institute on Drug Abuse (www.drugabuse.gov), March 2011.

What is comorbidity?

The term "comorbidity" describes two or more disorders or illnesses occurring in the same person. They can occur at the same time or one after the other. Comorbidity also implies interactions between the illnesses that can worsen the course of both.

Is drug addiction a mental illness?

Yes. Addiction changes the brain in fundamental ways, disturbing a person's normal hierarchy of needs and desires and substituting new priorities connected with procuring and using the drug. The resulting compulsive behaviors that weaken the ability to control impulses, despite the negative consequences, are similar to hallmarks of other mental illnesses.

How common are comorbid drug addiction and other mental illnesses?

Many people who are addicted to drugs are also diagnosed with other mental disorders and vice versa. For example, compared with the general population, people addicted to drugs are roughly twice as likely to suffer from mood and anxiety disorders, with the reverse also true.

Why do these disorders often co-occur?

Although drug use disorders commonly occur with other mental illnesses, this does not mean that one caused the other, even if one appeared first. In fact, establishing which came first or why can be difficult. However, research suggests the following possibilities for this common co-occurrence:

- Drug abuse may bring about symptoms of another mental illness. Increased risk of psychosis in vulnerable marijuana users suggests this possibility.

- Mental disorders can lead to drug abuse, possibly as a means of "self-medication." Patients suffering from anxiety or depression may rely on alcohol, tobacco, and other drugs to temporarily alleviate their symptoms.

These disorders could also be caused by shared risk factors, such as the following:

- **Overlapping genetic vulnerabilities:** Predisposing genetic factors may make a person susceptible to both addiction and other mental disorders or to having a greater risk of a second disorder once the first appears.

- **Overlapping environmental triggers:** Stress, trauma (such as physical or sexual abuse), and early exposure to drugs are common environmental factors that can lead to addiction and other mental illnesses.

- **Involvement of similar brain regions:** Brain systems that respond to reward and stress, for example, are affected by drugs of abuse and may show abnormalities in patients with certain mental disorders.

- **Drug use disorders and other mental illnesses are developmental disorders:** That means they often begin in the teen years or even younger—periods when the brain experiences dramatic developmental changes. Early exposure to drugs of abuse may change the brain in ways that increase the risk for mental disorders. Also, early symptoms of a mental disorder may indicate an increased risk for later drug use.

How are these comorbid conditions diagnosed and treated?

The high rate of comorbidity between drug use disorders and other mental illnesses calls for a comprehensive approach that identifies and evaluates both. Accordingly, anyone seeking help for either drug abuse/addiction or another mental disorder should be checked for both and treated accordingly.

Several behavioral therapies have shown promise for treating comorbid conditions. These approaches can be tailored to patients according to age, specific drug abused, and other factors. Some therapies have proven more effective for adolescents, while others have shown greater effectiveness for adults; some are designed for families and groups, others for individuals.

Effective medications exist for treating opioid, alcohol, and nicotine addiction and for alleviating the symptoms of many other mental disorders, yet most have not been well studied in comorbid populations. Some medications may benefit multiple problems. For example, evidence suggests that bupropion (trade names: Wellbutrin, Zyban), approved for treating depression and nicotine dependence, might also help reduce craving and use of the drug methamphetamine. More research is needed, however, to better understand how these medications work, particularly when combined in patients with comorbidities.

Section 31.2

Depression and Initiation of Alcohol and Drug Abuse in Teens

Excerpted from "Depression and the Initiation of Alcohol and Other Drug Use among Youths Aged 12 to 17," Substance Abuse and Mental Health Services Administration (www.samhsa.gov), July 11, 2008. Reviewed by David A. Cooke, MD, FACP, July 2013.

- In 2005, 8.8% of youths aged 12 to 17 (2.2 million persons) experienced at least one major depressive episode (MDE) in the past year.

- Among youths aged 12 to 17 who were at risk for alcohol initiation (i.e., those who had never used alcohol previously), those who experienced a past-year MDE were twice as likely to have initiated alcohol use in the past year as those who did not have a past-year MDE (29.2% vs. 14.5%).

- Among youths who were at risk for illicit drug initiation, those who experienced a past-year MDE were over twice as likely to have initiated use of an illicit drug as those who had not experienced an MDE in the past year (16.1% vs. 6.9%).

Research has shown that there is a strong association between mental health disorders and substance use disorders, but findings about the order of onset and direction of influence vary by substance and type of disorder. There is strong evidence, for example, that alcohol abuse can be a contributing factor to the development of depression, but more typically the mental condition occurs prior to the substance use disorder. Associations also exist between mental disorders and substance use behaviors that do not meet the criteria for substance use disorders. For example, research suggests that adults and adolescents with MDE in the past year were more likely than those without MDE to have used alcohol heavily or to have used an illicit drug in the past year.

The National Survey on Drug Use and Health (NSDUH) includes questions for youths aged 12 to 17 to assess lifetime and past-year MDE. For these estimates, MDE is defined using the diagnostic criteria set forth in the 4th edition of the *Diagnostic and Statistical Manual of Mental Disorders* (DSM-IV), which specifies a period of two weeks or longer during which there is either depressed mood or loss of interest or pleasure and at least four other symptoms that reflect a change in functioning, such as problems with sleep, eating, energy, concentration, and self-image.

NSDUH also asks youths aged 12 to 17 to report on their use of alcohol and illicit drugs in their lifetime and in the past year. Illicit drugs refer to marijuana/hashish, cocaine (including crack), inhalants, hallucinogens, heroin, or prescription-type drugs used nonmedically. Respondents who reported use of a given substance were asked when they first used it; responses to these questions were used to identify persons at risk for substance use initiation (i.e., persons who had not ever used the substance prior to the 12 months preceding the survey) and to identify recent initiates (i.e., persons who used the substance for the first time in the 12 months prior to the survey). In 2005 among youths aged 12 to 17, past-year initiates accounted for 29.8% of all past-year illicit drug users and 32.5% of past-year alcohol users.

This report examines past-year MDE, past-year initiation of alcohol and illicit drug use, and the association between MDE and the initiation of alcohol or other drug use in the past year among youths aged 12 to 17. All findings presented in this report are based on 2005 NSDUH data.

Past-Year Major Depressive Episode

In 2005, 8.8% of youths aged 12 to 17 (2.2 million persons) experienced at least one MDE in the past year. Females were three times as likely as males to have a past-year MDE (13.3% vs. 4.5%). Rates of past-year MDE varied by age, with youths aged 17 having the highest rate of past-year MDE (11.9%) and those aged 12 having the lowest rate (4.3%). Rates of past-year MDE were relatively similar across racial/ethnic groups.

Initiation of Alcohol and Illicit Drug Use in the Past Year

The 2005 NSDUH indicates that 2.7 million youths aged 12 to 17 were past-year initiates of alcohol use, representing 15.4% of youths who were at risk for initiation of alcohol use. An estimated 1.5 million youths were past-year initiates of illicit drug use, which represents 7.6% of youths at risk for initiation of illicit drug use.

Major Depressive Episode and Substance Use Initiation in the Past Year

Past-year MDE was associated with substance use initiation in the past year. Among youths aged 12 to 17 who had not previously used alcohol, those who experienced a past-year MDE were twice as likely to have initiated alcohol use in the past year as those who had not experienced a past-year MDE (29.2% vs. 14.5%). Similarly, among youths who had not previously used an illicit drug, those who experienced a past-year MDE were over twice as likely to have initiated use of an illicit drug in the past year as those who had not experienced a past-year MDE (16.1% vs. 6.9%). This pattern was relatively consistent across drugs.

Section 31.3

Reducing Drug Abuse among Patients with Mental Illness Complications

Excerpted from "New Therapy Reduces Drug Abuse among Patients with Severe Mental Illness," National Institute on Drug Abuse (www.drugabuse.gov), June 1, 2008. Reviewed by David A. Cooke, MD, FACP, July 2013.

A new intervention enhances prospects for substance abusers whose mental illness complicates the path to recovery. In a recent clinical trial, a six-month course of Behavioral Treatment for Substance Abuse in Severe and Persistent Mental Illness (BTSAS) reduced drug abuse, boosted treatment-session attendance, and improved the quality of life of outpatients with a wide spectrum of mental disorders.

A Focus on Extra Obstacles

Dr. Alan S. Bellack and colleagues at the University of Maryland School of Medicine in Baltimore designed BTSAS to counter the factors that make recovery from addiction especially difficult for people who have co-occurring severe and persistent mental illness. These factors include frequent failure to meet their own and others' expectations, inconsistent motivation, and social and personal pressure to appear normal.

Treatment outcomes comparing BTSAS to STAR (Supportive Treatment for Addiction Recovery) are as follows:

- **Drug-free urine samples:** 59% vs. 25%

- **Four weeks of abstinence:** 54% vs. 16%

- **Multiple four-week blocks:** 44% vs. 10%

- **Eight weeks of abstinence:** 33% vs. 8%

BTSAS therapy comprises six integrated components:

- Motivational interviews (directive counseling that explores and resolves ambivalence) to increase the desire to stop using drugs

393

- Contingency contracts linking drug-free urine samples with small financial rewards

- Realistic, short-term, structured goal-setting sessions

- Training in social and drug-refusal skills

- Information on why and how people become addicted to drugs and the dangers of substance use for people with mental illness

- Relapse-prevention training that inculcates behavioral strategies for coping with cravings, lapses, and high-risk situations

Twice-weekly sessions begin with urine tests. Patients who have provided drug-free urine samples are praised by the therapists and group members. They also receive financial incentives that start at $1.50 for the first drug-free sample and increase in $0.50 increments for every consecutive one thereafter, up to $3.50. The amount is set back to $1.50 after a drug-positive sample or an absence.

When participants submit drug-positive samples, the group takes a nonaccusatory approach by focusing on problem solving to help them achieve future abstinence. Each participant agrees upon a personal goal for drug abuse reduction or abstinence that he or she believes is achievable during the coming week and signs a contract stating that he or she will strive for it. The rest of the session consists of drug abuse education plus training in social skills and relapse-prevention strategies.

Superior Results

Substance abuse is common among the mentally ill. For example, surveys estimate that 48% of those with schizophrenia, 56% with bipolar disorder, and as many as 65% with severe and persistent mental illness have abused substances.

Dr. Bellack's research team recruited 175 patients from community clinics and a Veterans Affairs medical center in Baltimore. All had a dual diagnosis of severe and persistent mental illness and an addiction to cocaine, heroin, or marijuana. Among the participants, 38.3% met the diagnostic criteria for schizophrenia or schizoaffective disorders, 54.9% for major affective disorders, and the remainder for other mental disorders. Cocaine was the predominant drug abused by 68.6% of participants, opiates by 24.6%, and marijuana by 6.8%.

The researchers assigned half the trial participants to BTSAS group therapy and half to the program STAR, which is the typical treatment at the University of Maryland clinics. Unlike participants in BTSAS, those in STAR do not follow a structured format but instead select their own topics and work at their own pace. Patient interaction with other patients is encouraged but not required as it is with BTSAS. Although urine samples are collected before each session, results are not discussed in the group, and no systematic feedback is provided to the patient.

Assignments to the BTSAS and STAR groups were balanced for gender, psychiatric diagnosis, type of drug dependency, and number of substance use disorders. Treatment groups of four to six participants met twice a week for six months. BTSAS and STAR group sessions were all led by trained therapists and lasted from 60 to 90 minutes. Group meetings were videotaped weekly and then reviewed and assessed by independent reviewers to verify that the therapists were following the programs' parameters correctly.

The BTSAS group fared better than the STAR group on a wide range of treatment-related criteria. For example, more people in the BTSAS group stayed in treatment throughout the six-month trial period (57.4% versus 34.7%). The BTSAS group produced more drug-free urine samples and had longer periods of abstinence. They also had better clinical and general living outcomes than people in the STAR group and reported larger improvements in their ability to perform the activities of daily living.

"It was apparent from watching videotapes of treatment sessions that subjects in BTSAS valued the intervention and were learning important skills for reducing drug use," says Dr. Bellack. "We were very gratified that the data supported our clinical observations."

The researchers reported that the extra costs of running the BTSAS program were modest. For the six-month trial, monetary rewards averaged roughly $60 per patient; total per-patient cost, including therapist time, was $372.

Ongoing Refinements

The trial data indicate that patients who remain in BTSAS for at least three sessions are much more likely to finish the six-month program than patients who do not make it through the third session. Because a third of individuals initially recruited for the study left before the third treatment session, the researchers are currently developing new intervention strategies to keep people in the program until they have truly given it a chance. The innovation has two key components: a structured intervention to help patients overcome obstacles to treatment and an intervention to enlist family and friends as partners to connect patients with treatment.

"The BTSAS program will help clinicians make a difference in the lives of a very difficult-to-treat population," says Dr. Dorynne Czechowicz of the National Institute on Drug Abuse (NIDA)'s Division of Clinical Neuroscience and Behavioral Research. "One of its key strengths is that it positively affects many aspects of patients' lives. Moreover, as an outpatient treatment, it is well-suited to the situation. Most mentally ill people who abuse drugs live in the community, not in a sheltered facility, and this is where the majority of clinicians must treat them."

Sources

Bellack, A.S., et al. A randomized clinical trial of a new behavioral treatment for drug abuse in people with severe and persistent mental illness. *Archives of General Psychiatry* 63(4):426–432, 2006.

Kinnaman, J.E., et al. Assessment of motivation to change substance use in dually-diagnosed schizophrenia patients. *Addictive Behaviors* 32(9):1798–1813, 2007.

Section 31.4

Substance Use Disorder and Serious Psychological Distress (SPD)

"Substance Use Disorder and Serious Psychological Distress, by Employment Status," Substance Abuse and Mental Health Services Administration (www.samhsa.gov), July 11, 2008. Reviewed by David A. Cooke, MD, FACP, July 2013.

Substance use disorders and psychological distress have been shown to have a negative impact on many aspects of the lives of affected persons, including their ability to hold jobs and be productive in the workplace. The National Survey on Drug Use and Health includes questions about respondents' employment status, substance use, and mental health problems. NSDUH defines full-time employment as usually working 35 or more hours per week and working in the past week or having a job despite not working in the past week. Part-time employment includes those who usually work fewer than 35 hours per week and who were working in the past week or have a job despite not working in the past week. The unemployed category includes those who reported that they did not have a job, were on layoff, and were looking for work and made specific efforts to find work in the past 30 days. Other employment categories include student, full-time homemaker, retired, disabled, or other miscellaneous work statuses.

NSDUH asks persons aged 12 or older to report on their use of alcohol and illicit drugs, as well as symptoms of substance dependence or abuse during the past year. Substance dependence or abuse includes such symptoms as withdrawal, tolerance, use in dangerous situations, trouble with the law, and interference in major obligations at work, school, or home during the past year. NSDUH respondents also are asked whether they have received treatment for a substance use problem. For these analyses, an individual is defined as receiving treatment only if he or she reported specialty treatment for alcohol or illicit drugs in the past year.

NSDUH includes questions to assess serious psychological distress (SPD). SPD is an overall indicator of past-year nonspecific psychological distress that is constructed from the K6 scale administered

397

to adults aged 18 or older in NSDUH. The K6 scale consists of six questions that gather information on how frequently a respondent experienced symptoms of psychological distress during the one month in the past year when he or she was at his or her worst emotionally. NSDUH respondents also are asked about their experiences with mental health treatment, which is defined as the receipt of treatment or counseling for any problem with emotions, nerves, or mental health in the 12 months prior to the interview in any inpatient or outpatient setting, or the use of prescription medication for treatment of a mental or emotional condition. For the purpose of this report, individuals with both SPD and a substance use disorder are said to have co-occurring SPD and a substance use disorder.

This section examines the prevalence of past-year substance use disorder, SPD, and co-occurring SPD and a substance use disorder among the U.S. working-age civilian population (i.e., those aged 18 to 64). It is noteworthy that 62.7% of adults in this age group who had a past-year substance use disorder were employed full time. Among adults aged 18 to 64 who experienced SPD in the past year, 50.7% were employed full time. Because of the negative effects of substance use disorders and SPD on the workplace (i.e., decreased productivity, increased accidents, absenteeism, job turnover, and medical costs), rates of past-year substance use disorder, SPD, and co-occurring SPD and a substance use disorder among full-time employed persons are highlighted.

Substance Use Disorder, SPD, and Co-Occurring SPD and a Substance Use Disorder, by Employment Status

Among adults aged 18 to 64 overall, 10.8% (20 million persons) were classified as having a past-year substance use disorder, 12.9% (23 million persons) experienced past year SPD, and 3% (5 million persons) had co-occurring SPD and a substance use disorder.

Adults aged 18 to 64 who were unemployed and those who were nonworking students had the highest rates of past-year substance use disorder (18.9% and 17.5%, respectively), while retired adults and full-time homemakers had the lowest rates (3.6% and 4.5%, respectively). Rates of past-year SPD were highest among disabled persons (34.3%), unemployed persons (21%), and nonworking students (18.5%). These same three groups (unemployed adults [7.3%], disabled adults [5.5%], and nonworking adult students [5.1%]) also had the highest rates of co-occurring SPD and a substance use disorder. Retired persons had the lowest rate of SPD (6.7%) and co-occurring SPD and a substance use disorder (0.6%).

Substance Use Disorder, SPD, and Co-Occurring SPD and a Substance Use Disorder among Adults Employed Full Time

In 2004–2005, 10.6% of adults aged 18 to 64 who were employed full time were classified as having a past-year substance use disorder, 10.2% experienced past-year SPD, and 2.4% had co-occurring SPD and a substance use disorder. Among full-time employed adults, males were nearly twice as likely to have a substance use disorder than their female counterparts (13.2% vs. 6.9%), but females were nearly twice as likely to have SPD (14.2% vs. 7.3%). Rates of co-occurring SPD and a substance use disorder were relatively similar across genders (2.3% and 2.6% among males and females, respectively). Full-time employed persons aged 18 to 25 had the highest rates of substance use disorder, SPD, and co-occurring SPD and a substance use disorder when compared with full-time employed adults in other age categories.

Treatment of Substance Use Disorder, SPD, and Co-Occurring SPD and a Substance Use Disorder among Full-Time Employed Adults

Among adults aged 18 to 64 who were employed full time and who had a past-year substance use disorder, less than 5% (4.2%) received substance use treatment at a specialty facility in the past year. Among adults aged 18 to 64 who were employed full time and who had SPD, 38.5% received treatment for their mental health problem. Adults with co-occurring SPD and a substance use disorder may seek treatment for just their substance use disorder, just their SPD, both problems, or neither problem. Of the 2.9 million adults aged 18 to 64 employed full time who had co-occurring problems, nearly 60% were not treated for either problem, and less than 5% were treated for both problems.

Chapter 32

Substance Abuse and Suicide Prevention

Suicide has been spotlighted as a national public health issue, and as such, its two most significant risk factors, mental and substance abuse disorders, must also be seen in that same light. While 95% of individuals with a mental illness and/or substance use disorder will never complete suicide, several decades of evidence consistently suggests that as many as 90% of individuals who do complete suicide experience a mental or substance use disorder, or both. The vast majority experience a mood disorder, such as depression; as many as 25% experience alcohol abuse disorders. Many experience co-occurring mental and substance use disorders.

Unfortunately, despite ongoing efforts to educate the public, the same social stigma that surrounds suicide also continues to stand between many people with mental and substance use disorders and the care they need—care that could help thwart potential suicide. According to Substance Abuse and Mental Health Services Administration (SAMHSA)'s 2006 National Survey on Drug Use and Health (NSDUH), of the 23.6 million people aged 12 or older in need of treatment for an illicit drug use or alcohol use problem, only 2.5 million received treatment at a specialty facility. In the same year, among the 24.9 million adults aged 18 or older reporting serious psychological distress (having a level of symptoms known to be indicative of a mental disorder), fewer than half, 10.9 million (44%), received treatment for a mental health problem.

Excerpted from "Substance Abuse and Suicide Prevention: Evidence & Implications," Substance Abuse and Mental Health Services Administration (www.samhsa.gov), 2008. Reviewed by David A. Cooke, MD, FACP, July 2013.

The significant gap between needing and getting care for mental disorders and substance use problems—and the role both play in suicide—underscores the public health imperative of preventing behavioral health problems in the first place where possible, and otherwise identifying and treating them early in their course. Independent of each other, mental illnesses, substance abuse, and suicide each have a profound impact on individuals and families, schools and workplaces, communities and society at large. The human and economic costs of these public health problems are significant. When each of these three problems is examined separately, it becomes clear that, in many instances and for many individuals, each one is related in some way to the other two. Thus, the co-occurrence of mental and substance abuse disorders today is the expectation rather than the exception.

Substance Use Disorders and Suicide: The Big Picture

A growing body of studies has demonstrated that alcohol and drug abuse are second only to depression and other mood disorders as the most frequent risk factors for suicide. Molnar, Berkman, and Buka's assessment (in *Psychological Medicine*, 31, no. 6, 2001) of data from the National Comorbidity Survey disclosed that alcohol and drug abuse disorders are associated with a risk 6.2 times greater than average risk of suicide attempts.

According to SAMHSA's Drug Abuse Warning Network report on drug-related emergency department (ED) visits, in 2005, over 132,500 visits to emergency rooms were for alcohol- or drug-related suicide attempts. Substantial percentages of suicide victims tested positive for alcohol or other drugs. The most frequently identified substance was alcohol, found in one-third of those tested; four other substances were identified in approximately 10% of tested victims. Illicit drugs were involved in approximately one-fifth (19%) of the ED visits for drug-related suicide attempts. Over 85% of individuals associated with these attempts were seriously ill enough to merit admission to a hospital or another health care facility.

The Drug Abuse Warning Network also has examined emergency department visits for drug-related suicide attempts by youth. In 2004, the most recent year for which data are available, reporting emergency departments handled over 15,000 drug-related suicide attempts by youth, ages 12–17, almost 75% of which were serious enough to warrant hospitalization. Around half of all of these suicide attempts involved the use of pain medications.

These data do not suggest that all of the individuals who attempted suicide, whether young or adult, were experiencing substance abuse disorders; rather the data inform only that alcohol or drugs of abuse were used in what was characterized as a suicide attempt. Nonetheless, the sheer numbers are compelling.

Field-based studies have been ongoing to understand the relationships between substances of abuse and suicide. Significant studies have been based on psychological autopsies; only in the last few years have increasing numbers of prospective studies been conducted. Research is complicated and sometimes confounded by the complex interrelationships among mental and substance use disorders, combined with other biological, behavioral, environmental, and social factors influencing suicide risk.

Alcohol

In 1938, Karl Menninger observed that alcohol dependence is a type of chronic suicide (in Hufford, "Alcohol and Suicidal Behavior," *Clinical Psychology Review*, 21, no. 5, 2001). His observation has been found to be accurate over the decades during which the relationship between suicide and alcohol consumption, alcohol use, and alcohol dependence has been studied. As many as one-fourth of individuals who die by suicide are intoxicated with alcohol.

Today, the literature bearing on the role alcohol plays in suicide risk is considerably more robust than that associated with drug abuse and suicide. The association between suicidal behavior and alcohol abuse has been long documented, dating back to the 1980s. An extensive body of literature—primarily retrospective studies—has established that active alcohol use or abuse is a powerful risk factor for suicide. One of the more significant reasons posited for this association is the disinhibition resulting from alcohol use that occurs shortly prior to a suicide attempt. Hufford's aforementioned literature review suggests alcohol intoxication appears to play a more significant role as a proximal, rather than distal, risk factor for suicide.

However, some caution needs to be exercised regarding the body of published studies bearing on alcohol and suicide. Cherpirtel, Borges, and Wilcox ("Acute Alcohol Use and Suicidal Behavior: A Review of the Literature," *Alcoholism: Clinical and Experimental Research*, 28, no. 5, 2004) note in their literature review that the majority of studies, whether cross-sectional or case-controlled, are subject to several sources of bias due to their focus on completed suicide and the tendency to report prevalence estimates. She and her colleagues suggest the effectiveness of adopting a case-crossover design to overcome the biases and limitations of existing studies. One such case-crossover study suggests that the role of acute alcohol in suicidal behavior may include promoting depression and hopelessness, impairing problem solving, and facilitating aggression.

Drugs

The study of the relationship between drug abuse and suicide risk is substantially less well-developed than that of either mental illnesses or alcohol and suicide. As researchers have pointed out in their articles beginning in the mid-1990s to this date, relatively little is known about the impact of different drugs, drug combinations, substance-induced effects, and self-medication on suicidal behavior. What is known is that there is some association between current drug use and suicidal ideation that is not entirely due to the effects of co-occurring mental disorders. The number of substances used appears to be more predictive of suicidal behavior than the types of substances used. Moreover, based on a few initial studies, it also appears that drug abuse treatment itself may have the capacity to help reduce the risk for future suicidality. However, in the main, causal relationships between drugs of abuse—both in the aggregate and in specific instances—have not been well established.

Co-Occurring Disorders

A substantial body of knowledge suggests that substance use—both drugs and alcohol—is associated with mental disorders. Moreover, some suggest that this linkage may be bidirectional. For example, depression may be associated with increased substance use and chronic substance abuse may be a factor in the development of depression or other mood disorders. In fact, it has been suggested that co-occurring disorders should be considered the expectation rather than the exception by clinicians, and should be treated concurrently to be most effective.

Further, both mental and substance use disorders are known risk factors for suicide. Secondary analysis of combined 2004 and 2005 data from SAMHSA's NSDUH sheds light not only on the magnitude of co-occurring mental and substance use disorders, but also on the considerable impact they have when they occur together. According to the NSDUH analysis, an estimated 16.4 million adults, age 18 and older, experienced a major depressive episode in the past year. During their worst or most recent experience of major depression, over half thought they would be better off dead; over 10% attempted suicide. When alcohol abuse or the use of illicit drugs was added to a major depressive episode, the proportion of suicide attempts rose to nearly 14% for alcohol abuse and nearly 20% for illicit drug use.

A growing number of case-control and longitudinal studies have sought to examine whether substance and mental disorders, when co-occurring, exacerbate suicide risk. One study points out that co-occurrence of mood disorders, in particular in concert with substance abuse, greatly increases the likelihood of attempted suicide. Indeed, further research perhaps is warranted to determine if co-occurrence is a necessary condition for suicide to occur, despite previous findings that, independent of depressed mood, alcohol and drug dependency were associated with high levels of suicidal ideation among 891 hospitalized patients with major depressive disorder.

Roy's study ("Characteristics of Drug Addicts Who Attempt Suicide," *Psychiatry Research*, 121, 2003) of suicidality among 449 drug-dependent patients found that the 175 who had attempted suicide had greater lifetime comorbidity with major depression than the patients who did not attempt suicide. The results, similar to two other studies of drug-dependent patients conducted by the same researcher, highlight the complicating role distal factors, such as childhood abuse and family history of suicide, play in concert with drug abuse and depression in suicidality.

Further, Goldston's review ("Conceptual Issues in Understanding the Relationship between Suicidal Behavior and Substance Use during Adolescence," *Drug and Alcohol Dependence*, 76, no. 1, 2004) of conceptual issues associated with the relationships between suicide and substance abuse has clarified that what is not known about these relationships is far greater than what is known with certainty. He posits, for example, that both suicide and substance use share a number of risk factors—including depression, impulsivity, and thrill-seeking/life-threatening behaviors. As such, they ultimately may be related to underlying primary mental health problems. Data from the NSDUH point out the significantly higher rates of illicit drug, cigarette and alcohol use among those who experience a major depressive episode in the last year compared to those who did not. Both sets of findings suggest the potential use of substances, whether drugs, cigarettes, or alcohol, as a means of "self-medicating" a mood disorder. Conner and colleagues (in *Journal of Psychoactive Drugs*, 32, no. 3, 2000) have noted that suicide risk remains among people in remission from alcohol use; older adults frequently experience ongoing depression and younger individuals more subtle forms of mood disorders, such as dysthymia, problems that may have given rise to the substance abuse in the first place.

These findings speak to the need for clinicians to be vigilant about both substance abuse history and history of mental health problems among patients being seen for either or both illness. They speak to the ongoing need to consider and treat both substance abuse and mental illnesses concurrently in persons with co-occurring disorders to help reduce the risk for suicide when one of the co-occurring disorders is left untreated. All too often this is a fact of life for people of all ages with both substance use and mental disorders.

Part Five

Drug Abuse Treatment and Recovery

Chapter 33

Recognizing Drug Use

Chapter Contents

Section 33.1

Signs of Drug Use

Excerpted from "Family and Friends Can Make a Difference," 2012, and "How Young Adults Can Help Themselves or Loved Ones Heal from Addiction," 2009, Substance Abuse and Mental Health Services Administration, Recovery Month (www.recoverymonth.gov).

Family and Friends Can Make a Difference

Recognize Substance Use Disorders

Like mental health conditions, substance use disorders affect families of every race, ethnicity, socioeconomic status, and location.

Learn the signs of substance use and misuse to help recognize the problem, so you can encourage your loved one to seek treatment and recovery support services. The following are signs that a friend or family member may be abusing drugs:

- **Physical signs:** Bloodshot eyes or pupils larger or smaller than usual; changes in appetite or sleep patterns; sudden weight loss or weight gain; deterioration of physical appearance or personal grooming habits; unusual smells on the breath, body, or clothing; and tremors, slurred speech, or impaired coordination

- **Behavioral signs:** Drop in attendance and performance at work or school; unexplained need for money or financial problems; engaging in secretive or suspicious behaviors; sudden change in friends, favorite hangouts, and hobbies; and frequently getting into trouble (fights, accidents, illegal activities)

- **Psychological signs:** Unexplained change in personality or attitude; sudden mood swings, irritability or angry outbursts; periods of unusual hyperactivity, agitation, or giddiness; lack of motivation; appearing lethargic; and appearing fearful, anxious, or paranoid, with no reason

In adolescents, specific signs of substance use include the following:

- Bloodshot eyes or dilated pupils, and use of eye drops to try to mask these signs

- Absenteeism from class and poor classroom performance
- Trouble/misconduct at school
- Missing money, valuables, or prescriptions from the home
- Uncharacteristic behaviors, including isolation, withdrawal, anger, or depression
- Secrecy about a new peer group
- Lost interest in old hobbies
- Dishonesty about new interests and activities
- Demands for more privacy and sneaking around

Myths and Facts: Substance Use Disorders

In 2010, 4.1 million people aged 12 or older (1.6% of the population) received treatment for a problem related to the use of alcohol or illicit drugs. Learn the facts and dispel the myths about substance use disorders so you can encourage your family or friend to acknowledge a problem and seek help:

Myth: Overcoming substance misuse is simply a matter of willpower. You can stop using drugs and alcohol if you really want to.

Fact: Prolonged exposure to drugs alters the brain in ways that result in powerful cravings and a compulsion to use the substance again and again. These brain changes make it extremely difficult to quit by sheer force of will.

Myth: Substance dependence isn't a disease; there's nothing you can do about it.

Fact: Substance dependence is a brain disease. The brain changes associated with dependence can be treated and reversed through therapy, medication, exercise, and other treatments.

Myth: Someone with a substance use disorder has to hit rock bottom before he or she can get better.

Fact: Recovery can begin at any point in the process—and the earlier, the better.

Myth: You can't force someone into treatment; a person has to want help.

Fact: Treatment doesn't have to be voluntary to be successful. People who are urged into treatment by their family, friends, employer, or the legal system are just as likely to benefit as those who choose to enter treatment on their own. As they become engaged in treatment and their thinking clears, many formerly resistant individuals decide they want to change.

Myth: Treatment didn't work before, so there's no point trying again.

Fact: Recovery from substance misuse and dependence is a long process that often involves setbacks. Relapse doesn't mean that treatment has failed or the cause is lost. Rather, it's a signal to get back on track, either by going back to treatment or adjusting the approach.

How Young Adults Can Help Themselves or Loved Ones Heal from Addiction

Prescription Drug Misuse

Prescription drug misuse has been on the rise over the past few decades. The 2006 National Drug Control Strategy issued by the White House Office of National Drug Control Policy identified the illegal use of pharmaceuticals as one of the fastest-growing forms of drug abuse and outlined a program to reduce the availability of such drugs for nonmedical use and get users into treatment. In addition, the director of the National Institute on Drug Abuse has called for further research to develop safe and effective pain management strategies and medications with less potential for abuse.

In 2007, 6% of young adults aged 18 to 25 were current nonmedical users of prescription drugs, greater than the percentage using any illicit drug except marijuana. In the past 12 months, among all those aged 12 or older, the number of people initiating the nonmedical use of prescription drugs was—at 2.5 million—higher than the number initiating marijuana use, which was 2.1 million.

Your friends and loved ones may access these medications through a variety of channels, including you—whether you are aware of it or not. In both 2006 and 2007, more than half of people aged 12 or older who used prescription-type pain relievers, tranquilizers, stimulants, and sedatives nonmedically said they got the drugs from a friend or relative for free.

Because prescription drugs are legal, it is easy to think you are helping friends if they have pain or an ailment. However, there are risks associated with taking prescription drugs that are not prescribed for you. Mixing them with alcohol, other prescription drugs, or illegal drugs can be particularly dangerous.

To be safe, store your medicines out of sight and away from predictable places, such as the bathroom, and know that sharing your prescription drugs with someone else is illegal and dangerous.

Also be aware of your friends' internet use, because now people can turn to online sources to fuel a prescription drug problem. In 2008, the National Center on Addiction and Substance Abuse at Columbia University (CASA) identified 365 websites that either advertised or offered controlled prescription drugs for sale online. Of those:

- Only two were registered internet pharmacy practice sites.

- 85% offered drugs for sale that required no prescription from a physician.

- Half of sites that did require a prescription asked that the prescription be faxed, increasing the chance of fraud and multiple use of the same prescription.

If you notice a friend or loved one carrying around multiple bottles of pills, or witness any kind of substance use problem, consider having a conversation with the person.

Section 33.2

Am I Drug Addicted?

"Am I an Addict?" Copyright © 1983, 1988 by Narcotics Anonymous World Services, Inc. All rights reserved. Reprinted with permission. For additional information, visit www.na.org. Despite its older publication date, the material in this section is considered accurate and relevant.

"Am I an addict?" *Only you can answer this question.*
This may not be an easy thing to do. All through our usage, we told ourselves, "I can handle it." Even if this was true in the beginning, it is not so now. The drugs handled us. We lived to use and used to live. Very simply, an addict is a person whose life is controlled by drugs.
Perhaps you admit you have a problem with drugs, but you don't consider yourself an addict. All of us have preconceived ideas about what an addict is. There is nothing shameful about being an addict once you begin to take positive action. If you can identify with our problems, you may be able to identify with our solution. The following questions were written by recovering addicts in Narcotics Anonymous.

If you have doubts about whether or not you're an addict, take a few moments to read the questions below and answer them as honestly as you can.

1. Do you ever use alone? Yes ❑ No ❑

2. Have you ever substituted one drug for another, thinking that one particular drug was the problem? Yes ❑   No ❑

3. Have you ever manipulated or lied to a doctor to obtain prescription drugs? Yes ❑   No ❑

4. Have you ever stolen drugs or stolen to obtain drugs? Yes ❑   No ❑

5. Do you regularly use a drug when you wake up or when you go to bed? Yes ❑   No ❑

6. Have you ever taken one drug to overcome the effects of another? Yes ❑   No ❑

7. Do you avoid people or places that do not approve of you using drugs? Yes ❑   No ❑

8. Have you ever used a drug without knowing what it was or what it would do to you? Yes ❑   No ❑

9. Has your job or school performance ever suffered from the effects of your drug use? Yes ❑   No ❑

10. Have you ever been arrested as a result of using drugs? Yes ❑   No ❑

11. Have you ever lied about what or how much you use? Yes ❑   No ❑

12. Do you put the purchase of drugs ahead of your financial responsibilities? Yes ❑   No ❑

13. Have you ever tried to stop or control your using? Yes ❑   No ❑

14. Have you ever been in a jail, hospital, or drug rehabilitation center because of your using? Yes ❑   No ❑

15. Does using interfere with your sleeping or eating? Yes ❑   No ❑

16. Does the thought of running out of drugs terrify you? Yes ❑   No ❑

17. Do you feel it is impossible for you to live without drugs? Yes ❑   No ❑

18. Do you ever question your own sanity? Yes ❏   No ❏

19. Is your drug use making life at home unhappy? Yes ❏   No ❏

20. Have you ever thought you couldn't fit in or have a good time without drugs? Yes ❏   No ❏

21. Have you ever felt defensive, guilty, or ashamed about your using? Yes ❏   No ❏

22. Do you think a lot about drugs? Yes ❏   No ❏

23. Have you had irrational or indefinable fears? Yes ❏   No ❏

24. Has using affected your sexual relationships? Yes ❏   No ❏

25. Have you ever taken drugs you didn't prefer? Yes ❏   No ❏

26. Have you ever used drugs because of emotional pain or stress? Yes ❏   No ❏

27. Have you ever overdosed on any drugs? Yes ❏   No ❏

28. Do you continue to use despite negative consequences? Yes ❏   No ❏

29. Do you think you might have a drug problem? Yes ❏   No ❏

"Am I an addict?" This is a question only you can answer. We found that we all answered different numbers of these questions "Yes." The actual number of "Yes" responses wasn't as important as how we felt inside and how addiction had affected our lives.

Some of these questions don't even mention drugs. This is because addiction is an insidious disease that affects all areas of our lives— even those areas which seem at first to have little to do with drugs. The different drugs we used were not as important as why we used them and what they did to us.

When we first read these questions, it was frightening for us to think we might be addicts. Some of us tried to dismiss these thoughts by saying:

"Oh, those questions don't make sense;"

Or,

"I'm different. I know I take drugs, but I'm not an addict. I have real emotional/family/job problems;"

Or,

"I'm just having a tough time getting it together right now;"

415

Or,

"I'll be able to stop when I find the right person/get the right job, etc."

If you are an addict, you must first admit that you have a problem with drugs before any progress can be made toward recovery. These questions, when honestly approached, may help to show you how using drugs has made your life unmanageable. Addiction is a disease which, without recovery, ends in jails, institutions, and death. Many of us came to Narcotics Anonymous because drugs had stopped doing what we needed them to do. Addiction takes our pride, self-esteem, family, loved ones, and even our desire to live. If you have not reached this point in your addiction, you don't have to. We have found that our own private hell was within us. If you want help, you can find it in the Fellowship of Narcotics Anonymous. "We were searching for an answer when we reached out and found Narcotics Anonymous. We came to our first NA meeting in defeat and didn't know what to expect. After sitting in a meeting, or several meetings, we began to feel that people cared and were willing to help. Although our minds told us that we would never make it, the people in the fellowship gave us hope by insisting that we could recover. [...] Surrounded by fellow addicts, we realized that we were not alone anymore. Recovery is what happens in our meetings. Our lives are at stake. We found that by putting recovery first, the program works. We faced three disturbing realizations:

1. We are powerless over addiction and our lives are unmanageable;

2. Although we are not responsible for our disease, we are responsible for our recovery;

3. We can no longer blame people, places, and things for our addiction. We must face our problems and our feelings.

The ultimate weapon for recovery is the recovering addict."[1]

1. *Basic Text*, Narcotics Anonymous

Section 33.3

How to Identify Drug Paraphernalia

Excerpted from "What Is Drug Paraphernalia?" and "What Kinds of Things Are Paraphernalia?" Get Smart About Drugs, U.S. Drug Enforcement Administration (www.getsmartaboutdrugs.com), 2009. Despite its older publication date, the material in this section is considered accurate and relevant.

What is drug paraphernalia?

The term "drug paraphernalia" refers to any legitimate equipment, product, or material that is modified for making, using, or concealing illegal narcotics. Many kinds of items can be identified as drug paraphernalia, including ordinary household products, or things disguised to resemble ordinary items that can be extremely challenging to identify. Under federal law, the term "drug paraphernalia" means "any equipment, product or material of any kind which is primarily intended or designed for use in manufacturing, compounding, converting, concealing, producing, processing, preparing, injecting, ingesting, inhaling or otherwise introducing into the human body a controlled substance."

What kinds of things are paraphernalia?

Drug paraphernalia typically used to smoke marijuana, crack, cocaine, and methamphetamine like pipes and bongs are easily identifiable drug paraphernalia. Syringes are also widely known to be used to inject a wide variety of drugs such as heroin, methamphetamine, ketamine, and steroids. These forms of drug paraphernalia are often marketed specifically to youth—with colorful logos, celebrity pictures, and designs like smiley faces on the products, the items are meant to look harmless and minimize the dangers of taking controlled substances.

Drug paraphernalia, like magic markers, can conceal pipes, and small, hand-painted blown glass items look more like pretty trinkets than pipes or stash containers. Parents need to be aware that these kinds of products often conceal drug use. Identifying drug paraphernalia can be extremely challenging because they are ordinary items, or things that are disguised to resemble ordinary items.

For example, a soda can, lipstick dispenser, felt-tip marker, or a pager—all normal things that you may find in your child's room—could be used as paraphernalia to hide or use drugs. The soda can could have a false bottom to hide drugs; the lipstick dispenser could hide a drug pipe; the felt-tip marker might be an internal drug pipe; and the pager could be hollowed out to conceal drugs.

Other items that can be used to conceal drugs include the following:

- Plastic baggies

- Small paper bags

- Makeup kits

- Change bottles

- Plastic film canisters

- Cigarette packs

- Small glass vials

- Pill bottles

- Breath mint containers

- Candy or gum wrappers

Are certain paraphernalia associated with using specific drugs?

Ecstasy paraphernalia includes the following:

- Pacifiers and lollipops are often used to help ecstasy users guard against the teeth grinding that comes from involuntary jaw clenching.

- Candy necklaces are sometimes used to hide ecstasy pills (bags of small candies also are good for this purpose).

- Glow sticks, mentholated rub, and surgical masks are often used by kids on ecstasy to overstimulate their senses.

- Water bottles are used to bring alcohol to parties or to transport liquid drugs, such as GHB (gamma hydroxybutyrate).

Cocaine paraphernalia includes the following:

- Pipes to smoke crack

- Small mirrors and short plastic straws or rolled-up paper tubes

- Razor blades
- Small spoons (coke spoons)
- Lighters

Marijuana paraphernalia includes the following:

- Rolling papers
- Cigars to make a "blunt"
- Small plastic baggies and "stash cans"
- Deodorizers, incense, room deodorizers used to disguise the smell of marijuana
- Pipes (metal, wooden, acrylic, glass, stone, plastic, or ceramic)
- Bongs
- Roach clips

Inhalant paraphernalia includes the following:

- Rags used for sniffing
- Empty spray cans
- Tubes of glue
- Plastic bags
- Balloons
- Nozzles
- Bottles or cans with hardened glue, sprays, paint, or chemical odors inside of them

Be on the lookout for common products that are out of place in your home, including items used to cover up drug use:

- Mouth washes, breath sprays, and mints are used to cover alcohol or drug odors.
- Eye drops are used to conceal bloodshot eyes and can occasionally be used to deliver acid or other drugs.
- Sunglasses worn at seemingly inappropriate times may cover up "red eyes" from smoking drugs or changes in pupil size or eye movements related to drug use.

- Paraphernalia, clothing, jewelry, temporary or permanent tattoos, teen jargon, publications, and other displays may reflect messages associated with the "drug culture" and may be designed to openly flaunt drug culture involvement or identify drug culture involvement to "insiders."

Chapter 34

First Aid for
Drug Abuse Emergencies

Drug abuse is the misuse or overuse of any medication or drug, including alcohol. This chapter discusses first aid for drug overdose and withdrawal.

Considerations

Many street drugs have no therapeutic benefits. Any use of these drugs is a form of drug abuse.

Legitimate medications can be abused by people who take more than the recommended dose or who intentionally take them with alcohol or other drugs.

Drug interactions may also produce adverse effects. Therefore, it is important to let your doctor know about all the drugs you are taking, including vitamins and other over-the-counter medications.

Many drugs are addictive. Sometimes the addiction is gradual. However, some drugs (such as cocaine) can cause addiction after only a few doses.

Someone who has become addicted to a drug usually will have withdrawal symptoms when the drug is suddenly stopped. Withdrawal is greatly assisted by professional help.

A drug dose that is large enough to be toxic is called an overdose. This may occur suddenly, when a large amount of the drug is taken at

---

one time, or gradually, as a drug builds up in the body over a longer period of time. Prompt medical attention may save the life of someone who accidentally or deliberately takes an overdose.

Causes

An overdose of narcotics can cause sleepiness, slowed breathing, and even unconsciousness.

Uppers (stimulants) produce excitement, increased heart rate, and rapid breathing. Downers (depressants) do just the opposite.

Mind-altering drugs are called hallucinogens. They include LSD [lysergic acid diethylamide], PCP (angel dust [phencyclidine]), and other street drugs. Using such drugs may cause paranoia, hallucinations, aggressive behavior, or extreme social withdrawal.

Cannabis-containing drugs such as marijuana may cause relaxation, impaired motor skills, and increased appetite.

Legal prescription drugs are sometimes taken in higher than recommended amounts to achieve a feeling other than the therapeutic effects for which they were intended. This may lead to serious side effects.

The use of any of the aforementioned drugs may result in impaired judgment and decision-making skills.

Symptoms

Drug overdose symptoms vary widely depending on the specific drug used, but may include:

- abnormal pupil size;
- agitation;
- convulsions;
- death;
- delusional or paranoid behavior;
- difficulty breathing;
- drowsiness;
- hallucinations;
- nausea and vomiting;
- nonreactive pupils (pupils that do not change size when exposed to light);
- staggering or unsteady gait (ataxia);

- sweating or extremely dry, hot skin;
- tremors;
- unconsciousness (coma);
- violent or aggressive behavior.

Drug withdrawal symptoms also vary widely depending on the specific drug used, but may include:

- abdominal cramping;
- agitation;
- cold sweat;
- convulsions;
- delusions;
- depression;
- diarrhea;
- hallucinations;
- nausea and vomiting;
- restlessness;
- shaking;
- death.

First Aid

1. Check the patient's airway, breathing, and pulse. If necessary, begin CPR. If the patient is unconscious but breathing, carefully place him or her in the recovery position. If the patient is conscious, loosen the clothing, keep the person warm, and provide reassurance. Try to keep the patient calm. If an overdose is suspected, try to prevent the patient from taking more drugs. Call for immediate medical assistance.

2. Treat the patient for signs of shock, if necessary. Signs include: weakness, bluish lips and fingernails, clammy skin, paleness, and decreasing alertness.

3. If the patient is having seizures, give convulsion first aid.

4. Keep monitoring the patient's vital signs (pulse, rate of breathing, blood pressure) until emergency medical help arrives.

5. If possible, try to determine which drug(s) were taken and when. Save any available pill bottles or other drug containers. Provide this information to emergency medical personnel.

Do Not

Do NOT jeopardize your own safety. Some drugs can cause violent and unpredictable behavior. Call for professional assistance.

Do NOT try to reason with someone who is on drugs. Do not expect them to behave reasonably.

Do NOT offer your opinions when giving help. You do not need to know why drugs were taken in order to give effective first aid.

Call Immediately for Emergency Medical Assistance

Drug emergencies are not always easy to identify. If you suspect someone has overdosed, or if you suspect someone is experiencing withdrawal, give first aid and seek medical assistance.

Try to find out what drug the person has taken. If possible, collect all drug containers and any remaining drug samples or the person's vomit and take them to the hospital.

The National Poison Control Center (800-222-1222) can be called from anywhere in the United States. They will give you further instructions.

This is a free and confidential service. All local poison control centers in the United States use this national number. You should call if you have any questions about poisoning or poison prevention. It does NOT need to be an emergency. You can call for any reason, 24 hours a day, 7 days a week.

Chapter 35

Drug Abuse Intervention

If you are a parent who suspects your child or teen is using drugs or alcohol, it's important to take action right away. Casual drug use can quickly turn into a long-term problem. There are ways you and other family members can intervene:

- Set tighter limits with clear consequences.

- Get outside help and support if necessary.

- Have productive conversations by remaining calm, sharing your concerns, and listening.

- Monitor behavior and activities.

When offering support to someone with a substance use disorder, refer to the following tips to guide the conversation with your family member or friend.

- Express your concern and provide examples of ways in which the person's substance use has caused problems—be sure to include the most recent incident.

- Don't cover up or make excuses for substance use-related accidents or occurrences.

Excerpted from "Family and Friends Can Make a Difference," Substance Abuse and Mental Health Services Administration, Recovery Month (www .recoverymonth.gov), 2012.

- Intervene as soon as possible after a substance use–related argument, incident, or accident, when the individual is no longer under the influence.

- Gather information on treatment options and offer to accompany the person to the first appointment or meeting.

- Recruit other friends, family members, or people in recovery to deliver the message that help is available and treatment is effective.

Most importantly, remind these individuals that recovery is possible and that millions of people just like them were able to regain their lives and live healthy, rewarding lives in recovery.

Mental and/or Substance Use Disorders Affect the Whole Family

Individuals with mental and/or substance use disorders aren't the only ones whose lives are impacted by these conditions. These disorders affect family members and friends emotionally, physically, spiritually, and economically.

If someone in your life is suffering from a mental illness, you may wonder what caused your loved one to become ill or worry what others think. These are normal feelings, and it is important to remember that there is hope. The following tips will help you cope with changes in your life:

Set limits, roles, and boundaries: It may be tempting to help your loved one in what are actually counterproductive ways. For instance, calling in sick for someone or bailing someone out of jail can make things worse by delaying the person from getting help. Setting personal limits instead can encourage people with behavioral health conditions to take action themselves, empowering them on their road to recovery.

Develop a coping strategy: Change is difficult, both for you and your loved one. As you develop new ways of dealing with your loved one's behavioral health condition, that person may respond to you with anger, hostility, or unusual behavior. Preparing in advance how you will deal with these behaviors and being consistent in your response will help the affected person see that you are serious about helping him or her. Consistency is essential.

Accept your feelings: You may find yourself denying warning signs, worrying that your family will be exposed to prejudices, or unable to understand how a loved one's behavioral health condition developed. These feelings are normal and common among families going through similar situations. Find out all you can about mental and/or substance use disorders by researching them and talking with health professionals. Seek your own support network and share what you have learned with others.

Support recovery: There are many ways to support recovery. Clearly let the affected individual know that you are there for him or her throughout the recovery process. Offer praise about positive change, attend support group meetings, and participate in family therapy. Ask the person about his or her progress and celebrate even small successes.

Simplify your approach by setting small goals: People with mental and/or substance use disorders must set small goals, such as "one day at a time." The same is true for families and friends who care about them. It is easy to become overwhelmed, so it is important to step back and set one small goal for yourself at a time.

Sustain your own physical, mental, and spiritual health: All three of these can decline for the person who suffers from substance use or a mental health condition, and the same often happens to those around them. Eating properly, getting exercise, taking breaks, and addressing spiritual needs are very important for family members. Taking time to focus on yourself is essential and will ultimately help you keep things in perspective and improve your patience and compassion for helping your loved one.

When family members and friends are involved and supportive of a person seeking treatment for substance misuse, the likelihood of success is improved. You can work toward making things better for yourself and also increase the chances of your loved one reaching and maintaining recovery.

Chapter 36

Drug Abuse Treatment in a Health Care Setting

Chapter Contents

Section 36.1

Medical Professionals Need to Identify Substance Use Disorders

"Early Intervention and Treatment" and excerpts from "Integrating Treatment and Healthcare," White House Office of National Drug Control Policy (www.whitehouse.gov/ondcp), accessed March 19, 2013.

Early Intervention and Treatment

Early intervention and treatment improves health and saves money. Substance abuse has devastating effects on individuals, families, and communities and impacts many Americans. Less visible, but still significant, is the impact substance abuse has on the health care system. Medical professionals spend a great deal of their time and resources treating patients with injuries and illnesses resulting from substance abuse.

The Affordable Care Act, signed into law by President Barack Obama in March 2010, includes substance use disorders as one of the 10 elements of essential health benefits. This is significant because it means that all health insurance sold on Health Insurance Exchanges or provided by Medicaid to certain newly eligible adults starting in 2014 must include services for substance use disorders.

Integrating Treatment and Health Care

Identifying substance use disorders early, in any health care setting, can prevent addiction and save money in the health care system and in the local economy and will save lives. It is critical for medical professionals to be able to identify the early signs of substance abuse in their patients and to intervene early.

Screening, Brief Intervention, and Referral to Treatment (SBIRT)

SBIRT is a tool that health care professionals can use to ask patients about substance use during routine medical visits.

It helps health care providers identify patients with substance use disorders, provide them with medical advice, help them understand the health risks and consequences, and refer patients with more severe substance use–related problems to treatment.

From 2004 through 2008, Washington State achieved cost savings by targeting SBIRT to at-risk patients in emergency care settings and saved the state Medicaid program almost $2 million dollars per one year for just 1,000 patients.

Screening and brief intervention is often as simple as a primary care doctor asking a few questions about a patient's substance abuse history and providing feedback on how the patient can build a healthier life. This may include brief counseling or brief treatment for the patient focused on his or her alcohol or other drug use and its consequences. Early, brief interventions also pave the way for a patient whose alcohol or drug use goes beyond occasional heavy use to accept additional counseling or other services.

Section 36.2

Addiction Treatment Neglected in the Health Care Setting

Forty million Americans ages 12 and older have addiction involving nicotine, alcohol, or other drugs, a disease affecting more Americans than heart conditions, diabetes, or cancer according to a five-year national study released today by The National Center on Addiction and Substance Abuse at Columbia University (CASA Columbia). Another 80 million people are risky substance users—using tobacco, alcohol, and other drugs in ways that threaten health and safety.

The report, *Addiction Medicine: Closing the Gap between Science and Practice*, reveals that while about 7 in 10 people with diseases like hypertension, major depression and diabetes receive treatment, only about 1 in 10 people who need treatment for addiction involving alcohol or other drugs receive it. Of those who do receive treatment, most do not receive anything that approximates evidence-based care.

The CASA Columbia report finds that addiction treatment is largely disconnected from mainstream medical practice. While a wide range of evidence-based screening, intervention, treatment, and disease management tools and practices exist, they rarely are employed. The report exposes the fact that most medical professionals who should be providing treatment are not sufficiently trained to diagnose or treat addiction, and most of those providing addiction treatment are not medical professionals and are not equipped with the knowledge, skills, or credentials necessary to provide the full range of evidence-based services.

"This report shows that misperceptions about the disease of addiction are undermining medical care," said Drew Altman, PhD, president, the Henry J. Kaiser Family Foundation, who chaired the report's National Advisory Commission. The report finds that while doctors routinely screen for a broad range of health problems like high blood pressure or high cholesterol, they rarely screen for risky substance use or signs of addiction and instead treat a long list of health problems that result, including accidents, unintended pregnancies, heart disease, cancers, and many other costly conditions, without examining the root cause.

This landmark report examines the science of addiction—a complex disease that involves changes in the structure and function of the brain—and the profound gap between what we know about the disease and how to prevent and treat it versus current health and medical practice.

Few Patients with Addiction Receive Quality Care

The CASA Columbia report found that while almost half of Americans say they would go to their health care providers if someone close needed help for addiction, less than 6% of all referrals to addiction treatment come from health professionals.

The report also found no clearly delineated, consistent, and regulated national standards that stipulate who may provide addiction treatment in the U.S.; standards vary by state and by payer. Addiction treatment facilities and programs are not adequately regulated or held accountable for providing treatment consistent with medical standards and proven treatment practices.

Most providers of addiction treatment are addiction counselors who are not required to have any medical training. CASA Columbia's analysis of minimum state requirements found:

- 14 states do not require all addiction counselors to be licensed or certified;

- 6 states do not mandate any educational degree to become credentialed;

- 14 states require only a high school diploma or GED;

- 10 states require an associate's degree;

- 6 states require a bachelor's degree; and

- 1 state requires a master's degree.

Physicians and other medical professionals who make up the smallest share of providers of addiction treatment receive little education in addiction science, prevention, and treatment. In fact, CASA Columbia's report cites other research that found that of patients who had visited a general medical provider in the past year only 29% were even asked about alcohol or other drug use.

"Right now there are no accepted national standards for providers of addiction treatment," said Susan Foster, CASA Columbia's vice president and director of policy research and analysis, who was the principal investigator for the report. "There simply is no other disease where appropriate medical treatment is not provided by the health care system and where patients instead must turn to a broad range of practitioners largely exempt from medical standards. Neglect by the medical profession has resulted in a separate and unrelated system of care that struggles to treat the disease without the resources or knowledge base to keep pace with science and medicine."

A Costly Disease

The CASA Columbia report reveals that addiction and risky use of tobacco, alcohol, and other drugs constitute the largest preventable and most costly health problems facing the U.S. today, responsible for more than 20% of deaths in the U.S., causing or contributing to more than 70 other conditions requiring medical care and a wide range of costly social consequences, and accounting for one-third of all hospital inpatient costs. Research suggests that effective health care interventions to prevent and treat addiction would significantly reduce these costs.

In 2010 only $28 billion was spent to treat the 40 million people with addiction. In comparison, the United States spent:

- $44 billion to treat diabetes which affects 26 million people;

- $87 billion to treat cancer which affects 19 million people;

- $107 billion to treat heart conditions which affect 27 million people.

"As our nation struggles to reduce skyrocketing health care costs, this report makes clear that there are few targets for cost savings that are as straightforward as preventing and treating risky substance use and addiction" said Commission Chairman Altman.

Other Notable Findings

- Although addiction is often a chronic disease, treatment typically addresses it as an acute condition and does not include the necessary long-term disease management.

- Public perceptions do not distinguish between risky substance use and the disease of addiction.

- Costs to federal, state, and local governments amount to 11% of total spending; 95 cents of every dollar pay for the consequences and only 2 cents go to prevention and treatment.

Recommendations

The report offers a comprehensive set of recommendations to overhaul current intervention and treatment approaches and to bring practice in line with the scientific evidence and with the standard of care for other public health and medical conditions.

"It is time for health care practice to catch up with the science. Failure to do so causes untold human suffering and is a wasteful misuse of taxpayer dollars," noted Director Foster.

For this study, CASA Columbia conducted a thorough review of more than 7,000 publications; in-depth analysis of five national data sets; focus groups and a nationally representative survey of 1,303 adults; state-wide surveys of addiction treatment directors and staff providers in New York State; an online survey of 1,142 members of professional treatment associations involved in addiction care; an online survey of 360 individuals with a history of addiction who are managing the disease; and an in-depth analysis of state and federal governments' and professional associations' licensing, certification and accreditation requirements. CASA Columbia also obtained comments and suggestions from 176 leading experts in a broad range of fields relevant to the report.

Chapter 37

Detoxification

Introduction

Prior to the 1970s, public intoxication was commonly treated as a criminal offense. People arrested for it were held in "drunk tanks" where they often underwent withdrawal without medical intervention. As society moved toward a more humanitarian view of people with substance use disorders, several methods of detoxification have evolved.

The "medical model" of detoxification is characterized by the use of physicians and nursing staff and the administration of medication to assist people through withdrawal safely. The "social model" relies more on a supportive non-hospital environment than on medication to ease the passage through withdrawal.

Definitions

Detoxification is a set of interventions aimed at managing acute intoxication and withdrawal. It denotes a clearing of toxins from the body of the patient who is acutely intoxicated and/or dependent on substances of abuse. Detoxification seeks to minimize the physical harm caused by the abuse of substances. Detoxification alone is not sufficient in the treatment and rehabilitation of substance use disorders.

Excerpted from "Quick Guide for Administrators Based on Tip 45: Detoxification and Substance Abuse Treatment," Substance Abuse and Mental Health Services Administration (www.samhsa.gov), 2006. Reviewed by David A. Cooke, MD, FACP, July 2013.

Evaluation entails testing for the presence of substances of abuse in the bloodstream, measuring their concentration, and screening for co-occurring mental and physical conditions. Evaluation also includes a comprehensive assessment of the patient's medical, psychological, and social situation.

Stabilization includes the medical and psychosocial process of assisting the patient through acute intoxication and withdrawal to the attainment of a medically stable, fully supported, substance-free state.

Fostering the patient's entry into treatment involves preparing a patient for entry into treatment by stressing the importance of following through with a complete continuum of care.

Guiding Principles/Assumptions

1. Detoxification alone is not sufficient treatment for substance dependence, but it is one part of a continuum of care for substance-related disorders.

2. The detoxification process consists of the following three components:

    • Evaluation

    • Stabilization

    • Fostering patient readiness for and entry into treatment

3. Detoxification can take place in a wide variety of settings and at a number of levels of intensity within these settings. Placement should be appropriate to the patient's needs.

4. Persons seeking detoxification should have access to the components of the detoxification process described here, no matter what the setting or the level of treatment intensity.

5. All persons requiring treatment for substance use disorders should receive treatment of the same quality and appropriate thoroughness and should be put into contact with a substance abuse treatment program after detoxification.

6. Ultimately, insurance coverage for the full range of detoxification services is cost-effective. If reimbursement systems do not provide payment for the complete detoxification process, patients may be released prematurely, leading to medically or socially unattended withdrawal.

7. Patients seeking detoxification services have diverse cultural and ethnic backgrounds as well as unique health needs and life situations. Organizations that provide detoxification services need to ensure that they have standard practices in place to address cultural diversity.

8. A successful detoxification process can be measured, in part, by whether an individual who is substance dependent enters, remains in, and is compliant with the treatment protocol of a substance abuse treatment/rehabilitation program after detoxification.

Overarching Principles for Care during Detoxification Services

- Detoxification services do not offer a "cure" for substance use disorders; they are often a first step toward recovery and a "first door" through which patients pass to treatment.

- Substance use disorders are treatable, and there is hope for recovery.

- Substance use disorders are brain disorders and not evidence of moral weakness.

- Patients are treated with respect and dignity at all times.

- Patients are treated in a nonjudgmental and supportive manner.

- Services planning is completed in partnership with the patient and his or her social support network, including family, significant others, or employers.

- All health professionals involved in the care of the patient will maximize opportunities to promote rehabilitation and maintenance activities and to link the patient to appropriate substance abuse treatment immediately after the detoxification phase.

- Active involvement of the family and other support systems, while respecting the patient's right to privacy and confidentiality, is encouraged.

- Patients are treated with due consideration for individual background, culture, preferences, sexual orientation, disability, vulnerabilities, and strengths.

Challenges to Providing Effective Detoxification

Effective detoxification includes not only the medical stabilization of the patient and the safe and humane withdrawal from substances of abuse, but also entry into treatment. There are several challenges to providing these linkages.

The Health Care Delivery System

- One of the greatest challenges to providing linkages to treatment services occurs when programs try to develop linkages to treatment services.

- Only about one-fifth of 300,000 people discharged from acute care hospitals for detoxification receive substance abuse treatment during hospitalization.

- A recent study conducted for Substance Abuse and Mental Health Services Administration (SAMHSA) found a pronounced need for better linkage between detoxification services and treatment services.

Reimbursement

- Third-party payors sometimes prefer to manage payment for detoxification separately from other phases of addiction treatment; this "unbundling" of services has promoted the separation of services into scattered segments.

- Some reimbursement and utilization policies dictate that only "detoxification" can be authorized, and "detoxification" for that policy or insurer does not cover the nonmedical counseling that is an integral part of substance abuse treatment. This is true in spite of the fact that such nonmedical counseling is widely perceived as useful for patients.

Chapter 38

Treatment Approaches for Drug Addiction

Chapter Contents

Section 38.1

Treatment for Drug Addiction Overview

"DrugFacts: Treatment Approaches for Drug Addiction," National Institute on Drug Abuse (www.drugabuse.gov), September 2009.

Drug addiction is a complex illness characterized by intense and, at times, uncontrollable drug craving, along with compulsive drug seeking and use that persist even in the face of devastating consequences. While the path to drug addiction begins with the voluntary act of taking drugs, over time a person's ability to choose not to do so becomes compromised, and seeking and consuming the drug becomes compulsive. This behavior results largely from the effects of prolonged drug exposure on brain functioning. Addiction is a brain disease that affects multiple brain circuits, including those involved in reward and motivation, learning and memory, and inhibitory control over behavior.

Because drug abuse and addiction have so many dimensions and disrupt so many aspects of an individual's life, treatment is not simple. Effective treatment programs typically incorporate many components, each directed to a particular aspect of the illness and its consequences. Addiction treatment must help the individual stop using drugs, maintain a drug-free lifestyle, and achieve productive functioning in the family, at work, and in society. Because addiction is typically a chronic disease, people cannot simply stop using drugs for a few days and be cured. Most patients require long-term or repeated episodes of care to achieve the ultimate goal of sustained abstinence and recovery of their lives.

Too often, addiction goes untreated: According to the Substance Abuse and Mental Health Services Administration (SAMHSA)'s National Survey on Drug Use and Health (NSDUH), 23.2 million persons (9.4% of the U.S. population) aged 12 or older needed treatment for an illicit drug or alcohol use problem in 2007. Of these individuals, 2.4 million (10.4% of those who needed treatment) received treatment at a specialty facility (i.e., hospital, drug or alcohol rehabilitation or mental health center). Thus, 20.8 million persons (8.4% of the population aged 12 or older) needed treatment for an illicit drug or alcohol use problem but did not receive it. These estimates are similar to those in previous years.

Principles of Effective Treatment

Scientific research since the mid-1970s shows that treatment can help patients addicted to drugs stop using, avoid relapse, and successfully recover their lives. Based on this research, key principles have emerged that should form the basis of any effective treatment programs:

- Addiction is a complex but treatable disease that affects brain function and behavior.

- No single treatment is appropriate for everyone.

- Treatment needs to be readily available.

- Effective treatment attends to multiple needs of the individual, not just his or her drug abuse.

- Remaining in treatment for an adequate period of time is critical.

- Counseling—individual and/or group—and other behavioral therapies are the most commonly used forms of drug abuse treatment.

- Medications are an important element of treatment for many patients, especially when combined with counseling and other behavioral therapies.

- An individual's treatment and services plan must be assessed continually and modified as necessary to ensure that it meets his or her changing needs.

- Many drug-addicted individuals also have other mental disorders.

- Medically assisted detoxification is only the first stage of addiction treatment and by itself does little to change long-term drug abuse.

- Treatment does not need to be voluntary to be effective.

- Drug use during treatment must be monitored continuously, as lapses during treatment do occur.

- Treatment programs should assess patients for the presence of HIV/AIDS, hepatitis B and C, tuberculosis, and other infectious diseases as well as provide targeted risk-reduction counseling to help patients modify or change behaviors that place them at risk of contracting or spreading infectious diseases.

Effective Treatment Approaches

Medication and behavioral therapy, especially when combined, are important elements of an overall therapeutic process that often begins with detoxification, followed by treatment and relapse prevention. Easing withdrawal symptoms can be important in the initiation of treatment; preventing relapse is necessary for maintaining its effects. And sometimes, as with other chronic conditions, episodes of relapse may require a return to prior treatment components. A continuum of care that includes a customized treatment regimen—addressing all aspects of an individual's life, including medical and mental health services—and follow-up options (e.g., community- or family-based recovery support systems) can be crucial to a person's success in achieving and maintaining a drug-free lifestyle.

Medications

Medications can be used to help with different aspects of the treatment process.

Withdrawal: Medications offer help in suppressing withdrawal symptoms during detoxification. However, medically assisted detoxification is not in itself "treatment"—it is only the first step in the treatment process. Patients who go through medically assisted withdrawal but do not receive any further treatment show drug abuse patterns similar to those who were never treated.

Treatment: Medications can be used to help reestablish normal brain function and to prevent relapse and diminish cravings. Currently, we have medications for opioids (heroin, morphine), tobacco (nicotine), and alcohol addiction and are developing others for treating stimulant (cocaine, methamphetamine) and cannabis (marijuana) addiction. Most people with severe addiction problems, however, are polydrug users (users of more than one drug) and will require treatment for all of the substances that they abuse.

Behavioral Treatments

Behavioral treatments help patients engage in the treatment process, modify their attitudes and behaviors related to drug abuse, and increase healthy life skills. These treatments can also enhance the effectiveness of medications and help people stay in treatment longer. Treatment for drug abuse and addiction can be delivered in many different settings using a variety of behavioral approaches.

Outpatient behavioral treatment encompasses a wide variety of programs for patients who visit a clinic at regular intervals. Most of the programs involve individual or group drug counseling. Some programs also offer other forms of behavioral treatment, such as the following:

- Cognitive-behavioral therapy, which seeks to help patients recognize, avoid, and cope with the situations in which they are most likely to abuse drugs

- Multidimensional family therapy, which was developed for adolescents with drug abuse problems—as well as their families—addresses a range of influences on their drug abuse patterns and is designed to improve overall family functioning

- Motivational interviewing, which capitalizes on the readiness of individuals to change their behavior and enter treatment

- Motivational incentives (contingency management), which uses positive reinforcement to encourage abstinence from drugs

Residential treatment programs can also be very effective, especially for those with more severe problems. For example, therapeutic communities (TCs) are highly structured programs in which patients remain at a residence, typically for 6 to 12 months. TCs differ from other treatment approaches principally in their use of the community—treatment staff and those in recovery—as a key agent of change to influence patient attitudes, perceptions, and behaviors associated with drug use. The focus of the TC is on the resocialization of the patient to a drug-free, crime-free lifestyle.

Treatment within the Criminal Justice System

Treatment in a criminal justice setting can succeed in preventing an offender's return to criminal behavior, particularly when treatment continues as the person transitions back into the community. Studies show that treatment does not need to be voluntary to be effective.

Section 38.2

Medication-Assisted Treatment for Opioid Addiction

"Medication-Assisted Treatment for Opioid Addiction,"
White House Office of National Drug Control Policy
(www.whitehouse.gov/ondcp), September 2012.

The U.S. Food and Drug Administration (FDA) has approved three medications for use in the treatment of opioid dependence: methadone, naltrexone, and buprenorphine. With an array of medications now available for addressing the emerging prescription painkiller epidemic, it is crucial that providers in both primary and specialty care settings become trained in medication-assisted treatment (MAT), an approach that uses FDA-approved pharmacological treatments, often in combination with psychosocial treatments, for patients with opioid use disorders. Equally important, insurers and policy makers must strive to learn about available medicines and promote policies that ensure that use of these medications is covered as part of a comprehensive approach to treating prescription and illicit drug dependence.

Medication Options

Medications for treating opioid addiction—including addiction to narcotic prescription painkillers such as oxycodone and hydrocodone as well as illegal opioids like heroin—work by interacting with some of the same receptors in the brain that are triggered by the abused drug. Three types of medications currently are used for treating opioid addiction: agonists, partial agonists, and antagonists.

The rapid onset and short duration of an abused drug's euphoric effects contribute to compulsive, escalating drug use. Oral agonists, therefore, are useful because their effects are less intense, come on more slowly, and last longer. Even when receptors are "turned on" by an agonist-type medication, the slower onset and longer duration of action help prevent withdrawal. Partial agonists, as the name implies, produce effects that are similar to but weaker than those of full agonists. Antagonists work by blocking the action of receptors. Should a patient undergoing treatment with an antagonist-type medication relapse and use the formerly abused substance, that drug's power to trigger the receptors is often blocked or greatly diminished.

The following medications are approved by the FDA for use in opioid addiction treatment in conjunction with behavioral therapy:

Methadone

Methadone, a synthetic opioid, is an agonist that mitigates opioid withdrawal symptoms and, at higher doses, blocks the effects of heroin and other drugs containing opiates. Maintenance of opioid addiction treatment with methadone is approved "in conjunction with appropriate social and medical services." Methadone can be dispensed only at an outpatient opioid treatment program (OTP) certified by SAMHSA and registered with the Drug Enforcement Administration (DEA) or to a hospitalized patient in an emergency.

Buprenorphine

Buprenorphine, approved by the FDA in 2002 to treat opioid dependence, is a partial opioid agonist that, when dosed appropriately, suppresses withdrawal symptoms. Although buprenorphine can produce opioid agonist effects and side effects, such as euphoria and respiratory depression, its maximal effects are generally milder than those of full agonists like heroin and methadone. Physicians are permitted to distribute buprenorphine at intensive outpatient treatment programs that are authorized to provide methadone if providers are trained in its use. Additionally, a special program has been set up so that buprenorphine can be prescribed by physicians in office settings and dispensed by pharmacists.

A buprenorphine/naloxone combination is sometimes referred to as Bup/Nx. Formulations approved for drug abuse treatment are intended to be taken sublingually (placed under the tongue and allowed to dissolve). When taken this way, the naloxone has little effect. However, if a patient injects Bup/Nx, the naloxone enters the bloodstream and will block the buprenorphine, causing the patient to enter opioid withdrawal. This combination formulation may deter abuse through injecting because abusers are motivated to avoid unpleasant withdrawal symptoms.

Buprenorphine without naloxone has been used routinely for inducting patients onto buprenorphine. Induction occurs in the provider's presence, where risk of intravenous use is low and injection deterrence is generally unnecessary. Once patients are stabilized on the mono-formulation, those who can tolerate naloxone are switched to the combination product for ongoing maintenance

Naltrexone

Naltrexone is a nonaddictive antagonist used in the treatment of opioid dependence. The medication blocks opioid receptors so they cannot be activated. This "blockade" action, combined with naltrexone's ability to bind to opioid receptors even in the presence of other opioids, helps keep abused drugs from exerting their effects when patients have taken or have been administered naltrexone. As an antagonist, naltrexone blocks opioid receptor sites so that other substances present in a patient's system cannot bind to them. If a patient who has been administered naltrexone attempts to continue taking opioids, he or she is unable to feel any of the opioid's effects due to naltrexone's blocking action.

Naltrexone is administered in an injectable long-acting formulation (marketed under the brand name Vivitrol), sometimes called "depot naltrexone," which is designed for once-monthly dosing.

Detoxification vs. Stabilization and Maintenance

Some treatment programs provide medically assisted detoxification services, which involve weaning patients off addictive substances and managing withdrawal. However, research shows such programs are closely associated with relapse. And because tolerance to opioids fades rapidly even during a short period of abstinence, one episode of opioid misuse following detoxification can result in a life-threatening or deadly overdose.

Before medications became available for addiction treatment, detoxification routinely took place at the beginning of treatment. This is still the case in programs that set complete drug abstinence as a goal and in the treatment of addictions for which medications are not yet approved. However, in the case of methadone, researchers formulated a "phased approach" that does not necessarily emphasize complete detoxification.

According to the phased approach, the first step in treatment is not detoxification. Rather, it involves intensive stabilization, including withdrawal management, assessment, medication induction, and involvement in psychosocial counseling. The middle phase of care emphasizes medication maintenance and deeper work in and out of counseling on patient goals. In the third phase, "ongoing rehabilitation," the patient and provider might choose to detoxify from all medication or pursue indefinite maintenance, depending on the patient's needs. Treatment in a phased model, regardless of how long medication is used, involves participation in psychosocial treatment, and engagement with the self-help community is recommended. As such, participants in MAT can transition to a lifestyle consistent with being "in recovery" while using FDA-approved medication to treat their substance use disorder.

Section 38.3

Treatment for Methamphetamine Addiction

"Treatment for Meth Addiction," Reprinted with
permission from the Illinois Attorney General's MethNet website,
http://www.illinoisattorneygeneral.gov/methnet, © 2010.

What is known about meth addiction?

Addiction is a disease marked by three primary symptoms:

1. The addict has difficulty controlling the drug use. The addict uses the drug excessively or frequently and has extreme difficulty making the choice not to use the drug.

2. Use of the drug causes problems in the addict's life. Addicts typically withdraw from family and friends and also experience job-related difficulty, financial drain, and other negative consequences.

3. The addict feels a strong craving to use the drug, which can be associated with psychological triggers as well as physical symptoms.

Methamphetamine is extremely addictive. Meth causes chemical reactions in the brain that trick the body into believing it has unlimited energy supplies and drain energy reserves needed for other parts of the body. This causes meth addicts to stay awake for long periods of time until they crash from exhaustion. Meth also reduces the levels of dopamine (a chemical in the brain that causes feelings of pleasure) produced by the brain. When the user stops taking the drug, the brain is unable to function normally for a period of days, weeks, or even months.

What is drug addiction treatment?

In the most general terms, drug addiction treatment refers to the broad range of services provided to people suffering from addiction. These services include identification, intervention, assessment, diagnosis, counseling, health care, psychiatric services, psychological services, social services, and follow-up procedures. The overall goal of treatment is to reduce or eliminate drug use and restore the addict to a productive life. Because addiction is a life-long, relapsing disease, the recovery process is also life-long. For this reason, we refer to former drug users as "recovering" addicts.

What is the best treatment for meth addicts?

Because traditional treatment models are not effective for meth addiction, meth-specific treatment programs have been developed.

Successful meth treatment requires the use of cognitive-behavioral therapy. The cognitive-behavioral therapy approach, which focuses on how the way we think affects our feelings and actions, helps patients identify and plan for the triggers associated with the substance abuse. This approach prepares the addict for life-long recovery.

A critical consideration in meth treatment is something known as the "wall." Around 45 to 120 days into treatment, recovering addicts experience physiological changes that often lead to a return to meth use. This period of increased depression and need for the drug is the single significant factor today to the false perception that meth addiction is "untreatable."

Although recovering from meth addiction is challenging, it is not impossible. For meth treatment to be successful, it simply must meet the demands of meth addiction. Research shows that recovering meth addicts require a longer and more intense outpatient program than is the case for many other drugs. These outpatient services should be very structured and include frequent contact between the treatment provider and the recovering addict.

What does meth treatment entail?

The goal of treatment is to teach the addict new skills that will help him or her cope with drug cravings and prevent relapses. Often, the process will begin with a short series of "pre-treatment" sessions used to motivate the user to commit to treatment and to assess the user's drug history, mental status, current drug usage, and relationships with significant others. These sessions progress according to the interest and commitment of the addict, as does the ensuing treatment.

Meth treatment involves both individual and small group approaches. Addicts talk about their experiences and are walked through a variety of exercises and worksheets designed to further their recovery by increasing self-awareness. A first step toward recovery is a thorough understanding of addiction and its effects on the mind and body. It is extremely important that the user understand his or her addiction and identify the "triggers" that may cause his or her drug use. Once common triggers are identified, the user can determine ways of avoiding high-risk trigger situations and learn new ways of coping with them.

Throughout treatment, returns to meth use are treated not as failures but as opportunities to learn. By analyzing what caused the addict to relapse, the addict can learn how to keep it from happening again. Extensive work is done to assist the addict in developing effective coping mechanisms to help him or her work past cravings.

Treatment encourages users to see beyond the immediate "positive" effects gained from drug use toward the negative consequences of drug use that inevitably follow. Alternative coping mechanisms are then devised that will provide positive effects without the negative consequences of drug use. Finally, recovering addicts learn to manage their lives more successfully, increase their confidence and self-esteem, and set positive personal goals.

Treatment also addresses other medical or mental health issues facing the user and includes education on the risks of HIV and AIDS associated with meth use.

Treatment is ended when the recovering addict reaches set treatment goals. To facilitate the recovering addict's continued abstinence from meth, treatment professionals help the recovering addict set up a system of support to help him or her stay drug free after treatment. Often, this includes lifetime involvement in support groups or 12-step programs.

Section 38.4

Cocaine Vaccine Helps Some Reduce Drug Abuse

"Cocaine Vaccine Helps Some Reduce Drug Abuse," National Institute on Drug Abuse (www.drugabuse.gov), December 1, 2010.

A vaccine to prevent cocaine abuse proved mildly effective in its first placebo-controlled test. Although their individual responses varied, vaccine recipients reduced their cocaine use more quickly than placebo recipients. A subgroup of vaccinated patients generated levels of antibodies that were sufficient to block cocaine's effects, and during the period of peak antibody production, they submitted more drug-free urine samples than participants in the placebo group or those who did not respond strongly to the vaccine. With further refinement to increase response, a vaccine might someday be available as a therapy for cocaine abuse, says lead investigator Dr. Thomas Kosten of Baylor College of Medicine in Houston.

Testing the Concept

The cocaine vaccine consists of a small amount of the drug chemically bonded to a protein, derived from cholera toxin, that stimulates the immune system to produce antibodies. Anti-cocaine antibodies latch onto cocaine molecules in the bloodstream, forming drug-antibody complexes that are too large to pass through the fine-grained tissue filter that enwraps and protects the brain. If the vaccinated person develops enough antibodies to capture and hold onto most of the cocaine molecules circulating in the blood, the drug will not produce the euphoria or other psychoactive effects that reinforce drug taking and addiction.

For the first placebo-controlled test of the vaccine's ability to reduce cocaine use among people who are addicted to the drug, Dr. Kosten and colleagues recruited 115 men and women who were seeking treatment at an outpatient clinic after having abused cocaine for about 15 years. The study participants were taking cocaine, on average, three times daily, three days per week. All were also addicted to opioids and had initiated methadone maintenance therapy two weeks prior to their first dose of the cocaine vaccine or placebo. The researchers chose this population because the patients came to the clinic daily to receive their doses of methadone, thereby increasing the likelihood that they would be available for injections, as well as urine and blood tests, and would remain in the study for its full 24-week duration.

Dr. Kosten and colleagues randomly assigned 58 patients to receive the cocaine vaccine in five intramuscular injections spaced over 12 weeks, a regimen that previous research had suggested should cumulatively produce enough antibodies to neutralize the amount of drug typically in the body during cocaine abuse. The remaining 57 patients received placebo injections on an identical schedule. All patients also attended weekly drug abuse counseling sessions focused on relapse prevention. The participants submitted urine samples for cocaine assay three times each week and gave blood samples for antibody level monitoring at the end of the second week and then at four-week intervals.

Antibody Level Crucial

Some of the patients noted that the vaccine achieved its desired effect of suppressing cocaine's psychoactive effects. These individuals said that they felt little difference even after taking large amounts of the drug—in some cases up to 10 times their normal intake—confirmed by levels of a cocaine metabolite in their urine. In most of these cases, loss of cocaine's psychoactive effects occurred after three to four injections of the vaccine.

The patients who received the vaccine and those given placebo both reduced their cocaine use, but the former did so more rapidly. During the period of highest antibody response to the vaccine—from the week following the fourth booster injection through the month following the final one—30% of the vaccinated patients, but only 15% of the placebo patients, achieved a 50% reduction in cocaine-positive urine samples compared with levels at the beginning of the study. In prior research, this measure of success corresponded with improvements in daily functioning among people addicted to cocaine, Dr. Kosten says. No further injections were given after the 12th week of the study, and the difference in cocaine use between the vaccine and placebo groups disappeared by week 16.

The vaccinated patients varied greatly in their antibody responses, and only 38% of the 55 who completed the entire series of injections produced anti-cocaine antibodies in the quantity that the researchers calculate will reliably block drug-induced euphoria. During the eight weeks of the greatest antibody response, this group provided cocaine-free urine samples 45% of the time, as compared with 35% for the placebo group and the group with a lesser response to the vaccine. Of the patients who produced euphoria-blocking antibody levels, 53% at least doubled the frequency with which their urine samples demonstrated no new cocaine use, compared with 23% of those who received the vaccine but produced lower levels of the antibodies.

"If a patient makes enough antibodies, this treatment works well," says Dr. Kosten. Among cocaine abusers who receive the full course of injections, those who are motivated to quit are expected to achieve abstinence with a lower level of antibody than those who are not motivated to quit, he adds. Dr. Kosten estimates that, with the current vaccine, about 70% of cocaine abusers would develop high enough levels of antibody to block cocaine's euphoric effects by more than 90%, an effect considered sufficient to prevent relapse in individuals motivated to quit. However, people not motivated to quit but who receive the antibody treatment, perhaps in response to family pressure or other reasons, would require an antibody level high enough to completely prevent euphoric effects from whatever amount of cocaine they typically take.

There were no serious adverse events related to the vaccine, and no patients dropped out of the study because of the treatment.

Improving the Vaccine

Dr. Kosten's team is currently planning to enroll 300 participants in a large NIDA-supported multisite trial to confirm the results of this proof-of-concept study and determine whether the vaccine can benefit the general population of cocaine abusers. The team expects the challenge of retaining patients for the entire course of vaccinations and assessments to be greater than in the just-completed trial, however, as none will be opiate abusers scheduled for daily clinic visits for methadone. To bolster participants' motivation, the researchers are supplementing relapse-prevention behavioral therapy with the opportunity to earn rewards for keeping clinic appointments.

In other ongoing research with different collaborators, Dr. Kosten is modifying the vaccine in hopes of producing a stronger, more sustained antibody response. The researchers have replaced the cholera toxin with a carrier molecule developed by Merck Pharmaceuticals from the *Neisseria meningitidis* bacteria coat protein, which has boosted the amount of antibodies produced by other vaccines. This carrier has been used in a human meningitis vaccine for over 10 years. The newly configured vaccine has reduced cocaine self-administration in animals but has yet to be tried in people.

Dr. Kosten envisions a two-year course of vaccine-aided therapy for cocaine addiction that will include behavioral therapy and a series of vaccine injections followed by bimonthly or quarterly boosters.

Dr. Jamie Biswas of NIDA's Division of Pharmacotherapies and Medical Consequences of Drug Abuse agrees with this proposed length of treatment: "Patients need a couple of years of blocking the cocaine high to get used to being off the drug, and they may benefit from appropriate behavioral therapies as well."

Source

Martell, B.A., et al. Cocaine vaccine for the treatment of cocaine dependence in methadone-maintained patients: A randomized double-blind placebo-controlled efficacy trial. *Archives of General Psychiatry* 66(10):1116–1123, 2009.

Chapter 39

Supporting Substance Abuse Recovery

Chapter Contents

Section 39.1

Mutual Support Groups

"An Introduction to Mutual Support Groups for Alcohol and
Drug Abuse," Substance Abuse and Mental Health Services Administration
(www.samhsa.gov), 2008. Reviewed by David A. Cooke, MD, FACP, July 2013.

Mutual support (also called self-help) groups are an important part of recovery from substance use disorders (SUDs). Mutual support groups exist both for persons with an SUD and for their families or significant others and are one of the choices an individual has during the recovery process.

Mutual Support Groups

Mutual support groups are nonprofessional groups comprising members who share the same problem and voluntarily support one another in the recovery from that problem. Although mutual support groups do not provide formal treatment, they are one part of a recovery-oriented systems-of-care approach to substance abuse recovery. By providing social, emotional, and informational support for persons throughout the recovery process, mutual support groups help individuals take responsibility for their alcohol and drug problems and for their sustained health, wellness, and recovery. The most widely available mutual support groups are 12-step groups, such as Alcoholics Anonymous (AA), but other mutual support groups such as Women for Sobriety (WFS), SMART Recovery (Self-Management and Recovery Training), and Secular Organizations for Sobriety/Save Our Selves (SOS) are also available.

12-Step Groups

Twelve-step groups emphasize abstinence and have 12 core developmental "steps" to recovering from dependence. Other elements of 12-step groups include taking responsibility for recovery, sharing personal narratives, helping others, and recognizing and incorporating into daily life the existence of a higher power. Participants often maintain a close relationship with a sponsor, an experienced member with long-term abstinence, and lifetime participation is expected. AA is the oldest and best known 12-step mutual support group. There are more than 100,000 AA groups worldwide and nearly 2 million members. The AA model has been adapted for people with dependence on drugs and for their family members. Some groups, such as Narcotics Anonymous (NA) and Chemically Dependent Anonymous, focus on any type of drug use. Other groups, such as Cocaine Anonymous and Crystal Meth Anonymous, focus on abuse of specific drugs. Groups for persons with co-occurring substance use and mental disorders also exist (e.g., Double Trouble in Recovery; Dual Recovery Anonymous). Other 12-step groups—Families Anonymous, Al-Anon/Alateen, Nar-Anon, and Co-Anon—provide support to significant others, families, and friends of persons with SUDs. Twelve-step meetings are held in locations such as churches and public buildings. Metropolitan areas usually have specialized groups, based on such member characteristics as gender, length of time in recovery, age, sexual orientation, profession, ethnicity, and language spoken. Attendance and membership are free, although people usually give a small donation when they attend a meeting.

Meetings can be "open" or "closed" that is, anyone can attend an open meeting, but attendance at closed meetings is limited to people who want to stop drinking or using drugs. Although meeting formats vary somewhat, most 12-step meetings have an opening and a closing that are the same at every meeting, such as a 12-step reading or prayer. The main part of the meeting usually consists of (1) members sharing their stories of dependence, its effect on their lives, and what they are doing to stay abstinent, (2) the study of a particular step or other doctrine of the group, or (3) a guest speaker. Twelve-step groups are not necessarily for everyone. Some people are uncomfortable with the spiritual emphasis and prefer a more secular approach. Others may not agree with the 12-step philosophy that addiction is a chronic disease, thinking that this belief can be a self-fulfilling prophesy that weakens the ability to remain abstinent. Still others may prefer gender-specific groups. Mutual support groups that are not based on the 12-step model typically do not advocate sponsors or lifetime member ship. These support groups offer an alternative to traditional 12-step groups, but the availability of in-person meetings is more limited than that of 12-step programs. However, many offer literature, discussion boards, and online meetings.

Women for Sobriety

WFS is the first national self-help group solely for women wishing to stop using alcohol and drugs. The program is based on Thirteen

Statements that encourage emotional and spiritual growth, with abstinence as the only acceptable goal. Although daily meditation is encouraged, WFS does not otherwise emphasize God or a higher power. The nearly 300 meetings held weekly are led by experienced, abstinent WFS members and follow a structured format, which includes reading the Thirteen Statements, an introduction of members, and a moderated discussion.

SMART Recovery

SMART Recovery helps individuals become free from dependence on any substance. Dependence is viewed as a learned behavior that can be modified using cognitive-behavioral approaches. Its four principles are to (1) enhance and maintain motivation to abstain, (2) cope with urges, (3) manage thoughts, feelings, and behaviors, and (4) balance momentary and enduring satisfactions. At the approximately 300 weekly group meetings held worldwide, attendees discuss personal experiences and real-world applications of these SMART Recovery principles. SMART Recovery has online meetings and a message board discussion group on its website.

Secular Organization for Sobriety/Save Our Selves

SOS considers recovery from alcohol and drugs an individual responsibility separate from spirituality and emphasizes a cognitive approach to maintaining lifelong abstinence. Meetings typically begin with a reading of the SOS Guidelines for Sobriety and introductions, followed by an open discussion of a topic deemed appropriate by the members. However, because each of the approximately 500 SOS groups is autonomous, the meeting format may differ from group to group. SOS also has online support groups, such as the SOS International E-Support Group (health.groups.yahoo.com/group/sossaveourselves) and the SOS Women E-Support Group (groups.yahoo.com/group/ SOSWomen).

LifeRing Secular Recovery

Originally part of SOS, LifeRing is now a separate organization for people who want to stop using alcohol and drugs. The principles of LifeRing are sobriety, secularity, and self-help. LifeRing encourages participants to develop a unique path to abstinence according to their needs and to use the group meetings to facilitate their personal recovery plan LifeRing meetings are relatively unstructured; attendees discuss what has happened to them in the past week, but some meetings focus on helping members create a personal recovery plan. Although there are fewer than 100 meetings worldwide, LifeRing has a chat room, e-mail lists, and an online forum that provide additional support to its members.

The Effectiveness of Mutual Support Groups

Research on mutual support groups indicates that active participation in any type of mutual support group significantly increases the likelihood of maintaining abstinence. Previous research has shown that participating in 12-step or other mutual support group is related to abstinence from alcohol and drug use. An important finding is that these abstinence rates increase with greater group participation. Persons who attend mutual support groups have also been found to have lower levels of alcohol- and drug-related problems.

Another benefit of mutual support group participation is that "helping helps the helper." Helping others by sharing experiences and providing support increases involvement in 12-step groups, which in turn increases abstinence and lowers binge drinking rates among those who have not achieved abstinence.

Facilitating Mutual Support Group Participation

If a health care or social service provider suspects that a patient or client has an SUD, the provider should ensure that the client receives formal treatment. Once the client receives formal treatment—or if he or she refuses or cannot afford treatment—the provider's next step is to facilitate involvement in a mutual support group. Matching clients to treatment based solely on gender, motivation, cognitive impairment, or other such characteristics has not been proved to be effective. Clients who are "philosophically well matched" to a mutual support group are more likely to actively participate in that group. Thus, the best way to help a client benefit from mutual support groups is to encourage increased participation in his or her chosen group. Providers can increase their knowledge of mutual support groups, and thus their ability to make informed referrals, by doing the following:

- Become familiar with the different types of support groups and their philosophies. Most groups' websites describe their philosophies and have online publications.

- Determine which groups are active locally. Most groups' websites have meeting locator services.

- Find out about the different types of meetings available within local mutual support groups (e.g., which meetings are for women only).

- Establish contacts in local mutual support groups. AA and NA in particular have committees whose members work with health care and social service providers to get clients to meetings and to provide information to providers.

- Attend open meetings to expand knowledge of mutual support groups and how local meetings are conducted.

Understanding the needs and beliefs of clients with SUDs helps providers make informed referrals. Providers should find out clients' experiences with mutual support groups, their concerns and misconceptions about mutual support groups, and their personal beliefs. Persons who agree with the group's belief system are more likely to participate and, thus, more likely to have better outcomes. For example, having strong religious beliefs is related to greater participation in the spiritually based 12-step programs and WFS. In contrast, religiosity was less effective in increasing participation in SMART Recovery groups and decreased participation in SOS. Whether the client is participating in medication-assisted treatment (MAT) is another consideration when making a referral to a mutual support group because some groups may be more supportive of MAT than others. For example, individuals being treated with methadone for opioid dependence may be more comfortable attending a meeting of Methadone Anonymous, whose members understand the benefits of opioid pharmacotherapy. To improve the client's chances of attending a meeting, providers can do the following:

- Present more than one choice when making referrals and encourage clients to attend several meetings before making any judgments about the groups. Clients should be encouraged to attend different groups until they find one in which they are comfortable.

- Initiate the first conversation between a client and a support group contact person. Having a mutual support group member speak to a client by phone during the office visit may increase the likelihood that the client will attend the support group meeting.

- Refer family members or others who may be affected by the client's substance use. Their involvement may encourage participation by providing social support.

Once clients are attending a group they are comfortable with, the provider should actively encourage the clients' support group experiences by scheduling follow-up visits to talk about their experiences and providing positive feedback. Clients should be asked about details—how many meetings are they attending, if they have a sponsor, and if they abstinent. Gentle, positive encouragement will likely increase participation. Providers should watch for signs of an impending relapse, such as a reluctance to discuss group participation or periods of extreme stress. By offering knowledgeable advice and informed referrals and taking an ongoing, active interest in clients' support group experiences, providers can make a difference in their clients' recovery.

Mutual Support Groups for People Who Have a Substance Use Disorder

Alcoholics Anonymous: www.alcoholics-anonymous.org

Chemically Dependent Anonymous: www.cdaweb.org

Cocaine Anonymous: www.ca.org

Crystal Meth Anonymous: www.crystalmeth.org

Heroin Anonymous: www.heroin-anonymous.org

LifeRing Secular Recovery: www.unhooked.com

Marijuana Anonymous: www.marijuana-anonymous.org

Methadone Anonymous: www.methadone-anonymous.org

Narcotics Anonymous: www.na.org

Secular Organizations for Sobriety/Save Our Selves: www.sossobriety.org

SMART Recovery: www.smartrecovery.org

Women for Sobriety: www.womenforsobriety.org

Mutual Support Groups for People with Co-Occurring Disorders

Double Trouble in Recovery: www.doubletroubleinrecovery.org

Dual Recovery Anonymous: www.dualrecovery.org

Mutual Support Groups for Families, Friends, and Significant Others

Al-Anon/Alateen: www.al-anon.alateen.org

Co-Anon: www.co-anon.org

Families Anonymous: www.familiesanonymous.org

Nar-Anon: nar-anon.org

Section 39.2

Peer Recovery Support Services

"What Are Peer Recovery Support Services?" HHS Publication No. (SMA)
09-4454, Substance Abuse and Mental Health Services Administration,
Center for Substance Abuse Treatment (www.samhsa.gov), 2009.

Research has shown that recovery is facilitated by social support,
and four types of social support have been identified in the literature: emotional, informational, instrumental, and affiliational support.
These four categories refer to types of social support, not discrete services or service models. For example, a project that is planning social
support services to address recovering people's employment needs
might consider whether a job referral (informational support) by itself
is adequate, or whether emotional support (such as supportive coaching to prepare for an interview) and/or instrumental support (such as
help cleaning up a criminal record) might also be needed. In general,
the more robust the types of social support available to address any
given recovery concern, the more likely that a person seeking help
will walk away with useful information, a new insight or skill, or more
confidence to help with the tasks ahead.

Peer Leaders and the Peer Service Alliance

Recovery Community Services Program (RCSP) projects through
Substance Abuse and Mental Health Services Administration/Center
for Substance Abuse Treatment (SAMHSA/CSAT) use the term *peer*
to refer to all individuals who share the experiences of addiction and
recovery, either directly or as family members or significant others. In
a peer-helping-peer service alliance, a peer leader in stable recovery
provides social support services to a peer who is seeking help in establishing or maintaining his or her recovery. Both parties are helped by
the interaction as the recovery of each is strengthened.

RCSP projects use many other titles besides peer leader and peer
to describe the parties to the peer service alliance. On the peer leader
side of the equation, titles include recovery (or peer) mentor, guide,
or coach; peer services interventionist; firestarter; and peer resource

specialist. (Firestarters are peer leaders responsible for building local recovery communities in Native American communities.) The peer who seeks help also is given different titles in different RCSP projects, such as member (of the peer services organization), mentee, or simply peer. Most project leaders have consciously sought to find and use identifying terms that distinguish their peer services and service providers from those in formal, professional treatment programs or in mutual aid groups conducted by lay persons. For this reason, terms such as counselor, case manager, or sponsor, as well as client, consumer, or patient, are avoided.

The RCSP projects' attention to language reflects the need to clearly distinguish the role of the peer leader from the role of the treatment counselor or other professional and the 12-step sponsor. RCSP projects are intended by CSAT to enhance—not duplicate, replace, or compete with—valuable services already available in a community. Thus, in addition to using language that is not associated with treatment or mutual aid programs, axioms such as the following are commonly heard: "Peers do not diagnose;" "Peers do not provide therapy;" "Peers do not give advice." Similarly, it is common to hear, "You need to ask your sponsor, not me, for help working the 12-steps," or "That's a question for the doctor or nurse."

Peer Recovery Support Service Activities

The RCSP peer recovery support service projects have developed a variety of peer services. Not all programs provide all services, and some peer leaders may provide more than one service. The following is a useful overview of the four major types of recovery support services emerging in RCSP projects: (1) peer mentoring or coaching, (2) recovery resource connecting, (3) facilitating and leading recovery groups, and (4) building community.

Peer mentoring or coaching: Although the name given to this service activity varies from project to project, the terms *mentoring* or *coaching* refer to a one-on-one relationship in which a peer leader with more recovery experience than the person served encourages, motivates, and supports a peer who is seeking to establish or strengthen his or her recovery.

The nature and functions of mentoring or coaching vary from one RCSP project to another. Generally, mentors or coaches assist peers with tasks such as setting recovery goals, developing recovery action plans, and solving problems directly related to recovery, including finding sober housing, making new friends, finding new uses of spare time, and improving one's job skills. They may also provide assistance with issues that arise in connection with collateral problems such as having a criminal justice record or coexisting physical or mental challenges.

The relationship of the peer leader to the peer receiving help is highly supportive, rather than directive. The duration of the relationship between the two depends on a number of factors such as how much recovery time the peer has, how much other support the peer is receiving, or how quickly the peer's most pressing problems can be addressed.

RCSP projects distinguish the role of the peer mentor or coach from that of a 12-step sponsor in several ways. For example, the sponsor works within the 12-step framework and is expected to help the person in early recovery understand and follow the specific guidance of the 12-step program. The typical RCSP recovery mentor or coach, on the other hand, is often described as helping peers in early recovery make choices about which recovery pathway(s) will work for them, rather than urging them to adopt the mentor's or coach's own program or any specific program of recovery. The mentor or coach is often described as devoting a greater amount of time than the typical 12-step sponsor to connecting the person in early recovery to community health, employment, housing, educational, and social services and resources and often has more specific knowledge about a larger range of available services and resources.

Peer recovery resource connecting: The service activities of peer leaders in connecting peers to recovery resources might be likened to case management in substance use disorder treatment. The purpose of resource connecting services is to connect the peer with professional and nonprofessional services and resources available in the community that can help meet his or her individual needs on the road to recovery. The peer leader working in a peer setting to provide recovery resource connecting services often has had personal experience navigating the service systems and accessing the resources to which referral is being made and can bring those personal experiences to bear.

Peer recovery support services provided in RCSP projects typically can help peers with their most pressing early recovery needs—finding a safe place to live and a job. Thus, peer leaders are likely to refer peers to safe housing or to sources of information about housing and to a wide variety of resources and services that provide assistance in developing job readiness or finding jobs. Peer leaders also help peers navigate the formal treatment system, advocating for their access and gaining admittance, as well as facilitating discharge planning, typically in collaboration with treatment staff.

Peer leaders also encourage and support participation in mutual aid groups and provide specific information about the various groups that exist in the community. They encourage and facilitate participation in educational opportunities. Depending on the particular needs of the population they serve, they also may focus on developing linkages to resources that address specialized needs, such as agencies providing services related to HIV infection or AIDS, mental health disorders, chronic and acute health problems, parenting young children, and problems stemming from involvement with the criminal justice system.

Facilitating and leading recovery groups: In addition to conducting one-on-one coaching or mentoring and resource connecting activities, many peer leaders facilitate or lead recovery-oriented group activities. Some of these activities are structured as support groups, while others have educational purposes. Many have components of both.

The group activities that are structured as support groups typically involve the sharing of personal stories and some degree of collective problem solving. Many of these groups are formed around shared identity, such as belonging to a common cultural or religious group, or shared experience related to the substance use disorder, such as the need to re-enter the community following incarceration, being HIV positive, or facing challenges in parenting. Many, but not all, group activities conducted by peer leaders have a spiritual component.

The group educational activities tend to focus on a specific subject or skill set and may involve the participation of an expert as well as peer leaders. Typical topics and activities include training in job skills, budgeting and managing credit, and preventing relapse, as well as courses particularly targeted to people in recovery, such as conflict resolution grounded in recovery skills.

Building community: A person in early recovery is often faced with the need to abandon friends and/or social networks that promote and help sustain a substance use disorder but has no alternatives to put in their place that support recovery. Peer recovery support service providers can help such peers make new friends and begin to build alternative social networks. Peer leaders in RCSP projects often organize recovery-oriented activities that range from opportunities to participate in team sports to family-centered holiday celebrations and to payday get-togethers that are alcohol- and drug-free. These activities provide a sense of acceptance and belonging to a group, as well as the opportunity to practice new social skills.

The Adaptability of Peer Recovery Support Services

One strength of peer recovery support services has been their adaptability to many stages and modalities of recovery, as well as to different service settings and organizational contexts. This adaptability makes them an effective vehicle for extending support for recovery beyond the treatment system and into the communities where people live and to people following different pathways to recovery. On the other hand, because of the variations in settings, organizational contexts, and recovery stages and pathways, identifying commonalities in peer recovery support services can be challenging.

Section 39.3

Recovery Services

"Supporting Recovery," White House Office of
National Drug Control Policy (www.whitehouse.gov/
ondcp), accessed March 19, 2013.

A wide range of services, program models, and supports are available to help individuals in recovery.

Mutual aid: Mutual aid groups, also referred to as "self-help" or "support groups," are run by people in recovery and support their members as they follow a recovery pathway. Examples of mutual aid groups include 12-step fellowships, Alcoholics Anonymous, Narcotics Anonymous, and Cocaine Anonymous. There is also other addiction recovery mutual aid options, including online resources.

Recovery support services: Recovery support services are nonclinical services that help people achieve, enrich, and maintain recovery. Services include transportation assistance, child care, mentoring, recovery coaching, traditional Native American healing practices, and housing and employment assistance. Services are offered by substance use disorder treatment providers as well as provider organizations, such as recovery community organizations, substance abuse ministries, and other grassroots community organizations.

Recovery-oriented systems of care (ROSC): ROSC is a system and service approach that supports long-term recovery. This approach supports recovery systems that are operational in the community at the local, state, or tribal level and makes it possible for recovery services to be individually tailored.

Recovery community organizations (RCOs): RCOs are independent, nonprofit organizations led and governed by people in recovery. Their purpose is to mobilize resources to increase the number of individuals who achieve and sustain recovery from addiction to alcohol and other drugs.

Recovery housing: Recovery housing provides an environment that is safe and supportive of those in recovery from addiction to alcohol or other drugs. Recovery housing typically makes use of single-family residences, although there are congregate models in apartment buildings and college dormitories. A recently formed national association is developing national standards that will include uniform language that best describes recovery housing.

Recovery high schools: Recovery high schools provide a service-enriched and supportive school environment for students recovering from drug and alcohol problems. These schools offer standard academic courses, combined with continuing care and/or recovery support services. Generally, recovery schools do not provide substance use or mental health disorder treatment. In the U.S., there are approximately 35 recovery high schools. The Association of Recovery Schools (ARS) website provides additional information on these schools.

Collegiate recovery programs: Collegiate recovery programs can be found on the campuses of community colleges, major state universities, and private institutions of various sizes. There are approximately 18 programs nationally.

Technology and services: Technology provides a cost-effective way of supporting recovery. Technology used can range from landline and mobile phones to internet-based social networking platforms, and virtual services to advanced physiological monitoring systems. It plays an ever-expanding role in addiction treatment and recovery support. Practices such as telephone monitoring and adaptive counseling (TMAC), peer telephone recovery checkups, online recovery support services and mutual aid, and virtual services are becoming increasingly prevalent in the addictions treatment and recovery arena.

Section 39.4

Recovery Services for Youth

Excerpted from "Youth In Recovery" by John de Miranda Ed.M. and Greg Williams, B.A., *The Prevention Researcher*, Volume 18(2), April 2011. Reprinted with permission. © 2011 Integrated Research Services Inc. All rights reserved. To view the complete text ofthis article including references, visit www.tpronline.org.

As a nation we have been focused on alcohol and drug problems among youth for a very long time. Our approach has focused on drug use and the deficits associated with young people who experiment or become problematic users. National youth drug policy and funding has been largely limited to criminalization strategies, prevention programs with limited evidence to support their effectiveness, and messaging aimed at exhorting youth to not use drugs and refrain from drinking until the age of 21. At time our concerns border on the melodramatic and catastrophic and serve to camouflage the fact that alcohol and drug experimentation is normative.

The 1934 release of the movie *Reefer Madness* (originally titled *Tell Your Children*) captured society's concern with newspaper headlines of "dope peddlers caught in high school" and characterizations of marijuana as "destroying the youth of American in alarmingly increasing numbers." This kind of dramatic characterization of drug dangers and youth is still evident today in a recent exhortation opposing the California citizen's ballot proposition to legalize marijuana.

...marijuana is harmful to a young person's brain development, affecting their motivation, memory, learning, judgment, and behavior control. It can also hurt their ability to succeed academically, is linked to violence and gang activity, and is the most prevalent illegal drug detected in fatally injured drivers, and motor vehicle crash victims.

—Community Anti-drug Coalitions of America, 2010
[*Proposition 19: A losing proposition for California's youth*, press release]

The overwhelming majority of what is written about alcohol, drugs, and youth focuses on the developmental danger to, drug use epidemiology

of, and professional treatment for young people. Our national preoccu-
pation with the negative aspects of drugs and youth obscures a lesser-
known but very positive development that young people are entering
long-term recovery probably in greater numbers than ever before. The
key word here is "probably" because we know precious little about the
phenomenon of young people who recover from alcohol and drug addiction. This section is intended as a preliminary exploration of the subject,
and a call for a redirection of policy and resources to underwrite more
funding for adolescent addiction treatment and recovery support services.

Recovery Support

12-Step Programs

Although Alcoholics Anonymous is generally regarded as oriented
towards adults, and in particular adults in middle age, the 2007 general
membership survey of more than 8,000 randomly selected members of
Alcoholics Anonymous revealed that 2.3% are below the age of 21 and
11.3% are age 21 to 30. With approximately 1.3 million members in the
United States, this translates to 30,000 members under the age of 21 and
150,000 who are 21 to 30. A similar survey conducted by Narcotics Anonymous in 2008 of 11,723 members produced similar results. Two percent
of members surveyed were under 21 and 14% were 21 to 30 years old.

There are several 12-step methodologies targeting youth. The oldest,
young people's groups within Alcoholics Anonymous (AA), began appearing in the mid-1940s and an International Conference of Young People in
AA has been meeting annually since 1958. This annual event now draws
more than 3,000 young AA members from all over the United States.
Currently there are 66 different annual localized young people's AA
conferences taking play in nearly every state and area across the country (www.ypaa.info). A few 12-step-related organizations and programs
are also available online, including Teen Addiction Anonymous (www.
teenaddictionanonymous.com) and Teen Anon (www.teen-anon.com),
however the majority of websites and resources devoted to youth and
addictions are oriented to marketing and outreach for adolescent treatment programs. Two-thirds (66%) of adolescent treatment programs
have adopted a 12-step model and philosophy as key parts of their treatment process, making it the most widely used model for young people.

Recovery Schools

Another youth recovery trend is the growth of recovery high schools
and collegiate recovery communities. "Recovery schools exist at both

the high school and collegiate level. They provide academic services and assistance for students in recovery from drug and alcohol addiction. With embedded recovery supports, recovery schools provide students in recovery the opportunity to receive credit towards a high school diploma or a college degree" (Bourgeois, 2010 [In My Own Words: Celebrating Students' Stories of Recovery... A compilation of essays by high school and college students, *Addiction Technology Transfer Center Network*], pg. 3).

There are currently 30–35 recovery high schools and 15–18 collegiate recovery communities across the United States. This innovation first occurred in 1977 in dormitories at Brown University and a few years later at Rutgers University. As the concept grew it was recognized that there was a need for "sober schooling" for high school age students as well. The high school programs were formed mainly for adolescents who had been through formal substance use disorder treatment, in an attempt to avoid discharging youth from residential treatment back into the same school and social environment they left. Returning back to these same environments can produce academic challenges, continued connections to negative peer networks, and the availability of substances which are all significant relapse-risk factors for youth after drug treatment. The specialized services and supports in a recovery school can be the critical difference in sustaining long-term recovery.

A 2008 study of 17 recovery high schools demonstrated a significant reduction in substance use as well as in mental health symptoms among participating students. A specialized school setting for students in recovery provides a positive social and educational environment for young people conducive to their recovery. As one student said (Travis, 2010, [In My Own Words: Celebrating Students' Stories of Recovery... A compilation of essays by high school and college students, *Addiction Technology Transfer Center Network*], pg. 140):

> I am a junior and I have been at Hope Academy High School since I was a freshman. When I try to explain it to people at my former school, most people do not understand it. Hope Academy is a normal high school that is just based off of recovery. I think it's the best thing that has ever happened to me when it comes to school ... I was able to manage my sobriety and school in one building. I love Hope Academy and I love going to school today. I think that is so amazing that I am around a group of people that understand my everyday life.

Prior to 2002, recovery schools were developed in isolation, but in 2002 the Association of Recovery Schools (www.recoveryschools.org)

was formed with the intention of advocating, promoting, and strengthening schools across the country. The organization works to expand the number of schools across the country, because only 12 states currently have a recovery high school or collegiate recovery community.

The expansion of public recovery schools into new locations faces funding and legislative barriers that vary from state to state despite their effectiveness and positive success rates.

Recovery-Focused School Programs

In addition to formal peer-based recovery schools, there are also various forms of recovery-focused programming in high schools across the country. One of the most promising is a peer-to-peer prevention and recovery support model called "The Leadership Group," taking place at Central High School in Bridgeport, Connecticut. "The Leadership Group" was established not for the mainstream successful students, but rather for those at-risk students who were struggling with alcohol or drugs and other related issues like attendance, discipline, and academic performance trouble. The program, which was witnessed and documented on film by one of the authors, started in 2005 with just three students, and mainly through peer-to-peer outreach, at the end of the school year in June of 2010 the group had over 500 participating students helping one another live drug and alcohol free. The faculty also reports that in May 2010 they celebrated reaching 100 students who had been abstinent from drug and alcohol continuously for over a year; only a handful of these students received formal substance use disorder treatment.

"The Leadership Group" model is voluntary and consists of re-occurring weekly group meetings (facilitated by trained counselors) for students with a history of drug and alcohol problems. There is a positive and open culture where students share their lived experience to their groups and are given an opportunity to discuss, relate, and support one another. The group meetings take place during the school day during study hall periods for most of the students and focus on an abstinence-encouraged model. A recent, albeit preliminary, study of the program demonstrates signification improvements in attendance and grades, while discipline infractions have been significantly reduced. Other high schools in Bridgeport have begun to consider "The Leadership Group" model. Two more distant efforts, in Rochester, New York, and New Bedford, Massachusetts, have now begun the process to replicate this model in their local high schools as well. This is an example of a school and peer-based recovery support service for adolescents that works across the prevention, treatment, and recovery spectrum.

Recovery Support Services for Youth

In recent years, recovery support services (RSSs) have become increasingly important as an adjunct to formal treatment, as well as to create "recovery friendly" communities for those in recovery who do not participate in a treatment program. RSSs are often delivered by peers both paid and volunteer, and consist of a variety of non-clinical activities designed to support the maintenance of an alcohol- and drug-free lifestyle. Pre-recovery services such as sober cyber-cafes and homework clubs can help engage young people in recovery. Sober leisure activities such as dances and picnics can provide safe alternatives to keg parties and raves for those in early recovery.

The federal Center for Substance Abuse Treatment's Recovery Community Support Program has identified four types of RSSs:

Emotional support: Demonstrations of empathy, love, caring, and concern in such activities as peer mentoring and recovery coaching, as well as in recovery support groups

Informational support: Provision of health and wellness information; educational assistance; and help in acquiring new skills, ranging from life skills to skills in employment readiness and citizenship restoration (voting rights)

Instrumental support: Concrete assistance in task accomplishment, especially with stressful or unpleasant tasks such as filling out applications and obtaining entitlements, providing child care, or providing transportation to support-group meetings and clothing assistance outlets (clothing closets)

Companionship: Helping people in early recovery feel connected and enjoy being with others, especially in recreational activities in alcohol- and drug-free environments; this assistance is particularly crucial in early recovery, when little about abstaining from alcohol or drugs is reinforcing

RSSs are often delivered by recovery community organizations and recovery networks that are established expressly for this purpose. One of the few such programs for adolescents in recovery is *FreeMind* based at the Pima Prevention Partnership in Tucson, Arizona. *FreeMind's* mission is to create safe meeting places and attendant support for youth in substance use disorder recovery. It is a voluntary, peer-led recovery support network for youth that regularly involves peers in program planning and providing feedback. Youth educate each other about substance use and participate in recovery events throughout Southern Arizona. *FreeMind* provides a variety of services including

472

groups sessions that follow a flexible life skills curriculum, harm reduction training, after school hours/Cyber Cafe, and movie nights, games, occasional weekend events and outings.

Evaluation findings from a federal Recovery Community Services Program grant demonstrate that the program produces significant outcomes. During a 21-month period, 197 predominantly minority participants completed both intake and 6-month follow-up evaluations. Overall, 82% of participating youth sustained or initiated the recovery process after starting *FreeMind*. Similarly, illegal activity decreased by 57%. Respondent data also demonstrates a significant increase in social connection improvements between intake and 6-month follow-up.

Research

There has been very little empirical study of any of the methodologies cited here. One of the few peer-reviewed studies of adolescent 12-step involvement was conducted at two privately funded, adolescent inpatient substance use disorder treatment centers in metropolitan San Diego (Kelly et al. [Social recovery model: An 8-year investigation of adolescent 12-step involvement following inpatient treatment, *Alcoholism: Clinical and Experimental Research*, 32(8)], 2008). An intriguing suggestion of the study focuses on the issue of 12-step dosage. "Our investigation of thresholds of AA/NA attendance in relation to outcomes suggests that youth may benefit from even limited exposure to treatment" (p. 8). The study reports that "highly intensive adult-derived clinical recommendations [of 12-step participation] may not be critical for this age group," and that "adolescents may not need to attend as frequently as their more chronically dependent older adult counterparts so as to obtain similar outcomes" (pp. 8–9).

Chapter 40

Know Your Rights When in Recovery from Substance Abuse

The Federal Nondiscrimination Laws That Protect You

I am in recovery from substance abuse, but I still face discrimination because of my addiction history. Does any law protect me? Yes. Federal civil rights laws prohibit discrimination in many areas of life against qualified "individuals with disabilities." Many people with past and current alcohol problems and past drug use disorders, including those in treatment for these illnesses, are protected from discrimination by the following:

- The Americans with Disabilities Act (ADA)
- The Rehabilitation Act of 1973
- The Fair Housing Act (FHA)
- The Workforce Investment Act (WIA)

Who Is Protected?

These nondiscrimination laws discussed protect individuals with a "disability." Under these federal laws, an individual with a "disability" is someone who has a current "physical or mental impairment" that "substantially limits" one or more of that person's "major life

---

Excerpted from "Know Your Rights," Substance Abuse and Mental Health Services Administration, Center for Substance Abuse Treatment (www.samhsa .gov), 2007. Reviewed by David A. Cooke, MD, FACP, July 2013.

activities," such as caring for one's self, working, etc.; has a record of such a substantially limiting impairment; or is regarded as having such an impairment.

- Whether a particular person has a "disability" is decided on an individualized, case-by-case basis.

- Substance use disorders (addiction) are recognized as impairments that can and do, for many individuals, substantially limit the individual's major life activities. For this reason, many courts have found that individuals experiencing or who are in recovery from these conditions are individuals with a "disability" protected by federal law.

- To be protected as an individual with a "disability" under federal nondiscrimination laws, a person must show that his or her addiction substantially limits (or limited, in the past) major life activities.

- People wrongly believed to have a substance use disorder (in the past or currently) may also be protected as individuals "regarded as" having a disability.

Who Is Not Protected?

- People who currently engage in the illegal use of drugs are not protected under these nondiscrimination laws, except that individuals may not be denied health services (including drug rehabilitation) based on their current illegal use of drugs if they are otherwise entitled to those services.

- People whose use of alcohol or drugs poses a direct threat—a significant risk of substantial harm—to the health or safety of others are not protected.

- People whose use of alcohol or drugs does not significantly impair a major life activity are not protected (unless they show they have a "record of" or are "regarded as" having a substance use disorder—addiction—that is substantially limiting).

What Is, and Is Not, Illegal Discrimination?

- Discriminating against someone on the basis of his or her disability—for example, just because he has a past drug addiction or she is in an alcohol treatment program—may be illegal discrimination.

- Acting against a person for reasons other than having a disability is not generally illegal discrimination, even if the disability is related to the cause of the adverse action.

For instance, it is not likely to be ruled unlawful discrimination if someone in substance abuse treatment or in recovery is denied a job, services, or benefits because he does not meet essential eligibility requirements; is unable to do the job; creates a direct threat to health or safety by his behavior, even if the behavior is caused by a substance use disorder; or violates rules or commits a crime, including a drug- or alcohol-related one, when that misconduct is cause for excluding or disciplining anyone doing it.

Since the basis for the negative action in these cases is not (or not solely) the person's disability, these actions do not violate federal nondiscrimination laws.

Employment

Are people in treatment for or in recovery from substance use disorders protected from job discrimination? The answer in many cases is yes. The Americans with Disabilities Act and the Rehabilitation Act prohibit most employers from refusing to hire, firing, or discriminating in the terms and conditions of employment against any qualified job applicant or employee on the basis of a disability.

- The ADA applies to all state and local governmental units, and to private employers with 15 or more employees.

- The Rehabilitation Act applies to federal employers and other public and private employers who receive federal grants, contracts, or aid.

Rights: In general, these employers must follow these criteria:

- May not deny a job to or fire a person because he or she is in treatment or in recovery from a substance use disorder, unless the person's disorder would prevent safe and competent job performance.

- Must provide "reasonable accommodations," when needed, to enable those with a disability to perform their job duties. Changing work hours to let an employee attend treatment is one kind of a reasonable accommodation. (But if an accommodation would cause the employer undue hardship—significant difficulty or expense—it is not required.)

- Must keep confidential any medical-related information they discover about a job applicant or employee, including information about a past or present substance use disorder.

Limits: The nondiscrimination laws protect only applicants and employees. Remember, people who pose a direct threat to health or safety, or have committed misconduct warranting job discipline, are not protected.

Medical Inquiries and Examinations

As a general rule, employers must follows these specifics:

- May not use information they learn about an individual's disability in a discriminatory manner—they may not deny or treat anyone less favorably in the terms and conditions of employment if he or she is qualified to perform the job

- Must maintain the confidentiality of all information they obtain about applicants' and employees' health conditions

Before making a job offer, employers may not ask the following:

- Questions about whether a job applicant has or has had a disability, or about the nature or severity of an applicant's disability—pre-offer medical examinations also are illegal

- Whether a job applicant is or has ever abused or been addicted to drugs or alcohol, or if the applicant is being treated by a substance abuse rehabilitation program or has received such treatment in the past

Employers may ask job applicants these things:

- Whether the applicant currently is using drugs illegally

- Whether the applicant drinks alcohol

- Whether the applicant can perform the duties of the job

After making a job offer, employers may do the following:

- Make medical inquiries and require an individual to undergo a medical examination (including ones that reveal a past or current substance use disorder), as long as all those offered the position are given the same exam

- Condition employment on the satisfactory results of such medical inquiries or exams

478

After employment begins, employers may make medical inquiries or require an employee to undergo a medical examination, but only when doing this is job related and justified by business necessity.

Such exams and inquiries may be permitted if the employer has a reasonable belief, based on objective evidence, that an employee has a health (including substance use–related) condition that impairs his or her ability to perform essential job functions or that poses a direct threat to health or safety.

Workplace Drug Testing

Employers are permitted to test both job applicants and employees for illegal use of drugs and may refuse to hire—or may fire or discipline—anyone whose test reveals such illegal use.

Employers may not fire or refuse to hire any job applicant or employee solely because a drug test reveals the presence of a lawfully used medication (such as methadone).

Employers must keep confidential information they discover about an employee's use of lawfully prescribed medications.

Medical Leave

Do I have the right to take medical leave from my job if I need it for substance abuse treatment? Yes, in many workplaces, you do.

Rights: The Family and Medical Leave Act (FMLA) gives many employees the right to take up to 12 weeks of unpaid leave in a 12-month period when needed to receive treatment for a "serious health condition" —which, under the FMLA, may include "substance abuse." The leave must be for treatment; absence because of the employee's use of the substance does not qualify for leave.

Neither the FMLA nor federal non-discrimination laws make it illegal for an employer to fire or discipline an employee for a legitimate non-discriminatory reason, even when the employee is granted or entitled to leave under these laws or under the employer's personnel policy. This means an employee who violates workplace rules or who uses drugs illegally still can be fired for those reasons.

Housing

Am I also protected from discrimination when it comes to renting or buying housing? The Fair Housing Act (FHA) makes discrimination in housing and real estate transactions illegal when it is based on a disability. The FHA protects people with past and current alcohol addiction and past drug addiction—although other federal laws sometimes limit their rights. The FHA does not protect people who currently engage in illegal drug use.

Rights: Landlords and other housing providers may not refuse to rent or sell housing to people in recovery or who have current alcohol disorders, and may not discriminate in other ways against them in housing transactions solely on the basis of their disability.

Limits on public housing eligibility: Federal law limits some people's eligibility for public and other federally assisted housing because of past or current substance use–related conduct. The Quality Housing and Work Responsibility Act requires the following of public housing agencies, Section 8, and other federally assisted housing providers:

- They must exclude any person evicted from public housing because of drug-related criminal activity (including possession or sale). A public housing agency can lift of shorten the three-year bar if the individual successfully completes a rehabilitation program.

- They must exclude any household with a member who is abusing alcohol or using drugs in a manner that may interfere with the health, safety, or right to peaceful enjoyment of the premises by other residents. Exceptions can be made if the individual demonstrates that he or she is not currently abusing alcohol or using drugs illegally and has successfully completed a rehabilitation program.

- Applicants for public housing may be denied admission if a member of the household has engaged in any drug-related criminal activity (or certain other criminal activity) within a "reasonable time" of the application.

How You Can Protect Your Rights

Is there anything I can do to protect my rights under these federal non-discrimination laws? Yes. If you believe you are being or have been discriminated against because of your past or current alcohol disorder or past drug use disorder, you can challenge the violation of your rights in two ways:

- You may file a complaint with the Office of Civil Rights, or similar office, of the federal agency(s) with power to investigate and remedy violations of the disability discrimination laws. You do not need a lawyer to do this. Filing with the government can be faster and easier than a lawsuit and get you the same remedies. However, the deadline for filing these complaints can be as soon as 180 days after the discriminatory act—or even sooner, with federal employers.

- In most (but not all) cases, you also may file a lawsuit in federal or state court, in addition to or instead of filing an administrative complaint. Deadlines for lawsuits vary from one to three years following the discriminatory act.

- You must file employment discrimination claims under the ADA with the U.S. Equal Opportunity Employment Commission (EEOC). You may not file a lawsuit first or instead of filing with the EEOC.

If your complaint is upheld, the persons or organizations that discriminated against you may be required to correct their actions and policies, compensate you, or give you other relief.

Chapter 41

Employee Assistance Programs (EAPs) for Substance Abuse

Chapter Contents

Section 41.1

Employee Assistance Programs Overview

"Drug-Free Workplace Advisor: Employee Assistance Program," Department of Labor Office of the Assistant Secretary for Policy (www.dol.gov/elaws/asp/drugfree), 2003. Reviewed by David A. Cooke, MD, FACP, July 2013.

How does an EAP (Employee Assistance Program) support your drug-free workplace program?

An Employee Assistance Program offers other valuable services to the organization that go beyond those of a drug-free workplace program. An EAP can complement and support your drug-free workplace program in a unique way. By encouraging employees to seek assistance with a variety of emotional issues and day-to-day problems, employee assistance professionals are in a position to identify employees who have developed problems with drugs and/or alcohol before there are problems at work. Furthermore, an EAP gives supervisors tools for dealing with troubled employees, while allowing them to remain focused on employees' work performance, rather than on employees' personal lives.

The EAP component of a drug-free workplace program maximizes the health and efficiency of the workforce while conveying a caring attitude on the part of the employer. Organizations that have EAPs as part of their drug-free workplace program have adopted a prevention and treatment approach to alcohol and drug problems. This means that employees are encouraged to come forward on their own to seek help, and those who are identified as using prohibited drugs are offered treatment and education. By addressing personal problems early, EAPs can help prevent employees from starting to use alcohol or drugs in misguided attempts to relieve pressure and stress. The EAP can help to properly assess and refer the employee who has problems to the most appropriate level of help.

The EAP supports three important ideas in a drug-free workplace:

1. Employees are a vital part of business and valuable members of the team.

2. It is better to offer assistance to employees than to fire them.

3. Recovering employees can, once again, become productive and effective members of the workforce.

Including an EAP as part of your drug-free workplace reflects a concern about the well-being of employees and represents a distinctly different approach from that of "test and terminate." Employers who adopt the "test and terminate" approach attempt to achieve a drug-free workplace by eliminating and discarding drug-using employees without offering treatment or opportunities for recovery.

In addition to offering an EAP, employers can choose to help employees by allowing a reasonable period of time off the job to participate in treatment as well as adequate benefits coverage for the treatment of addiction. Even in the absence of a formal EAP, employers may make such benefits available and maintain a list of qualified therapists and treatment facilities that specialize in the treatment of alcoholism and drug addiction.

What are the goals of an EAP?

Employers implement EAPs to accomplish a variety of goals:

- Identify employee personal problems at an early stage before there is a serious impact on the job

- Motivate employees to seek help through easy access to assessment and referral

- Direct employees to the best source of help and high-quality providers

- Limit health insurance costs through early intervention

- Reduce workers' compensation claims by encouraging easy access to help

- Decrease employee turnover

- Offer an alternative to firing valuable employees

- Provide employees with support and demonstrate that a company is a caring employer

What are the essential components of an EAP?

An EAP should include these essential components:

- A policy statement that defines how employees access the EAP, the services provided, and how confidentiality is protected
- Consultation and training services for supervisors and managers on how to manage and refer troubled employees to the EAP
- Promotional activities to ensure the EAP is highly visible and easily accessible to employees.
- Educational programs for employees on relevant issues such as alcohol and drug addiction
- Problem identification and referral services provided directly to individual employees (and often to family members)
- Identification and maintenance of a current, annotated directory of qualified providers of treatment or assistance to enable prompt referral of employees to appropriate resources

Some EAPs also offer short-term counseling by licensed professionals.

What services does an EAP offer?

EAPs provide services to a variety of "customers" within the work organization. EAPs provide distinct but complementary services to each customer group—the employer or work organization, the supervisors/managers, and the employees.

Organizational services include the following:

- Assistance in developing alcohol and drug policies
- Consultation regarding legal compliance issues
- Design and selection of health benefit plans
- Evaluation of health care providers
- Compliance with drug-free workplace policies

Guidance to managers and supervisors includes these elements:

- How to make supervisor referrals based on declining job performance
- Separating performance issues from behavioral health issues
- Determining the need to intervene with troubled employees
- Following up on an employee's progress

486

Assistance provided directly to individual employees includes the following:

- General information and referral resources
- Crisis intervention
- Easy access to help
- Timely problem identification
- Short-term problem resolution
- Substance abuse assessments
- Referral for diagnosis and treatment or other kinds of help
- Follow-up contacts or sessions to provide support
- Educational seminars and workshops

In addition to addressing alcohol and drug addiction problems and at no additional cost, most EAPs also help employees with these concerns:

- Marital/relationship problems
- Job stress
- Child care issues
- Grief
- Financial problems
- Legal concerns
- Elder care issues

How does an EAP help employees?

EAPs target both employees whose performance shows a pattern of decline that is not readily explained by job circumstances and employees who are aware of personal problems that may or may not be affecting their performance.

Any employee can seek assistance from the EAP to get information or to discuss a personal problem. Approximately 4% to 6% of employees will contact the EAP on their own every year. In fact, most employees who use the EAP seek these services on their own. However, employees with job performance problems who do not contact the EAP are of most concern to supervisors. When a supervisor refers a troubled employee to the EAP, the supervisor does not have to wait until the problem is job threatening. Having an EAP allows supervisors to combine their offers of assistance with early disciplinary measures to help restore performance.

The EAP systematically and effectively approaches workplace and personal problems. The employee assistance professional meets privately with the employee, discusses the issues with the employee, and helps identify the problem. The EAP then explores available options and refers the employee to appropriate resources that may be available in the community or professional services covered under the employee benefit plan.

Most EAPs offer services not only to employees but also to their dependent family members. This proves to be a wise investment because the work performance of an employee can be affected when a parent, spouse, or child is abusing alcohol and other drugs.

How does an EAP work?

Employees can directly access the EAP voluntarily or be referred by their supervisor in cases of job-performance problems. When an employee uses EAP services voluntarily, there is no need for involvement on the part of the supervisor. However, when a supervisor refers an employee to the EAP because of job performance, the offer of help may be combined with progressive discipline, and the supervisor will need to continue to monitor the employee's performance.

How is confidentiality protected?

Employees will support and have faith in your program only if their confidentiality is protected. The assurance of confidentiality means that an employee's private and personal information will not be released to anyone other than with whom the employee confides.

As with any performance problem, the employee needs to be aware that the issue of his/her performance problems will not be made public. Although his/her supervisors may share information about disciplinary action with other managers or the human resources department, all information about performance issues, constructive confrontation, and disciplinary actions should be maintained in the employee's personnel file. In addition, access should be strictly limited to those in management with a need to know.

The EAP should assure employees that their personal information and details of their personal problems will not go beyond the EAP. Private conversations with the EAP should not be shared with supervisors and EAP records must be kept completely separate from personnel records. These records should be protected by the EAP's confidentiality policy and should not be released without the employee's expressed, written permission.

In some instances, it may be in the employee's best interest for information to be shared; however, this information should not be shared without a written release. Some examples of circumstances when an employee may request release of information include these:

- Releasing information so that benefits can be accessed or insurance companies can conduct reviews.

- Releasing information regarding EAP participation if the employee was referred by the supervisor based on declining job performance.

- Releasing information to support a request for accommodation or recovery support.

- Releasing information of assessment, evaluation, and follow-through following a positive drug test when the employee will be given an opportunity to return to the job.

- Releasing information according to company policy for verification for treatment release time, leave requests, and disability.

There also are limited areas where state laws require disclosure. These are circumstances where someone is in imminent danger, such as in cases of child abuse, elder abuse, or serious threats of homicide or suicide.

The EAP policy must be very clear about the limits of what information can be shared and with whom it can be shared. If an employee chooses to tell co-workers about his or her private concerns, that is a personal decision. However, when an employee tells a supervisor something in confidence, the supervisor is obligated to protect that disclosure.

Section 41.2

Employer Benefits for EAPs for Substance Abuse

"Issue Brief #9: An EAP that Addresses Substance Abuse Can Save You Money," Substance Abuse and Mental Health Services Administration, Center for Substance Abuse Treatment (www.samhsa.gov), 2008. Reviewed by David A. Cooke, MD, FACP, July 2013.

Substance use disorders can negatively affect an employer's bottom line by increasing health care costs and reducing productivity. But employers have a simple and cost-effective tool available for addressing these risks: a workplace substance abuse program administered through an EAP.

EAPs are designed to help identify and resolve productivity problems affecting employees who are impaired by personal concerns. EAPs come in many different forms, from telephone-based to on-site programs. Face-to-face programs provide more comprehensive services for employees with substance use disorders, including confidential screening, treatment referrals, and follow-up care. Assuring that workers with substance use disorders receive treatment can help employers save money. Intervening early can prevent the need for more intensive treatment and hospitalizations down the road.

Employers See Savings When EAPs Address Substance Abuse

Through the Federal Occupational Health EAP, 80% of federal workers and their family members who received treatment for alcohol or drug problems reported improvements in work attendance. A majority also reported improvements in both work performance and social relationships. ChevronTexaco found that from 1990 to 1996, 75% of employees who entered the company EAP with alcohol problems were able to retain their employment, saving the company the cost of recruiting and training new employees. Gillette Company saw a 75% drop in inpatient substance abuse treatment costs after implementing an EAP. A large international holding company found that employees who used

490

an EAP for help with mental health and substance use problems had fewer inpatient medical days than those who only participated in the company's medical insurance plan. In addition, the company saved an average of $426,000 each year on mental health and substance abuse treatment as a result of employees' participation in the EAP.

How Substance Abuse Impacts the Workplace

Substance abuse costs the nation an estimated $276 billion a year. Lost work productivity and excess health care expenses account for the majority of those costs. The magnitude of the cost, coupled with the fact that 76% of people with drug or alcohol problems are in the workforce, gives employers a major stake in ensuring that employees have access to treatment.

Substance abuse by employees results in the following:

- Higher health care expenses for injuries and illnesses

- More absenteeism

- Reductions in job productivity and performance

- More workers' compensation and disability claims

- Increased safety, and other, risks for employers

Conducting random drug testing and firing offending employees can have a short-term impact but may ultimately be more costly because the cost of replacing employees is high and the risk remains that new employees may also abuse drugs or alcohol.

How to Hire an EAP

1. Develop specifications and request proposals from several EAP vendors.

2. Evaluate their capabilities, for example, the range of services they offer, the types of clients they currently serve, and their ability to meet your company's specific needs.

3. Include performance standards in your EAP contract so you can measure the effectiveness of your investment.

EAPs Can Reduce Costs Related to Substance Abuse

EAPs address a wide variety of concerns that may negatively affect job performance, including mental health issues, financial and legal problems, career advancement, and other personal problems. EAPs can do the following:

- Screen for risky behaviors involving alcohol and drugs
- Educate employees about the health consequences of substance use
- When necessary, refer employees for appropriate treatment
- Provide support services that address recovery and the chronic nature of addiction

Incorporating a substance abuse component into an EAP can help reduce absenteeism, improve employee health and job performance, and reduce medical costs, all of which save employers money.

Chapter 42

Drug Abuse Treatment in the Criminal Justice System

Chapter Contents

Section 42.1

Drug Courts

Excerpted from "Drug Courts," White House Office of National
Drug Control Policy (www.whitehouse.gov/ondcp), October 2011.

Drug courts, which combine treatment with incentives and sanctions, mandatory and random drug testing, and aftercare, are a proven tool for improving public health and public safety. They provide an innovative mechanism for promoting collaboration among the judiciary, prosecutors, community corrections agencies, drug treatment providers, and other community support groups. These special courts have been operating in the United States for more than 20 years, and their effectiveness is well documented. In times of serious budget cuts, the drug court model offers state and local governments a cost-effective way to increase the percentage of addicted offenders who achieve sustained recovery, thereby improving public safety and reducing costs associated with re-arrest and additional incarceration. Every dollar spent on drug courts yields more than two dollars in savings in the criminal justice system alone. With more than 2,600 drug courts in operation today, approximately 120,000 Americans annually receive the help they need to break the cycle of addiction and recidivism.

Drug court programs have a tangible effect on criminal recidivism. In a recent Department of Justice study, drug court participants reported 25% less criminal activity and had 16% fewer arrests than comparable offenders not enrolled in drug courts. In addition, 26% fewer drug court participants reported drug use and were 37% less likely to test positive for illicit substances.

Additionally, an analysis of drug court cost-effectiveness conducted by the Urban Institute found that drug courts provided $2.21 in benefits to the criminal justice system for every $1 invested. When expanding the program to all at-risk arrestees, the average return on investment increased even more, resulting in a benefit of $3.36 for every $1 spent.

A review of five independent meta-analyses concluded that drug courts significantly reduce crime by an average of 8 to 26 percentage points; well-administered drug courts were found to reduce crime rates by as much as 35%, compared to traditional case dispositions.

The Drug Court Model: Best Practices

Drug court participants are provided intensive treatment and other services for a minimum of one year. There are frequent court appearances and random drug testing, with sanctions and incentives to encourage compliance and completion. Successful completion of the treatment program results in dismissal of the charges, reduced or set-aside sentences, lesser penalties, or a combination of these. Most important, graduating participants gain the necessary tools to rebuild their lives.

Because the problem of drugs and crime is much too broad for any single agency to tackle alone, drug courts rely upon the daily communication and cooperation of judges, court personnel, probation, treatment providers, and providers of other social services. Drug courts vary somewhat in terms of their structure, scope, and target populations, but they all share three primary goals:

1. Reduced recidivism rates

2. Reduced substance use among participants

3. Rehabilitation of participants

Achieving these goals requires adherence to the core organizational structure and attributes of the drug court model. This model, which has successfully been replicated in thousands of courtrooms nationwide, includes the following key components:

- Integration of alcohol and other drug treatment services within justice system case processing

- A non-adversarial approach, through which prosecution and defense counsel promote public safety while protecting participants' due process rights

- Early identification of eligible participants and prompt placement in the drug court

- Access to a continuum of alcohol, drug and other treatment, and rehabilitation services

- Frequent alcohol and other drug testing to monitor abstinence

- A coordinated strategy governing drug court responses to participants' compliance or noncompliance

- Ongoing judicial interaction with each participant

- Monitoring and evaluation to measure achievement of program goals and gauge effectiveness

- Continuing interdisciplinary education to promote effective drug court planning, implementation, and operations

- Forging of partnerships among drug courts, public agencies, and community-based organizations to generate local support and enhance drug court program effectiveness

Drug courts following these tenets reduce recidivism and promote other positive outcomes. The magnitude of a court's impact may depend upon how well the practitioners address and balance these core components and adapt to the needs of their clients and court staff.

Connecting Drug Courts to Law Enforcement

A strong partnership with local law enforcement is a critical component of a successful drug court. Street-level enforcement officers provide a unique perspective and benefit to drug court teams. Law enforcement can improve referrals to the court and extend the connection of the drug court team into the community for further information gathering and monitoring of participants. Law enforcement personnel play important roles not only in the day-to-day operations of the drug court, but also in showing other government and community leaders the public safety efficacy of these courts.

A comprehensive study of the key attributes of successful drug courts reinforces the importance of this relationship. In the 18 adult drug courts studied, researchers found the following:

- Having a member from law enforcement on the team was associated with higher graduation rates, compared to teams without a law enforcement member (57% versus 46%).

- Drug court teams that included law enforcement personnel reduced costs an additional 36% over the reductions achieved by traditional drug courts.

In recognition of the importance of law enforcement participation in the drug court process, the National Association of Drug Court Professionals' (NADCP) National Drug Court Institute (NDCI) has created a National Law Enforcement Task Force. This task force is designed to increase the involvement of law enforcement personnel in the drug court process and gather critical input from key law enforcement leaders across the country. The task force has representatives from a number of law enforcement organizations.

To further educate and expand law enforcement involvement in drug courts, NDCI is developing a curriculum for law enforcement personnel. This curriculum will include information on the medical aspects of addiction, treatment, and recovery and how to engage substance abuse service providers.

Section 42.2

Alternatives to Incarceration for Substance Abuse Offenders

"Alternatives to Incarceration," White House Office of National Drug Control Policy (www.whitehouse.gov/ondcp), August 2011.

Nearly seven million American adults are under supervision of the state and federal criminal justice systems. Approximately two million of these individuals are incarcerated for their crimes, while the remaining five million are supervised through probation or parole. For states and localities across the country, the costs of managing these populations have grown significantly. More important, these offenders can place a burden on the health, safety, and well-being of their families, their communities, and themselves. Despite the significant costs, too many offenders are unable to remain drug and crime free upon their reentry into society.

Federal, state, and local leaders are looking for innovative ways to improve public health and public safety outcomes while reducing the costs of criminal justice and corrections. The administration's National Drug Control Strategy recognizes that addiction is a disease and that the criminal justice system can play a vital role in reducing the costs and consequences of crimes committed by drug-involved offenders. With an increasing body of evidence suggesting the right combination of policies and strategies can break the cycle of arrest, incarceration, release, and rearrest, the strategy promotes several alternatives to incarceration that can save public funds and improve public health by keeping low-risk, nonviolent, drug-involved offenders out of prison or jail, while still holding them accountable and ensuring the public safety of our communities.

Smart Probation Strategies

Probation officers often find themselves with large, unmanageable caseloads, while judges are forced to choose between sending repeat offenders away for long periods of time or ignoring probation or parole violations altogether. "Smart" justice systems now offer better, cheaper, and more effective options. More states and localities are implementing strategies to improve outcomes and reduce the burden of drug-involved offenders on their criminal justice and corrections systems. These innovative new programs include Alaska's Probationer Accountability with Certain Enforcement (PACE), Delaware's "Decide Your Time," and Arizona's "Swift, Accountable, Fair Enforcement" (SAFE) program.

Smart Probation—Project HOPE: Hawaii's Opportunity Probation with Enforcement (HOPE) program has shown promising results in reducing drug use and recidivism. Started in 2004, the HOPE program uses drug testing and swift, certain sanctions to change a probationer's drug using and criminal behavior, all under the supervision of a single judge. Researchers compared HOPE participants to probationers in a control group and after one year, the HOPE probationers were the following:

- 55% less likely to be arrested for a new crime

- 61% less likely to skip appointments with their supervisory officer

- 72% less likely to use drugs

- 53% less likely to have their probation revoked

HOPE costs approximately $2,500 per probationer. This is a minor increase over traditional probation, but it can realize considerable savings in incarceration, treatment, and other criminal justice costs.

Smart Probation—The 24/7 Sobriety Project: The 24/7 Sobriety Project is a court-based program designed to reduce the re-offense rates of repeat Driving Under the Influence (DUI) offenders. Started as a pilot in South Dakota in 2005, the 24/7 Project requires participants to maintain full sobriety, meaning no use of alcohol or illegal drugs, in order to keep their driving privileges and stay out of jail. The South Dakota attorney general's evaluation found offenders enrolled in 24/7 for at least 30 consecutive days are nearly 50% less likely to commit another DUI offense. Research also indicates these results are sustained over periods longer than those of more traditional interventions (i.e., ignition interlock devices).

Drug Courts

Operating in the U.S. for over 20 years, drug courts combine treatment with incentives and escalating sanctions, mandatory and random drug testing, and aftercare to reduce substance use and prevent crime among participants. These courts provide an intensive intervention that is well-suited for high-risk/high-need offenders, effectively meeting the public health and public safety needs of both the community and the drug-involved offender. In times of serious budget cuts for state and local governments, drug courts are another cost-effective investment that helps offenders on the road to recovery and reduce costs associated with incarceration and recidivism.

Part Six

Drug Abuse Testing and Prevention

Chapter 43

Effective Public Health Responses to Drug Abuse

The United States has historically suffered from some of the highest rates of drug abuse in the world and, as a result, has made unparalleled investments in demand reduction research and programming. Through hard experience, we have learned much about the nature of addiction and what works in prevention and treatment. Our policies are still evolving as we seek to incorporate components that deliver sustained, measurable results. The United States National Drug Control Strategy seeks to put resources where research and experience have proven that they can have the greatest effect in reducing the demand for drugs in America.

Anti-Drug Media Campaigns

Media campaigns work. Any country that intends to reduce drug abuse among its youth should dedicate resources to project consistent anti-drug messages out to their youth through the media. All over the world, parents, teachers, religious leaders, and others are struggling to compete with the volume of misleading messages and negative influences that young people are exposed to through the media, especially when it comes to drug use. Anti-drug media campaigns are an effective way to push back against these negative messages and "unsell" the idea of drug use to young people. Private corporations spend money on

Excerpted from "What Works? Effective Public Health Responses to Drug Use," National Criminal Justice Reference Service, U.S. Department of Justice (ncjrs.gov), March 2008. Revised by David A. Cooke, MD, FACP, July 2013.

advertising because they know it works. Anti-drug media campaigns, properly executed, will reduce drug use.

In the United States, the National Youth Anti-Drug Media Campaign has sought to turn youth attitudes against drug use and encourage increased parental engagement through national paid advertising and public communications outreach. The intent is to deliver clear, consistent, credible, and sustained anti-drug messages. Most of the advertising is created by the Partnership for a Drug-Free America [now Partnership at Drugfree.org], one of our most creative and effective advertising agencies.

The teen brand "Above the Influence" inspires young people to reject drug use by appealing to their sense of individuality and independence. All television advertisements are subject to a rigorous process of qualitative and quantitative testing, ensuring, before they are ever broadcast, that the advertisements are credible and have the intended effect on awareness, attitudes, and behaviors.

Since 2002, the campaign has been strategically focused on marijuana, as that is often the first illegal drug a young person will try, and studies show that preventing or delaying the onset of illegal drug use during youth significantly reduces the likelihood of substance abuse problems later in life. However, the abuse of prescription drugs by young people has increased over the past several years. In response, the campaign is addressing this emerging drug threat through a national effort to inform parents about the risky and growing abuse of prescription drugs by young people.

Drug-Free Communities Coalitions

In every country, drug problems vary from community to community, creating the need for local solutions to local problems. In the United States, the formation of Drug Free Communities (DFC) coalitions has proven to be an effective catalyst for reduced drug use among youth and increased citizen participation. The federally funded Drug Free Communities Support Program enables such coalitions to strengthen their coordination and prevention efforts, encourage citizen participation in substance abuse reduction efforts, and disseminate information about effective programs. The federal government is currently supporting 736 (FY 2007) local drug free community coalitions though this program, reaching 31% of all youth in grades 6–12 in the United States, Puerto Rico, and the U.S. Virgin Islands.

This initiative primarily targets youth, but there is also support for a number of local coalitions that focus on young adults aged 18–25, as well as support for efforts that assist parents and youth in mobilizing their communities to prevent youth alcohol, tobacco, prescription, and other drug abuse.

In order to support the growth and development of community-based coalitions, the Office of National Drug Control Policy contracts with a nongovernmental organization, Community Anti-Drug Coalitions of America (CADCA), to provide training and technical assistance through its National Coalition Institute. Originally formed in 1992 in response to the dramatic growth in the number of community coalitions and their need to share ideas, problems, and solutions, CADCA's National Coalition Institute not only supports emerging community coalitions, but it also works in partnership with ONDCP to help strengthen DFC-funded communities.

Understanding that there is no one-size-fits-all approach to protecting youth and strengthening communities to prevent drug use, Drug Free Communities promote creative local solutions. The result is that communities who receive funding and support through the Drug Free Communities program experience lower rates of substance use among their youth through their comprehensive, community-wide approach to substance abuse and its related problems.

Drug Testing in Schools and in the Workplace

Substance abuse problems take a terrible toll on the productivity of any country's population, undermining the role of the school as a place of learning and of the workplace as an engine of the economy. Random drug testing holds great promise both as a prevention tool and as an effective means of reducing the costs of drug abuse to society.

In schools, random student drug testing programs satisfy two important public health goals: the prevention and treatment of substance abuse. Student drug-testing programs are non-punitive. They are designed to 1) deter students from initiating drug use, 2) help identify students who have just begun to use drugs before a dependency begins, and 3) help identify students with a dependency so that they may be referred to appropriate treatment. Random student drug testing programs serve to both prevent substance abuse and expand the reach of treatment.

The power of random student drug testing as a prevention tool cannot be understated. The spread of drug use throughout a school often closely mirrors the way a disease is spread—from student-to-student contact, multiplying rapidly as more and more students are affected. Random testing can provide young people with a reason to never start using drugs that will be accepted by their peers—protecting them during a time when they are most vulnerable both to peer pressure and to the adverse health effects of drug use.

In the United States, the Supreme Court has upheld the authority of public schools to test students for illegal drugs, allowing random drug tests for all middle and high school students participating in competitive extracurricular activities, as well as those who, with a parent or guardian, consent to testing. In addition, in order for a student drug testing program to receive federal support, it must be part of a comprehensive drug prevention program, provide for referral to treatment or counseling, as appropriate, and ensure the confidentiality of its testing results.

The concept of testing for drug use as a prevention tool has been proven effective in the workplace, as well. The U.S. Department of Defense began testing its military personnel more than 25 years ago, and during that time the rate of positive tests among service members has fallen from nearly 30% to less than 2%. Drug testing has also proven effective in the broader workforce. As drug-free workplace programs have expanded, positive test rates have fallen, reaching the lowest point since 1988, according to Quest Diagnostics' Drug Testing Index.

However, workplace safety is the reason most commonly cited by employers for implementing drug testing programs. In fact, one study found that construction companies that tested for drug use experienced a 51% reduction in injury rates within two years of implementing their drug testing programs. Studies have also clearly demonstrated the impact that drug abuse can have on workplace productivity if left unchecked. A 2000 Substance Abuse and Mental Health Services Administration (SAMHSA) study revealed that workers who reported past-month illicit drug use were more likely than those who did not report such use to say the following: they had more than three employers in the past year (5.7% vs. 2.3%), they had missed work for more than two days in the past month due to illness or injury (11.6% vs. 6.5%), and they had skipped work more than two days in the past month (4.4% vs. 1.6%).

Screening, Brief Intervention, and Referral to Treatment

Millions of people around the world suffer from serious problems with addiction, but the vast majority likely are not aware that they need help. In the United States alone, the National Survey on Drug Use and Health estimates that there are more than 20 million individuals who meet the medical definition of abuse or addiction to alcohol or drugs. Of this number, more than 94% do not realize they need help and have not sought treatment or other professional care.

It is estimated that 180 million Americans age 18 or older see a health care provider at least once a year, which gives the health care community the potential to become a powerful tool in identifying substance abuse problems—or potential problems—and intervening as appropriate. With a few carefully worded questions using an evidence-based questionnaire, health care providers can learn a great deal about whether a patient is at risk for problems related to substance abuse. Depending on the answers to these questions, physicians can intervene with a brief, nonjudgmental motivational conversation about the dangers of substance abuse and ways to overcome it—or, on the other end of the spectrum, if a patient's screening score falls in the range associated with addiction, the patient can be referred to specialty treatment for a more extensive and longer period of care.

The great promise of screening is not just in that it is highly effective, it also does not require an expensive or new comprehensive mechanism to institute. Screening can be added, or "mainstreamed," into the existing medical infrastructure of each country. Although it is always true that it takes more than one initiative to cause sustained positive change, screening in and of itself has tremendous potential to transform an entire nation's drug abuse problem.

In the United States, the federal government is actively supporting the adoption of screening and brief intervention practices in the medical community through a demonstration program administered by SAMHSA. The federally funded Screening, Brief Intervention, and Referral to Treatment (SBIRT) program is supporting screening and brief intervention activities in hospitals, primary care settings, colleges, and one tribal council. As of December 2007, more than 577,436 clients in 11 states had been screened. Approximately 23% received a score that triggered the need for further assistance. Of this number, 15.9% received a brief intervention, 3.1% received brief drug treatment, and only 3.6% required referral to specialized drug treatment programs.

Outcome measures from the federal program reveal that screening and brief intervention helps reduce substance abuse and related consequences, including emergency room and trauma center visits and deaths. By encouraging health care professionals to identify at-risk populations and intervene early, we can significantly reduce alcohol and drug abuse and possibly prevent an individual in need of help from ever reaching the point of addiction.

Improving Access to Treatment and Recovery

As screening and brief intervention services bring more of those in need into contact with the treatment system, we must ensure that treatment providers have the capacity to serve these individuals. The United States has tried to close this "treatment gap" through an initiative known as "Access to Recovery," or ATR. ATR expands substance abuse treatment capacity, promotes choices in both recovery paths and services, increases the number and types of providers, allows clients through the use of voucher systems to play a more significant role in the development of their treatment plans, and links clinical treatment with important recovery support services such as transportation, mentoring, and child care.

Flexibility is one of the hallmarks of the Access to Recovery initiative. A grant program administered by SAMHSA, ATR allows states and tribal organizations to tailor programs to meet their primary treatment needs. In Texas, ATR has been used to target the state's criminal justice population, which generally has been underserved in the area of drug treatment. Tennessee has used its ATR funds to target those whose primary addiction is methamphetamine. The voucher component of the program allows individuals to choose among eligible clinical treatment and recovery support providers—including, for the first time, faith-based and community-based providers—thereby empowering Americans to be active in their recovery.

How ATR Works in the United States

- Those individuals seeking drug and alcohol treatment and recovery support are assessed and receive a voucher to pay for a range of appropriate services.

- The states work with a consortium of public and private entities to jointly administer the program, distribute vouchers, and deliver alcohol and drug treatment and other services.

- States are required to monitor client outcomes and to make adjustments based on the cost-effectiveness of services received.

- Accountability is achieved by linking reimbursement for services to demonstrated abstinence from drug and alcohol use by clients after discharge.

As of September 30, 2007, more than 190,000 people with substance use disorders had received clinical treatment and/or recovery support services through ATR, exceeding the three-year target of 125,000. Approximately 65% of the clients for whom status and discharge data are available have received recovery support services, which, though critical for recovery, are not typically funded through other federal grant programs. As a result of ATR, states and tribal organizations have expanded the number of providers of treatment and recovery support services. Faith-based organizations, which generally do not receive funding from state governments for substance abuse treatment, have received approximately 32% of ATR funds. These organizations offer a unique and compassionate approach to people in need.

Drug Courts

As in the rest of the world, substance abuse problems in the United States often go hand in hand with criminal behavior. For nonviolent drug offenders whose underlying problem is substance use, drug treatment courts combine the power of the justice system with effective treatment services to break the cycle of criminal behavior, alcohol and drug use, child abuse and neglect, and incarceration. Drug courts have proven to be one of the most successful demand reduction initiatives in the United States. Today, there are more than 2,000 drug courts in operation in the United States, and additional drug courts have been established in 10 other countries.

The objective of drug courts is to stop alcohol abuse, drug abuse, and related criminal activity by offenders. Drug courts handle cases involving drug-addicted offenders through an extensive supervision and treatment program. In exchange for successful completion of the program, the court may dismiss the original charge, reduce or set aside a sentence, offer some lesser penalty, or offer a combination of these. Some drug courts are co-located on the grounds of residential treatment facilities, reducing additional barriers to recovery.

Chapter 44

Drug Abuse Prevention Begins at Home

Chapter Contents

Section 44.1

Talking to Your Child about Drugs

Just as you inoculate your kids against illnesses like measles, you can help "immunize" them against drug use by giving them the facts before they're in a risky situation.

When kids don't feel comfortable talking to parents, they're likely to seek answers elsewhere, even if their sources are unreliable. Kids who aren't properly informed are at greater risk of engaging in unsafe behaviors and experimenting with drugs. Parents who are educated about the effects of drug use and learn the facts can help correct any misconceptions children may have.

Make talking about drugs a part of your general health and safety conversations with your child. Parents are role models for their children so your views on alcohol, tobacco, and drugs can strongly influence the views of your child.

Preschool to Age 7

Before you get nervous about talking to young kids, take heart. You've probably already laid the groundwork for a discussion. For instance, whenever you give a fever medication or an antibiotic to your child, you have the opportunity to discuss the benefits and the appropriate and responsible use of those drugs. This is also a time when your child is likely to be very attentive to your behavior and guidance.

Start taking advantage of "teachable moments" now. If you see a character on a billboard or on TV with a cigarette, talk about smoking, nicotine addiction, and what smoking does to a person's body. This can lead into a discussion about other drugs and how they can potentially cause harm.

Keep the tone of these discussions calm and use terms that your child can understand. Be specific about the effects of the drugs: how they make a person feel, the risk of overdose, and the other long-term damage they can cause. To give your kids these facts, you might have to do a little research.

Ages 8 to 12

As your kids grow older, you can begin conversations with them by asking them what they think about drugs. By asking the questions in a nonjudgmental, open-ended way, you're more likely to get an honest response.

Kids this age usually are still willing to talk openly to their parents about touchy subjects. Establishing a dialogue now helps keep the door open as kids get older and are less inclined to share their thoughts and feelings.

Even if your question doesn't immediately result in a discussion, you'll get your kids thinking about the issue. If you show your kids that you're willing to discuss the topic and hear what they have to say, they might be more willing to come to you for help in the future.

News, such as steroid use in professional sports, can be springboards for casual conversations about current events. Use these discussions to give your kids information about the risks of drugs.

Ages 13 to 17

Kids this age are likely to know other kids who use alcohol or drugs, and to have friends who drive. Many are still willing to express their thoughts or concerns with parents about it.

Use these conversations not only to understand your child's thoughts and feelings, but also to talk about the dangers of driving under the influence of drugs or alcohol. Talk about the legal issues—jail time and fines—and the possibility that they or someone else might be killed or seriously injured.

Consider establishing a written or verbal contract on the rules about going out or using the car. You can promise to pick your kids up at any time (even 2:00 a.m.!) no questions asked if they call you when the person responsible for driving has been drinking or using drugs.

The contract also can detail other situations: For example, if you find out that someone drank or used drugs in your car while your son or daughter was behind the wheel, you may want to suspend driving privileges for six months. By discussing all of this with your kids from the start, you eliminate surprises and make your expectations clear.

513

Laying Good Groundwork

No parent, child, or family is immune to the effects of drugs. Some of the best kids can end up in trouble, even when they have made an effort to avoid it and even when they have been given the proper guidance from their parents.

However, certain groups of kids may be more likely to use drugs than others. Kids who have friends who use drugs are likely to try drugs themselves. Those feeling socially isolated for whatever reason may turn to drugs.

So it's important to know your child's friends—and their parents. Be involved in your children's lives. If your child's school runs an anti-drug program, get involved. You might learn something! Pay attention to how your kids are feeling and let them know that you're available and willing to listen in a nonjudgmental way. Recognize when your kids are going through difficult times so that you can provide the support they need or seek additional care if it's needed.

Role-playing can help your child develop strategies to turn down drugs if they are offered. Act out possible scenarios they may encounter. Helping them construct phrases and responses to say no prepares them to know how to respond before they are even in that situation.

A warm, open family environment—where kids are encouraged to talk about their feelings, where their achievements are praised, and where their self-esteem is bolstered—encourages kids to come forward with their questions and concerns. When censored in their own homes, kids go elsewhere to find support and answers to their most important questions.

Make talking and having conversations with your children a regular part of your day. Finding time to do things you enjoy together as a family helps everyone stay connected and maintain open communication.

If you are looking for more resources for yourself or your child, be sure to also talk to your doctor.

Section 44.2

Parents' Influence on Children's and Teens' Drug Use

Adolescent substance use is a widely researched topic as well as the focus of various prevention programs. Alcohol and drug use is considered a risky behavior for teens due to its potential for negative consequences. Substance use puts teens at an increased risk for suicide, homicide, car crashes, and other unintentional injuries (National Institute on Alcohol Abuse and Alcoholism, 2005). Substance use can also lead to academic problems or risky sexual behavior and has even shown to have negative effects on brain development. Furthermore, early initiation of drinking is shown to increase the risk of alcoholism later in life (McGue & Iacono, 2008). Factors leading to a youth's decision to engage in underage drinking or other substance use are complex and likely include influences from multiple domains. While social environment and peer influences are often recognized as contributing factors to an individual's decision to engage in underage drinking or illegal drug usage, the effect of family factors should not be ignored.

Support and control have been identified by researchers as two complementary components of parenting (Barnes and Farrell, 1992). The construct of support includes areas such as nurturance, attachment, acceptance, and love, whereas the construct of control includes discipline, supervision, and monitoring. Monitoring has further been defined as parental knowledge of their child's companions, whereabouts, and activities. Another dichotomy that has been used to conceptualize parenting is parental attitudes or values, which includes perceived permissiveness, and parental behaviors, which includes perceived monitoring.

Each of these areas can be examined in relation to adolescent alcohol, tobacco, and other drug (ATOD) use (e.g. does the degree of

515

closeness an adolescent feels within the family impact their alcohol or drug use?; do strict family rules prevent adolescents from drinking?). In addition to relating these general constructs to adolescent ATOD use, recent research has investigated how alcohol-specific socialization by the family impacts adolescents' substance use. Alcohol-specific socialization refers to any activities that parents undertake specifically to manage their children's drinking behaviors and may include things such as making alcohol-specific rules, showing disapproval of drinking, and talking about alcohol use (Van der Vorst, Engels, Dekovic, Meeus, & Vermulst, 007). Research by Kuntsche and Kuendig (2006) focused on the support construct of parenting as it relates to ATOD use. They found that a lack of family bonding was a predictor of alcohol use by adolescents. Family bonding is defined as a feeling of closeness and intimacy toward one's parents and included behaviors such as listening to a child's worries, spending free time with the child, and providing help to the child when needed. Mothers and fathers may not have the same impact on children's substance use as illustrated by Zhang, Welte, & Wieczorek (1999); their research showed that the closeness to mothers but not fathers predicted adolescent drinking. On the other hand, Barnes and Farrell (1992) showed that high levels of support by both mothers and fathers were associated with lower levels of regular drinking and illicit drug use. Also, mother's support had a stronger effect on deviance for girls than for boys. Other research has found that family bonds influence substance use indirectly through peers (Bahr, Marcos, & Maughan, 1995). Youth with stronger family bonds are less likely to have friends involved with substance use. It is suggested that spending time with parents helps the children to adopt their values and thus abstain from alcohol use. Another possible explanation for this effect is that spending more time with the family means that adolescents spend less time with their peers, and thus experience less peer pressure and limited opportunities to access substances apart from supervision.

Key Findings

- There is a strong association between rules about alcohol use and actual consumption. Alcohol-specific rules lower the likelihood of drinking initiation (Van der Vorst, Engels, Meeus, & Dekovic, 2006; Van der Vorst et al., 2007).

- High levels of parental monitoring are associated with low frequencies of drinking and illicit drug use (Barnes & Farrell, 1992).

- Parents are stricter toward younger adolescents than older; parents become more permissive of alcohol use as the adolescents get older (Van der Vorst et al., 2007).

- Parents feel more confident about influencing their younger child rather than their older child, which coincides with a belief that parents have less control over their children as they get older; however, data showed that parents were equally effective for adolescents at all ages (Van der Vorst, Engels, Meeus, Dekovic, & Leeuwe, 2005).

- Alcohol-specific rules by parents are less effective once an adolescent's drinking pattern has been established, meaning that parents can impact their children's alcohol use during the initiation phase of drinking (Van der Vorst et al., 2007).

- Prohibiting alcohol use in the home reduces children's involvement in underage alcohol use (Yu, 2003).

- Parental influences on drinking behavior moderate the peer influences; when parents are more involved, peer influences on drinking are not as influential (Wood, Read, Mitchell, & Brand, 2004).

- When mothers reported on family rules, there was no relationship with adolescent drinking or drug use; however, when the adolescents reported on parental rules, there were significant relationships. Along with the finding that adolescents identified fewer parental rules for their behavior than the parents identified, this indicates that it is the adolescents' perception of having rules that is critical. A distinction must be made between verbally provided rules and an assumption by parents that their children know the rules (Barnes & Farrell, 1992; Van der Vorst et al., 2006).

- Adolescents imitate the consumption of their parents, especially their father (Van der Vorst et al., 2005).

- Parents that drink are more permissive about their children drinking and parents that are strict about their children drinking are less likely to drink themselves. It is possible that parents who drink feel less credible in providing rules about the behaviors or are more accepting of drinking in general (Van der Vorst et al., 2006).

Similar to the findings with alcohol-specific rules, Jackson & Henriksen (1997) found that children whose parents engage in antismoking socialization (setting rules to eliminate cigarettes smoking in the home, awareness of children's smoking behaviors, and making disciplinary consequences of smoking clear) are less likely to begin smoking. This study also found that children are more likely to begin smoking if they see the parents modeling the behavior.

In summary, though pathways to adolescent alcohol and drug use are complex, parents are an important influence on their children's decision-making about substance use. Nurturing and supportive relationships between parents and their children as well as strict parental monitoring and clearly communicated parental rules specific about substance use can prevent adolescents from engaging in this illegal and dangerous behavior. Various studies have indicated that it is not the adolescent's age that matters as much as whether or not the adolescent has an established pattern of behavior; older children can still be impacted if they have not yet established a drinking pattern. Parents should clearly communicate their rules and expectations regarding the child's behavior, and parents should continue to set and enforce alcohol-specific rules and to monitor their children's whereabouts and activities. As the adolescent ages, parents should not assume that they lose credibility or that ATOD use by their teenager is inevitable. In addition to findings of direct effects between parenting and adolescent substance use, family influences can also impact how peer relationships impact the adolescents. Finally, parental substance use is an important factor both directly through modeling and indirectly through parent's willingness to set rules about ATOD use.

References

Bahr, S. J., Marcos, A. C., & Maughan, S. L. (1995). Family, educational, and peer influences on the alcohol use of female and male adolescents. *Journal of Studies on Alcohol, 56*, 457–469.

Barnes, G. M., & Farrell, M. P. (1992). Parental support and control as predictors of adolescent drinking, delinquency, and related problem behaviors. *Journal of Marriage and the Family, 54*, 763–776.

Jackson, C., & Henriksen, L. (1997). Do as I say: parent smoking, antismoking socialization, and smoking onset among children. *Addictive Behaviors, 22*, 104–114.

Kuntsche, E. N., & Kuendig, H. (2006). What is worse? A hierarchy of family-related risk factors predicting alcohol use in adolescence. *Substance Use & Misuse, 41*, 71–86.

McGue, M., & Iacono, W. G. (2008). The adolescent origins of substance use disorders. *International Journal of Methods in Psychiatric Research, 17*, S30–S38.

National Institute on Alcohol Abuse and Alcoholism (2005). Alcohol development in youth—A multidisciplinary overview. *Alcohol Research & Health*, 28(3). Retrieved May 21, 2009, from http://pubs.niaaa.nih.gov/publications/arh283/toc28-3.htm.

Van der Vorst, H., Engels, R.C.M.E., Dekovic, M., Meeus, W., & Vermulst, A. A. (2007). Alcohol-specific rules, personality and adolescents' alcohol use: a longitudinal person-environment study. *Addiction*, 102, 1064–1075.

Van der Vorst, H., Engels, R.C.M.E., Meeus, W., & Dekovic, M. (2006). The impact of alcohol-specific rules parental norms about early drinking and parental alcohol use on adolescents' drinking behavior. *Journal of Child Psychology and Psychiatry*, 47, 1299–1306.

Van der Vorst, H., Engels, R.C.M.E., Meeus, W., Dekovic, M., & Van Leeuwe, J. (2005). The role of alcohol-specific socialization in adolescents' drinking behavior. *Addiction*, 100, 1464–1476.

Wood, M. D., Read, J. P., Mitchell, R. E., & Brand, N. H. (2004). Do parents still matter? Parent and peer influences on alcohol involvement among recent high school graduates. *Psychology of Addictive Behaviors*, 18, 19–30.

Yu, J. (2003). The association between parental alcohol-related behaviors and children's drinking. *Drug and Alcohol Dependence*, 69, 253–262.

Zhang, L., Welte, J. W., & Wieczorek, W. F. (1999). The influence of parental drinking and closeness on adolescent drinking. *Journal of Studies on Alcohol*, 60, 245–251.

Section 44.3

Protecting Your Children from Prescription Drugs in Your Home

"What to Do: 3 Steps" © 2013 www.drugfree.org / The Partnership at Drugfree.org. All rights reserved. Reprinted with permission.

Step 1: Monitor

Parents are in an influential position to immediately help reduce teen access to prescription drugs because these drugs are found in the home. But how aware are you? Think about this: would you know if some of your pills were missing? From this day forward, make sure you can honestly answer, "yes."

- Start by taking note of how many pills are in each of your prescription bottles or pill packets.

- Keep track of your refills. This goes for your own medication, as well as for your teens and other members of the household. If you find you need to refill your medication more often than expected, that could indicate a problem.

- If your teen has been prescribed a drug, be sure you control the medication, and monitor dosages and refills.

- Make sure your friends and relatives—especially grandparents—are also aware of the risks. Encourage them to regularly monitor their own medicine cabinets.

- If there are other households your teen has access to, talk to those families as well about the importance of helping safeguard their medications.

Step 2: Secure

Teens abuse prescription drugs because they are easily accessible and either free or inexpensive. In fact, 64% of kids age 12 to 17 who have abused pain relievers say they got them from their friends or relatives, typically without their knowledge. Approach securing your prescriptions the same way you would other valuables in your home, like jewelry or cash. There's no shame in helping protect those items. The same holds true for your medications.

- Take prescription medications out of the medicine cabinet and hide them in a place only you know about.

- If possible, keep all medicines, both prescription and over-the-counter, in a safe place, such as a locked cabinet your teen cannot access.

- Tell relatives, especially grandparents, to lock their medications or keep them in a safe place.

- Talk to the parents of your teenager's friends. Encourage them to secure their prescriptions.

Step 3: Dispose

Safely disposing of expired or unused prescription medications is a critical step in helping protect your teens. Here's how to help safeguard your family and home, and decrease the opportunity for your teens or their friends to abuse your medications.

- Take an inventory of all of the prescription drugs in your home. Start by discarding expired or unused prescription drugs, when your teens are not home.

- Unbelievable though it may seem, teenagers will retrieve discarded prescription drugs from the trash. To help prevent this from happening, mix the medication with an undesirable substance, such as used coffee grounds or kitty litter. Put the mixture into an empty can or bag and discard.

- Unless the directions on the packaging say otherwise, do not flush medication down the drain or toilet.

- To help prevent unauthorized refills and protect your and your family's privacy, remove any personal, identifiable information from prescription bottles or pill packages before you throw them away.

Section 44.4

How to Protect Children from Inhalant Abuse

"A Parent's Guide to Preventing Inhalant Abuse," Consumer
Product Safety Commission (www.cpsc.gov), undated. Reviewed
by David A. Cooke, MD, FACP, July 2013.

Inhalant Abuse: It's Deadly

Inhalant abuse can kill. It can kill suddenly, and it can kill those
who sniff for the first time. Every year, young people in this country
die of inhalant abuse. Hundreds suffer severe consequences, including
permanent brain damage, loss of muscle control, and destruction of
the heart, blood, kidney, liver, and bone marrow.

Today more than 1,000 different products are commonly abused.
The National Institute on Drug Abuse reported in 1996 that one in
five American teenagers have used inhalants to get high.

Many youngsters say they begin sniffing when they're in grade
school. They start because they feel these substances can't hurt them,
because of peer pressure, or because of low self-esteem. Once hooked,
these victims find it a tough habit to break.

What is inhalant abuse?

Inhalant abuse is the deliberate inhalant or sniffing of common
products found in homes and schools to obtain a "high."

What are the effects of inhalant abuse?

Sniffing can cause sickness and death. For example, victims may
become nauseated, forgetful, and unable to see things clearly. Victims
may lose control of their body, including the use of arms and legs. These
effects can last 15 to 45 minutes after sniffing.

In addition, sniffing can severely damage many parts of the body,
including the brain, heart, liver, and kidneys.

Even worse, victims can die suddenly—without any warning. "Sudden sniffing death" can occur during or right after sniffing. The heart
begins to overwork, beating rapidly but unevenly, which can lead to

cardiac arrest. Even first-time abusers have been known to die from sniffing inhalants.

What products are abused?

Ordinary household products, which can be safely used for legitimate purposes, can be problematic in the hands of an inhalant abuser. The following categories of products are reportedly abused: glues/adhesives, nail polish remover, marking pens, paint thinner, spray paint, butane lighter fluid, gasoline, propane gas, typewriter correction fluid, household cleaners, cooking sprays, deodorants, fabric protectors, whipping cream aerosols, and air conditioning coolants.

How can you tell if a young person is an inhalant abuser?

If someone is an inhalant abuser, some or all these symptoms may be evident:

- Unusual breath odor or chemical odor on clothing
- Slurred or disoriented speech
- Drunk, dazed, or dizzy appearance
- Signs of paint or other products where they wouldn't normally be, such as on the face or fingers
- Red or runny eyes or nose
- Spots and/or sores around the mouth
- Nausea and/or loss of appetite
- Chronic inhalant abusers may exhibit such symptoms as anxiety, excitability, irritability, or restlessness

Inhalant abusers also may exhibit the following signs:

- Sitting with a pen or marker near nose
- Constantly smelling clothing sleeves
- Showing paint or stain marks on the face, fingers, or clothing
- Hiding rags, clothes, or empty containers of the potentially abused products in closets and other places

What is a typical profile of an inhalant abuser in the U.S.?

There is no typical profile of an inhalant abuser. Victims are represented by both sexes and all socioeconomic groups throughout the

U.S. It's not unusual to see elementary and middle-school age youths involved with inhalant abuse.

How does a young person who abuses inhalants die?

There are many scenarios for how young people die of inhalant abuse. Here are some of them:

- A 13-year-old boy was inhaling fumes from cleaning fluid and became ill a few minutes afterwards. Witnesses alerted the parents, and the victim was hospitalized and placed on life support systems. He died 24 hours after the incident.

- An 11-year-old boy collapsed in a public bathroom. A butane cigarette lighter fuel container and a plastic bag were found next to him. He also had bottles of typewriter correction fluid in his pocket. CPR failed to revive him, and he was pronounced dead.

- A 15-year-old boy was found unconscious in a backyard. According to three companions, the four teenagers had taken gas from a family's grill propane tank. They put the gas in a plastic bag and inhaled the gas to get high. The victim collapsed shortly after inhaling the gas. He died on the way to the hospital.

What can you do to prevent inhalant abuse?

One of the most important steps you can take is to talk with your children or other youngsters about not experimenting even a first time with inhalants. In addition, talk with your children's teachers, guidance counselors, and coaches. By discussing this problem openly and stressing the devastating consequences of inhalant abuse, you can help prevent a tragedy.

If you suspect your child or someone you know is an inhalant abuser, what can you do to help?

Be alert for symptoms of inhalant abuse. If you suspect there's a problem, you should consider seeking professional help. Contact a local drug rehabilitation center or other services available in your community, or the following:

National Inhalant Prevention Coalition: 800-269-4237 or www .inhalants.org

National Drug and Alcohol Treatment Referral Service: 800-662-HELP

National Clearinghouse for Alcohol and Drug Information:
800-729-6686

Section 44.5

Information for Parents about Club Drugs

Excerpted from "Tips for Parents: The Truth about Club
Drugs," Federal Bureau of Investigation (www.fbi.gov),
accessed August 12, 2013.

What are raves?

"Raves" are high-energy, all-night dances that feature hard pounding techno music and flashing laser lights. Raves are found in most metropolitan areas and, increasingly, in rural areas throughout the country. The parties are held in permanent dance clubs, abandoned warehouses, open fields, or empty buildings.

Raves are frequently advertised as "alcohol free" parties with hired security personnel. Internet sites often advertise these events as "safe" and "drug free." However, they are dangerously overcrowded parties where your child can be exposed to rampant drug use and a high-crime environment. Numerous overdoses are documented at these events.

Raves are one of the most popular venues where club drugs are distributed. Club drugs include MDMA (more commonly known as "ecstasy"), GHB (gamma hydroxybutyrate) and Rohypnol (also known as the "date rape" drugs), ketamine, methamphetamine (also known as "meth"), and LSD (lysergic acid diethylamide).

Because some club drugs are colorless, odorless, and tasteless, they can be added without detection to beverages by individuals who want to intoxicate or sedate others in order to commit sexual assaults.

Rave promoters capitalize on the effects of club drugs. Bottled water and sports drinks are sold at raves, often at inflated prices, to manage hyperthermia and dehydration. Also found are pacifiers to prevent involuntary teeth clenching, menthol nasal inhalers, surgical masks, chemical lights, and neon glow sticks to increase sensory perception and enhance the rave experience.

Cool-down rooms are provided, usually at a cost, as a place to cool off due to increased body temperature of the drug user.

Don't risk your child's health and safety. Ask questions about where he or she is going and see it for yourself.

What are the signs?

The following are effects of stimulant club drugs, such as MDMA and methamphetamine:

- Increased heart rate
- Convulsions
- Extreme rise in body temperature
- Uncontrollable movements
- Insomnia
- Impaired speech
- Dehydration
- High blood pressure
- Grinding teeth

Effects of sedative/hallucinogenic club drugs, such as GHB, ketamine, LSD, and Rohypnol, are as follows:

- Slow breathing
- Decreased heart rate (except LSD)
- Respiratory problems
- Intoxication
- Drowsiness
- Confusion
- Tremors
- Nausea

Effects common to all club drugs can include anxiety, panic, depression, euphoria, loss of memory, hallucinations, and psychotic behavior. Drugs, traces of drugs, and drug paraphernalia are direct evidence of drug abuse. Pacifiers, menthol inhalers, surgical masks, and other such items could also be considered indicators.

Where do you go for help?

If you suspect your child is abusing drugs, monitor behavior carefully. Confirm with a trustworthy adult where your child is going and what he or she is doing. Enforce strict curfews. If you have evidence of club drug use, approach your child when he or she is sober and, if necessary, call on other family members and friends to support you in the confrontation.

Once the problem is confirmed, seek the help of professionals. If the person is under the influence of drugs and immediate intervention is necessary, consider medical assistance. Doctors, hospital substance programs, school counselors, the county mental health society, members of the clergy, organizations such as Narcotics Anonymous, and rape counseling centers stand ready and waiting to provide information and intervention assistance.

Section 44.6

Parental Intervention for Teenage Drug Abuse

"How to Know? I Think My Child Is Using Alcohol and/or Drugs" and "What to Do? I Know My Child Is Using Alcohol and/or Drugs," © 2011 New York State Office of Alcoholism and Substance Abuse Services (www.oasas.ny.gov). Reprinted with permission.

How to Know? I Think My Child Is Using Alcohol and/or Drugs

Take Action

When you suspect your child may be using alcohol and/or drugs, it is important to take action.

Prepare yourself: Work with what happened rather than why it happened. Don't blame someone else, yourself, or your child. Don't be shocked or judgmental because there are many innovative ways to conceal use. Don't be afraid and/or hesitate to investigate your son/daughter's belongings such as cell phones, computers, etc.

Confront the issue: Don't let anger or fear overwhelm your effectiveness in dealing with your child. Cool down or take a walk before you begin the conversation.

Have a conversation: Putting your head in the sand is counterproductive. Accept that your son/daughter may be using so that you can begin the conversation.

Set standards: Take a stand. Say "NO" clearly and firmly. Carry through on consequences.

Ask for help: There are many confidential resources available for parents—if you ask! Ask your school health professional for help or seek assistance from a mental health or substance abuse counselor.

Facts

There is no greater influence on a young person's decisions about alcohol or drug use than his/her own parents or guardians. To successfully keep kids drug-free, parents must provide active support and positive role modeling.

Parents are key in preventing underage drinking and drug use. Be a parent, not a friend. Establish boundaries that take a clear stand against alcohol and other drug use.

Current brain research shows that the brain is not fully developed until the mid-twenties. Adding chemicals to a developing brain is a very risky endeavor—and one that can lead to health problems and places kids at high risk for addiction, even death.

Signs and Symptoms

Any one of the following behaviors can be a symptom of normal adolescence. However, keep in mind that the key is change. It is important to note any significant changes in your child's physical appearance, personality, attitude, or behavior.

Physical Signs

- Loss or increase in appetite; unexplained weight loss or gain
- Inability to sleep or unusual laziness
- Smell of substance on breath or clothes
- Nausea, vomiting, sweating, shakes of hands, feet, or head
- Red, watery eyes; pupils larger or smaller than usual; blank stare, thick tongue, slurred speech

Behavioral Signs

- Change in attitude/personality
- Change in friends; new hangouts
- Change in activities, hobbies or sports
- Drop in grades or work performance
- Isolation and secretive behavior
- Moodiness, irritability, nervousness, giddy

Why Teens Use

Acceptance: To fit in with friends, to become popular or be where the action is.

Curiosity: Youth hear about "highs" and want to find out for themselves.

Easy access: If pills, alcohol, or other drugs are easy to obtain they are more likely to experiment.

Modeling: When parents or older siblings use alcohol, drugs, and/or tobacco, youth are more eager to try.

Self-medication: To cope with pressures of problems or as an antidote to deal with issues.

Seeking independence: Some students believe using is a way of self-expression and a way to test their individuality.

Widely Used Drugs

- Tobacco
- Alcohol
- Prescription painkillers
- Marijuana
- Inhalants

What to Do? I Know My Child Is Using Alcohol and/or Drugs

Introduction

If you know your child is using drugs, you have good reason to be concerned. You may feel helpless, fearful, and even ashamed, but you

CAN do something. You can try a variety of ways that will make your child's drug use less appealing for them. It is important to note that getting help for your child is a process, never an event. This means that you will have to try a variety of techniques over time, while never giving up. This section will offer ideas and tips for you to begin to help your child, but it is most important that you educate yourself and get help for yourself as well.

Knowledge Is Power

If you know your child is using alcohol, drugs, or tobacco, remember knowledge is power. The more information you have about discussing substance use with your child, the more comfortable and prepared you will be. Finding the right time, when you both are available, to discuss your concerns is the first step toward a positive discussion. Be ready for avoidance and denial. Prepare for some possible questions about your own use.

Outline for an Intervention

Seek professional help. School counselors/health care professionals are trained to assist with referrals to trained counselors who are equipped to properly assess your child's alcohol and/or drug use.

Don't shy away from addressing this. Be prepared to discuss and take appropriate action.

Express concern over a particular incident and relate this to the chemical use.

Be factual and specific.

Describe how you felt.

Set limits and arrange an outcome.

Example:

- *I know you would not have (insert behavior).*
- *I am so concerned about you and I am afraid for what is happening to our family.*
- *I have arranged an appointment for you so you can get help.*

Sample Contract

Terms: No use of alcohol, drugs, or tobacco. No hanging with users.

Privileges: Anything that is a perk for your child.

Consequences: Loss of privileges and seek out professional help.

Signatures: Yours and your child's.

Steps You Can Take

Keep yourself and your child surrounded by loving support.

- Talk to your child when he/she is not under the influence of alcohol and/or drugs.

- Express concern not blame.

- It is important to use your knowledge of your child and trust your own instincts about how to approach the subject.

- Don't cover up your child's alcohol and/or drug seeking behaviors from family members.

- Establish guidelines for behaviors, as well as curfews and type of friends. Put these into a contract that has both consequences and privileges.

- Always have your child assume responsibility for his/her actions.

- It is important to not let shame or anger prevent you from getting help from someone who knows addiction.

- Make sure that you and other caregivers are on the same page so you can show your child a united front.

- If your child needs treatment, you can prepare a formal intervention that would involve significant others and have treatment as the outcome.

- Keep in mind, treatment is voluntary, and your child may refuse to go. It is important to have some type of leverage such as: legal consequences, removal from extra-curricular activities, or placement outside the home.

Section 44.7

Healthy Family Relationship and Religious Involvement Protect Adolescents from Drug Use

American-Indian adolescents continue to have the highest rates of illicit drug use among all ethnic groups. Although previous research has found that increasing adolescent exposure to protective factors can reduce their risk for substance abuse, this has not been thoroughly examined in American-Indian adolescents. Recent findings from a University of Missouri study reveal that positive family relationships and religious affiliation can counteract risk factors—including addicted family members, exposure to violence, and deviant peers—associated with drug use.

"For American-Indian youths, our study suggests that intervention and prevention programs should consider a supportive family environment as an important focus," said ManSoo Yu, assistant professor in the MU [Missouri University] School of Social Work and Public Health Program. "Healthy relationships protect adolescents against exposure to violence and negative social environments, and therefore, may lower their risk for drug involvement. Practitioners also can encourage adolescents to connect with religious organizations, which can reduce negative peer influence and increase positive family relationships."

In the study, Yu examined the mediating roles of positive environment (healthy families and religious affiliation) on the associations between negative environment (addicted family members, deviant peers, and negative school environment) and illicit drug symptoms. Identifying mediators can help clarify interrelationships among various risk and protective factors in predicting health-risk behaviors, Yu said.

Yu found that positive family relationships mediated the impact of addicted family members, violence victimization, and negative school environment on illicit drug symptoms. The findings expand prior research that indicates healthy families protect adolescents from delinquent behaviors, including drug problems. Further, religious affiliation mediated the impact of deviant peers and negative school environment on positive family relationships.

Yu also found that addicted family members and deviant peers directly predicted illicit drug use, while positive family relationships and religious affiliation mediated their impact on drug use. The results are consistent with previous findings that poor familial environment (notably, family members' substance problems) and misbehaving friends are strong predictors of substance problems in youths.

"Establishing effective treatment and prevention plans requires a greater understanding of the complex associations between negative and positive variables in predicting substance use disorders such as nicotine dependence and alcohol and drug abuse," Yu said. "It is clear that strategies to help youths with drug problems can be more effective by addressing family, school, and peer contexts."

The rate of illicit drug use among American-Indian adolescents age 12–17 is approximately 19%, significantly higher than rates for Whites, Blacks, and Hispanics (around 10%) and Asians (6.7%), according to the U.S. Department of Health and Human Services.

The study, "Positive family relationships and religious affiliation as mediators between negative environment and illicit drug symptoms in American Indian adolescents," was published in the July issue of *Addictive Behaviors*. This study was funded by the National Institute on Drug Abuse, the University of Missouri System Research Board, and the MU Margaret W. Mangel Faculty Research Catalyst Fund.

Chapter 45

Drug Abuse Testing and Prevention in Schools

Chapter Contents

Section 45.1

Drug Testing in Schools

"Frequently Asked Questions About Drug Testing in Schools," National
Institute on Drug Abuse (www.drugabuse.gov), December 2012.

What is drug testing?

Some schools, hospitals, or places of employment conduct drug
testing. There are a number of ways this can be done, including:
pre-employment testing, random testing, reasonable suspicion/cause
testing, post-accident testing, return to duty testing, and follow-up
testing. This usually involves collecting urine samples to test for
drugs such as marijuana, cocaine, amphetamines, PCP (phencyclidine), and opiates.

Following models established in the workplace, some schools have
initiated random drug testing and/or reasonable suspicion/cause testing. During random testing, schools select, using a random process (like
flipping a coin), one or more individuals from the student population
to undergo drug testing. Currently, random drug testing can only be
conducted among students who participate in competitive extracurricular activities. Reasonable suspicion/cause testing involves a school
requiring a student to provide a urine specimen when there is sufficient evidence to suggest that the student may have used an illicit
substance. Typically, this involves the direct observations made by
school officials that a student has used or possesses illicit substances,
exhibits physical symptoms of being under the influence, and has patterns of abnormal or erratic behavior.

Why do some schools want to conduct random drug tests?

Schools that have adopted random student drug testing are hop-
ing to decrease drug abuse among students via two routes. First,
schools that conduct testing hope that random testing will serve
as a deterrent and give students a reason to resist peer pressure to
take drugs. Secondly, drug testing can identify adolescents who have
started using drugs so that interventions can occur early, or identify
adolescents who already have drug problems, so they can be referred

for treatment. Drug abuse not only interferes with a student's ability to learn, but it can also disrupt the teaching environment, affecting other students as well.

Is student drug testing a standalone solution, or do schools need other programs to prevent and reduce drug use?

Drug testing should never be undertaken as a standalone response to a drug problem. If testing is done, it should be a component of broader prevention, intervention, and treatment programs, with the common goal of reducing students' drug use.

If a student tests positive for drugs, should that student face disciplinary consequences?

The primary purpose of drug testing is not to punish students who use drugs but to prevent drug abuse and to help students already using become drug-free. The results of a positive drug test should be used to intervene with students who do not yet have drug problems, through counseling and follow-up testing. For students that are diagnosed with addiction, parents and a school administrator can refer them to effective drug treatment programs to begin the recovery process.

Why test teenagers at all?

Teens are especially vulnerable to drug abuse, when the brain and body are still developing. Most teens do not use drugs, but for those who do, it can lead to a wide range of adverse effects on the brain, the body, behavior, and health.

Short term: Even a single use of an intoxicating drug can affect a person's judgment and decision making—resulting in accidents, poor performance in a school or sports activity, unplanned risky behavior, and the risk of overdosing.

Long term: Repeated drug abuse can lead to serious problems, such as poor academic outcomes, mood changes (depending on the drug: depression, anxiety, paranoia, psychosis), and social or family problems caused or worsened by drugs.

Repeated drug use can also lead to the disease of addiction. Studies show that the earlier a teen begins using drugs, the more likely he or she will develop a substance abuse problem or addiction. Conversely, if teens stay away from drugs while in high school, they are less likely to develop a substance abuse problem later in life.

How many students actually use drugs?

Drug use among high school students has dropped significantly since 2001. In December, the 2007 Monitoring the Future study of 8th, 10th, and 12th graders showed that drug use had declined by 24% since 2001.

Despite this marked decline, much remains to be done. Almost 50% of 12th graders say that they've used drugs at least once in their lifetime, and 18% report using marijuana in the last month. Prescription drug abuse is high—with nearly 1 in 10 high school seniors reporting nonmedical use of the prescription painkiller Vicodin in the past year.

What testing methods are available?

There are several testing methods available that use urine, hair, oral fluids, and sweat (patch). These methods vary in cost, reliability, drugs detected, and detection period. Schools can determine their needs and choose the method that best suits their requirements, as long as the testing kits are from a reliable source.

Which drugs can be tested for?

Various testing methods normally test for a "panel" of drugs. Typically, a drug panel tests for marijuana, cocaine, opioids, amphetamines, and PCP. If a school has a particular problem with other drugs, such as MDMA ("ecstasy"), GHB (gamma hydroxybutyrate), or steroids, they can include testing for these drugs as well.

What about alcohol?

Alcohol is a drug, and its use is a serious problem among young people. However, alcohol does not remain in the blood long enough for most tests to detect recent use. Breathalyzers and oral fluid tests can detect current use. Adolescents with substance abuse problems are often polydrug users (they use more than one drug) so identifying a problem with an illicit or prescription drug may also suggest an alcohol problem.

How accurate are drug tests? Is there a possibility a test could give a false positive?

Tests are very accurate but not 100% accurate. Usually samples are divided so if an initial test is positive a confirmation test can be conducted. Federal guidelines are in place to ensure accuracy and fairness in drug testing programs.

Can students "beat" the tests?

Many drug-using students are aware of techniques that supposedly detoxify their systems or mask their drug use. Popular magazines and internet sites give advice on how to dilute urine samples, and there are even companies that sell clean urine or products designed to distort test results. A number of techniques and products are focused on urine tests for marijuana, but masking products increasingly are becoming available for tests of hair, oral fluids, and multiple drugs.

Most of these products do not work, are very costly, are easily identified in the testing process, and need to be on hand constantly, because of the very nature of random testing. Moreover, even if the specific drug is successfully masked, the product itself can be detected, in which case the student using it would become an obvious candidate for additional screening and attention. In fact, some testing programs label a test "positive" if a masking product is detected.

Is random drug testing of students legal?

In June 2002, the U.S. Supreme Court broadened the authority of public schools to test students for illegal drugs. Voting five to four in *Pottawatomie County v. Earls*, the court ruled to allow random drug tests for all middle and high school students participating in competitive extracurricular activities. The ruling greatly expanded the scope of school drug testing, which previously had been allowed only for student athletes.

A school or school district that is interested in adopting a student drug testing program should seek legal expertise so that it complies with all federal, state, and local laws. Individual state constitutions may dictate different legal thresholds for allowing student drug testing. Communities interested in starting student drug testing programs should become familiar with the law in their respective states to ensure proper compliance.

What has research determined about the utility of random drug tests in schools?

There is not very much research in this area, and the early research shows mixed results. A study published in 2007 (Goldberg et al, *J. Adolesc Health*, 41: 421–29, 2007) found that student athletes who participated in randomized drug testing had overall rates of drug use similar to students who did not take part in the program, and in fact some indicators of future drug abuse increased among those participating in the drug testing program. Because of the limited number of studies on this topic more research is warranted.

Section 45.2

Drug Use Prevention Education in Schools

Excerpted from "Alcohol- or Other Drug-Use Prevention,"
Centers for Disease Control and Prevention (www.cdc.gov), 2006.
Reviewed by David A. Cooke, MD, FACP, July 2013.

Health Education

The following were true of the two years preceding the study:

- 82.0% of states and 71.0% of districts provided funding for staff development or offered staff development on alcohol- or other drug-use prevention to those who teach health education.

- 26.6% of elementary school classes and required middle school and high school health education courses had a teacher who received staff development on alcohol- or other drug-use prevention.

Health Services and Mental Health and Social Services

- The percentage of states that required districts or schools to provide alcohol- or other drug-use treatment services increased from 8.2% in 2000 to 17.6% in 2006, whereas the percentage of districts that required schools to provide these services decreased from 46.2% in 2000 to 33.6% in 2006.

- The percentage of states that required districts or schools to provide alcohol- or other drug-use prevention services in one-on-one or small-group sessions increased from 22.0% in 2000 to 42.0% in 2006.

The following were true of the two years preceding the study:

- The percentage of states that provided funding for staff development or offered staff development to school mental health or social services staff on alcohol- or other drug-use prevention services and alcohol- or other drug-use treatment services increased from 82.6% to 93.3%, and from 77.8% to 89.4%, respectively.

Table 45.1. Percentage of Schools in Which Teachers Taught Alcohol- or Other Drug-Use Prevention Topics as Part of Required Instruction, by School Level

Topic	Elementary	Middle	High
Benefits of not using alcohol	68.8	80.4	91.4
Benefits of not using illegal drugs	70.7	79.4	90.3
Distinguishing between medical and nonmedical drug use	66.4	75.1	83.1
Drink equivalents and blood alcohol content	17.1	62.9	87.5
Effects of alcohol or other drug use on decision making	70.2	81.5	92.8
Long-term health consequences of alcohol use and addiction	61.9	80.2	92.8
Long-term health consequences of illegal drug use and addiction	63.8	78.1	90.6
Making a personal commitment not to use alcohol or other drugs	70.2	72.2	79.9
Resisting peer pressure to use alcohol or other drugs	71.4	81.6	92.2
Short-term health consequences of alcohol use and addiction	68.8	79.7	90.9
Short-term health consequences of illegal drug use and addiction	66.9	77.5	89.8
Social or cultural influences on alcohol or other drug use	54.9	76.8	87.3

- The percentage of school mental health or social services coordinators who served as study respondents who received staff development on alcohol- or other drug-use prevention services decreased from 68.2% in 2000 to 54.9% in 2006.

- The percentage of school health services coordinators who served as study respondents who received staff development on alcohol- or other drug-use treatment services during the two years preceding the study decreased from 49.9% in 2000 to 39.4% in 2006.

Healthy and Safe School Environment

- Among the 25.5% of districts containing middle schools or high schools that had adopted a student drug-testing policy, 56.1%

conducted student drug testing randomly among members of specific groups of students (e.g., athletes, students who participate in other extracurricular activities, or student drivers), 63.9% conducted student drug testing when it was suspected that a student was using drugs at school, 37.6% had voluntary drug testing for all students, 3.6% had voluntary drug testing for specific groups of students, and 13.4% used some other unspecified criteria.

• 11.4% of middle schools and 19.5% of high schools conducted drug testing on students.

• The percentage of districts that provided model policies to schools during the two years preceding the study increased from 64.0% in 2000 to 76.2% in 2006 for illegal drug-use prevention and from 64.9% to 75.4% for alcohol-use prevention.

• The percentage of schools that had or participated in a community-based alcohol-use prevention program decreased from 49.6% in 2000 to 38.5% in 2006, and the percentage of schools that had or participated in a community-based illegal drug-use prevention program decreased from 60.0% in 2000 to 46.8% in 2006.

Chapter 46

Drug Testing

Chapter Contents

Section 46.1

Overview of Drug Testing

"Drugs of Abuse Testing: Test Sample, The Test," © 2013 American Association for Clinical Chemistry. Reprinted with permission. For additional information about clinical lab testing, visit the Lab Tests Online website at www.labtestsonline.org.

The Test Sample

What is being tested?

Drugs of abuse testing is the detection of one or more illegal and/or legal substances in the urine or, more rarely, in the blood, saliva, hair, or sweat. It usually involves an initial screening test followed by a second test that identifies and/or confirms the presence of a drug or drugs. Most laboratories use commercially available tests that have been developed and optimized to screen urine for the "major drugs of abuse."

For most drugs of abuse testing, results of initial screening testing are compared with a predetermined cutoff. Anything below that cutoff is considered negative; anything above is considered a positive screening result.

Within each class of drug that is tested, there may be a variety of chemically similar drugs. Legal substances that are chemically similar to illegal ones can produce a positive screening result. Therefore, screening tests that are positive for one or more classes of drugs are frequently confirmed with a secondary test that identifies the exact substance present using a very sensitive and specific method, such as gas chromatography/mass spectrometry (GC/MS).

Some of the most commonly screened drug classes are listed in Table 46.1.

Substances that are not similar to the defined classes can produce false negative results. Some drugs may be difficult to detect with the standardized assays, either because the test is not set up to detect the drug, such as methylenedioxy-methamphetamine (MDMA, Ecstasy), oxycodone (Oxycontin), or buprenorphine, or because the drug does not remain in the body long enough to be detected, such as gamma-hydroxybutyrate (GHB).

Table 46.1. Commonly Screened Drug Classes

Drug class screened	Examples of specific drugs identified during confirmation
Amphetamines	Methamphetamine, amphetamine
Barbiturates	Phenobarbital, secobarbital, pentobarbital
Benzodiazepines	Diazepam, lorazepam
Cannabinoids	Marijuana
Cocaine	Cocaine and/or its metabolite (benzoylecognine)
Opiates	Codeine, morphine, metabolite of heroin
Phencyclidine (PCP)	PCP

(See a more comprehensive list of drug classes and drugs of abuse [at http://labtestsonline.org/understanding/analytes/drug-abuse/drug-table].)

For sports testing of hormones and steroids, each test performed is usually specific for a single substance and may be quantitative. Athletes, especially those at the national and international level, are tested for illegal drugs and are additionally governed by a long list of prohibited substances called performance enhancers.

Groups of drug tests are typically ordered for medical or legal reasons, as part of a "drug-free workplace," or as part of a sports testing program. People who use these substances ingest, inhale, smoke, or inject them into their bodies. The amounts that are absorbed and the effects that they have depend on which drugs are taken, how they interact, their purity and strength, the quantity, timing, method of intake, and the individual person's ability to metabolize and excrete them. Some drugs can interfere with the action or metabolism of other medications, have additive effects such as taking two drugs that both depress the central nervous system (CNS), or have competing effects such as taking one drug that depresses the CNS and another that stimulates it. The drugs tested for are not normally found in the body, with the exception of some hormones and steroids measured as part of sports testing.

How is the sample collected for testing?

Urine is the most frequently tested sample, but other body samples such as hair, saliva, sweat, and blood also may be used for drug abuse screening but not interchangeably with urine.

Urine and saliva are collected in clean containers. A blood sample is obtained by inserting a needle into a vein in the arm. Hair is cut close to the scalp to collect a sample. A sweat sample is typically collected by applying a patch to the skin for a specified period of time.

Is any test preparation needed to ensure the quality of the sample?

No test preparation is needed.

The Test

How is it used?

Drug of abuse testing may be used in one of several different ways:

- Medical screening
- Legal or forensic testing
- Employment drug testing
- Sports/athletic testing

Medical screening: Medical screening for drugs of abuse is primarily focused on determining what drugs or combinations of drugs a person may have taken so that he can receive the proper treatment. The overall effect on a particular person depends on the response of his body to the drugs, on the quantity and combination he has taken, and when each was taken. For instance, MDMA is initially a stimulant with associated psychedelic effects, but it also causes central nervous system (CNS) depression as it is metabolized and cleared from the body. In many cases, drugs have been combined and/or taken with ethanol (alcohol). If someone drinks ethanol during this time period, they will have two CNS depressants in their system, a potentially dangerous combination.

Those who may be tested for drugs for medical reasons include:

- someone in the emergency room who is having acute health problems that the doctor thinks may be drug-related: unconsciousness, nausea, delirium, panic, paranoia, increased temperature, chest pain, respiratory failure, seizures, and/or headaches;
- someone in the emergency room who has been in an accident, when the doctor suspects that drugs and/or alcohol may have been involved;
- a youth or adult who the doctor suspects may be using drugs;

- those who are being monitored for known drug use (this may include both legal and illegal drug use); it may be general testing or specific for the substance that has been abused;

- pregnant women thought to be at risk for drug abuse or neonates exhibiting certain characteristic behaviors.

Legal or forensic testing: Drug testing for legal purposes is primarily concerned with the detection of illegal or banned drug use in a variety of situations. Sample collection procedures for this type of testing are strictly controlled and documented to maintain a legal "chain-of-custody." The donor provides a sample that is sealed and secured with a tamperproof seal in his or her presence. Specific chain-of-custody paperwork then accompanies the sample throughout the testing process; each person who handles and/or tests the sample provides their signature and the reason for the sample transfer. This creates a permanent record of each step of the process. Examples of legal drug abuse screening include:

- court-mandated drug testing usually involves the random monitoring of someone who has been convicted of illegal drug use; testing may also be ordered in custody cases to rule out drug use by one or both parents;

- government child protective services may sometimes require extended monitoring of a parent with a known drug problem to ensure that they have not returned to drug use;

- law enforcement drug testing may be done when someone has an accident that is suspected to be alcohol- or drug-related;

- forensic testing utilizes a variety of body fluids and tissues that may be tested for numerous drugs during a crime investigation; the goal may be to determine whether drugs were a contributing factor to an accident or crime, such as a DUI or rape—testing may also be done to determine whether someone died of a drug overdose or drug-related condition;

- insurance companies may perform drug screening on their applicants; this may include a test for cocaine and a test for nicotine, even though tobacco is a legal substance;

- schools may have programs that incorporate random drug testing; this may include illegal drugs of abuse and, with competitive sports, may include testing for performance-enhancing substances.

Employment drug testing: Employment drug testing may be done prior to employment, on a random basis, following an accident, or if the employer has a reasonable suspicion that their employee is using illegal drugs. The major drugs of abuse are tested, and any positives are confirmed by another method. Employment drug testing is commonplace. It is required in some industries, such as those that involve the U.S. Department of Transportation or federal employees, and accepted practice in many other industries.

As with legal or forensic drug testing, the sample collection and testing procedures for employment drug testing are often strictly controlled and documented to maintain a legal "chain-of-custody." A sample is obtained (usually a urine sample) from the employee in a container that is secured with a tamperproof seal in his or her presence. Specific chain-of-custody paperwork then accompanies the sample throughout the testing process and documents each person who handles and/or tests the sample. This creates a permanent record of each step of the process.

Sports/athletic screening: While conventional drug testing is performed on competitive athletes, the primary focus is on doping—drugs and/or supplements that are taken to promote muscle growth and/or to improve strength and endurance. On a local level, sports testing may be limited, but on a national and international level, it has become highly organized.

The World Anti-Doping Agency (WADA), U.S. Anti-Doping Agency (USADA), and the International Association of Athletics Federations (IAAF) work together to monitor athlete drug use on a national, international, and Olympic level. WADA has a written code, which establishes uniform drug testing rules and sanctions for all sports and countries, and a substantial list of prohibited substances. Athletes are responsible for any banned substances that are found in their body during testing. Most of the compounds tested are considered positive if they are detected in any quantity while others, such as caffeine, are only prohibited when they are present in large amounts. Some of the substances, such as anabolic steroids (testosterone) and peptide hormones such as erythropoietin, growth hormone, and Insulin-like Growth Factor-1, are banned but are difficult to measure as they are produced by the body. Testing methods must be able to distinguish between endogenous (that produced by the athlete's body) and supplemented compounds.

Screening programs randomly perform out-of-competition drug tests on athletes during the training season to look for anabolic steroids, such as testosterone, that promote increased muscle growth. During competitions, testing is frequently done both randomly and on all winners and includes categories such as: stimulants, narcotics, anabolic agents, and peptide hormones. Sports such as archery, gymnastics, and shooting add additional testing for substances like beta blockers, which are prohibited in these sports because they decrease blood pressure and heart rate.

While professional sports organizations, such as the NFL (National Football League), NHL (National Hockey League), and NBA (National Basketball Association), are not covered by the WADA code, they have programs in place to test their athletes for panels of drugs that combine aspects of sports and employment testing. Those professional athletes who also take part in the Olympics, however, are subject to the same out-of-competition (pre-game) and in-competition testing as other competing athletes.

When is it ordered?

Drug testing is performed whenever a doctor, employer, legal entity, or athletic organization needs to determine whether a person has illegal or banned substances in his body. It may be ordered prior to the start of some new jobs and insurance policies, at random to satisfy workplace and athletic drug testing programs, as mandated when court ordered, as indicated when ordered by a doctor to monitor a known or suspected substance abuse patient, and whenever a person has symptoms that suggest drug use.

What does the test result mean?

If a result is positive during initial drug screening, then it means that the person has a substance in his body that falls into one of the drug classes and is above the established cutoff level. If the sample is confirmed as positive after secondary testing, such as positive for marijuana, then the person has taken this drug. In some cases, this result can be tied to a window of time that the person took the substance and roughly to the quantity but, in most circumstances, that information is not necessary. Interpretation of when and how much drug was consumed can be challenging because the concentration of many drugs varies, as does their rate of metabolism from person to person.

If the drug or drugs is not present or is below the established cutoff, then the result is usually reported as "not detected" or "none detected." A negative result does not necessarily mean that the person did not take a drug at some point. The drug may be present below the established cutoff, the drug may have been already metabolized and eliminated from the body, or the test method does not detect the particular drug present in the sample.

Urine testing shows drug use over the last two or three days for amphetamines, cocaine, and opiates. Marijuana and its metabolites, cannabinoids, may be detectable for several weeks. Hair samples, which test the root end of the hair, reflect drug use within the last two to three months but not the most recent two to three weeks—the amount of time it takes for the hair to grow. Saliva detects which drugs have been used in the last 24 hours. Samples of sweat may be collected on an absorbent patch worn for several days to weeks and therefore can indicate drug use at any point during that extended period of time. These other types of samples are often used for specific purposes. For instance, hair samples may be used as an alternative to urine testing for employment or accident drug testing. Sweat testing may be used as a court-ordered monitoring tool in those who have been convicted of drug use, while saliva is often used by the insurance industry to test insurance applicants for drug use. Blood is most frequently used for alcohol testing.

Interpretation of sports testing results for hormones and steroids should be done by someone who is familiar with the test methods. A negative result indicates that there is a "normal" amount of the substance present in the body. Positive results reflect the presence of the substance above and beyond what is normally produced by the athlete's body. This can be complicated by the fact that each person will have their own normal baseline concentration and will produce varying amounts of hormones and steroids, depending upon the circumstances.

Is there anything else I should know?

Symptoms associated with drug abuse and drug overdose will vary from person to person, from time to time, and do not necessarily reflect drug concentrations in the body.

Ethanol may be measured in both the blood and the breath. This is the basis for the breathalyzer test used by law enforcement.

For some types of testing, such as workplace testing of federal employees, there are many regulations that cover the test from collection through interpretation and reporting of results. It is important for the ordering physician, law enforcement representative, forensic professional, government entity, insurance agent, employer, and sports organization as well as for the person being tested to understand what exactly is included in the testing, how it is done, and how the results may or may not be interpreted. This process is not nearly as simple or straightforward as collecting a sample and requesting "drug testing."

Certain prescription and over-the-counter drugs may give a positive screening result. You should declare any medications that you have taken and/or for which you have prescriptions when you have a drug test so that your results can be interpreted correctly. Also, poppy seeds that have not been washed can cause a positive opiate screening result if eaten, for example, with a bagel or muffin. You may want to avoid these foods if you have drug testing done.

Section 46.2

Home Use Drug Testing

"Drugs of Abuse Home Use Test," U.S. Food and Drug Administration (www.fda.gov), June 1, 2011.

What do these tests do?

These tests indicate if one or more prescription or illegal drugs are present in urine. These tests detect the presence of drugs such as marijuana, cocaine, opiates, methamphetamine, amphetamines, PCP, benzodiazepine, barbiturates, methadone, tricyclic antidepressants, ecstasy, and oxycodone.

The testing is done in two steps. First, you do a quick at-home test. Second, if the test suggests that drugs may be present, you send the sample to a laboratory for additional testing.

What are drugs of abuse?

Drugs of abuse are illegal or prescription medicines (for example, oxycodone or Valium) that are taken for a nonmedical purpose. Non-medical purposes for a prescription drug include taking the medication for longer than your doctor prescribed it for or for a purpose other than what the doctor prescribed it for. Medications are not drugs of abuse if they are taken according to your doctor's instructions.

What type of test are these?

They are qualitative tests—you find out if a particular drug may be in the urine, but not how much is present.

When should you do these tests?

You should use these tests when you think someone might be abusing prescription or illegal drugs. If you are worried about a specific drug, make sure to check the label to confirm that this test is designed to detect the drug you are looking for.

How accurate are these tests?

The at-home testing part of this test is fairly sensitive to the presence of drugs in the urine. This means that if drugs are present, you will usually get a preliminary (or presumptive) positive test result. If you get a preliminary positive result, you should send the urine sample to the laboratory for a second test.

It is very important to send the urine sample to the laboratory to confirm a positive at-home result because certain foods, food supplements, beverages, or medicines can affect the results of at-home tests. Laboratory tests are the most reliable way to confirm drugs of abuse.

Many things can affect the accuracy of these tests, including (but not limited to) the following:

- The way you did the test
- The way you stored the test or urine
- What the person ate or drank before taking the test
- Any other prescription or over-the-counter drugs the person may have taken before the test

Note that a result showing the presence of an amphetamine should be considered carefully, even when this result is confirmed in the laboratory testing. Some over-the-counter medications will produce the same test results as illegally abused amphetamines.

Does a positive test mean that you found drugs of abuse?

No. Take no serious actions until you get the laboratory's result. Remember that many factors may cause a false positive result in the home test.

Remember that a positive test for a prescription drug does not mean that a person is abusing the drug because there is no way for the test to indicate acceptable levels compared to abusive levels of prescribed drugs.

If the test results are negative, can you be sure that the person you tested did not abuse drugs?

No. No drug test of this type is 100% accurate. There are several factors that can make the test results negative even though the person is abusing drugs. First, you may have tested for the wrong drugs. Or, you may not have tested the urine when it contained drugs. It takes time for drugs to appear in the urine after a person takes them, and they do not stay in the urine indefinitely; you may have collected the urine too late or too soon. It is also possible that the chemicals in the test went bad because they were stored incorrectly or they passed their expiration date.

If you get a negative test result, but still suspect that someone is abusing drugs, you can test again at a later time. Talk to your doctor if you need more help deciding what steps to take next.

How soon after a person takes drugs will they show up in a drug test? And how long after a person takes drugs will they continue to show up in a drug test?

The drug clearance rate tells how soon a person may have a positive test after taking a particular drug. It also tells how long the person may continue to test positive after the last time he or she took the drug. Clearance rates for common drugs of abuse are given in Table 46.2. These are only guidelines, however, and the times can vary significantly from these estimates based on how long the person has been taking the drug, the amount of drug they use, or the person's metabolism.

How do you do a drugs of abuse test?

These tests usually contain a sample collection cup, the drug test (it may be test strips, a test card, a test cassette, or other method for testing the urine), and an instruction leaflet or booklet. It is very important that the person doing the test reads and understands the instructions first, before even collecting the sample. This is important because with most test kits, the result must be visually read within a certain number of minutes after the test is started.

Table 46.2. Clearance Rates for Common Drugs of Abuse

Drug	How soon after taking drug will there be a positive drug test?	How long after taking drug will there continue to be a positive drug test?
Marijuana/pot	1–3 hours	1–7 days
Crack (cocaine)	2–6 hours	2–3 days
Heroin (opiates)	2–6 hours	1–3 days
Speed/uppers (amphetamine, methamphetamine)	4–6 hours	2–3 days
Angel dust/PCP	4–6 hours	7–14 days
Ecstasy	2–7 hours	2–4 days
Benzodiazepine	2–7 hours	1–4 days
Barbiturates	2–4 hours	1–3 weeks
Methadone	3–8 hours	1–3 days
Tricyclic antidepressants	8–12 hours	2–7 days
Oxycodone	1–3 hours	1–2 days

You collect urine in the sample collection cup and test it according to the instructions. If the test indicates the preliminary presence of one or more drugs, the sample should be sent to a laboratory where a more specific chemical test will be used in order to obtain a final result. Some home use kits have a shipping container and preaddressed mailer in them. If you have questions about using these tests, or the results that you are getting, you should contact your health care provider.

Chapter 47

Preventing Drug Abuse in the Workplace

Chapter Contents

Section 47.1

Drug-Free Workplace Policies

"Drug-Free Workplace Advisor: Program Planning and Philosophy," U.S. Department of Labor (www.dol.gov/elaws/asp/drugfree), accessed March 20, 2013, and "Drug-Free Workplaces: Employer Rights and Responsibilities," U.S. Small Business Administration (www.sba.gov), February 17, 2011.

Program Planning and Philosophy

An organization's philosophy concerning alcohol and drugs sets the tone for its drug-free workplace policy and program. Some organizations focus on detection, apprehension, and discharge and apply a strong law enforcement model that treats employees who use drugs as criminals. Other organizations focus on performance and emphasize deterrence and assistance because they view alcohol and drug use as causing impairment of otherwise capable employees. The most effective drug-free workplace programs strike a balance between these two philosophies. They send a strong clear message and, at the same time, encourage employees to seek assistance if they are struggling with alcohol or drug problems.

The following are some philosophies and practices that can undermine the effectiveness of drug-free workplace programs:

- Focusing only on illicit drug use and failing to include alcohol—the number one drug of abuse in our society

- Accepting drug use and alcohol abuse as part of modern life and a cost of doing business

- Overreliance on drug testing

- Focusing on termination of users rather than rehabilitation

- Reluctance of supervisors to confront employees on the basis of poor performance

- Reinforcing an individual's denial regarding the impact of his or her alcohol and drug use

- Restricting benefits and/or access to treatment of alcoholism and addiction

- Allowing insurers to restrict access to treatment programs

The characteristic common to all effective drug-free workplace programs is balance. A successful drug-free workplace program must strike a delicate balance between a number of sometimes competing elements, including the following:

- The rights of employees and the rights of employers
- The need to know and rights to privacy
- Detection and rehabilitation
- Respect for employees and the safety of all

Drug-Free Workplaces: Employer Rights and Responsibilities

Most private employers have rights when it comes to testing for illegal substances in the workplace. Although employee drug testing is generally not required by law, if you choose to exercise your testing rights, you must comply with federal and state regulations.

The first step to establishing a drug-free workplace is understanding what's considered an acceptable and reasonable drug-testing policy.

Employer Rights

The Drug-Free Workplace Act of 1988 does not require employers to create a drug-free workplace policy or implement drug testing for applicants or employees. For many businesses, however, this has become a standard practice. The Americans with Disabilities Act (ADA) and the Rehabilitation Act of 1973 establish several important federal rights for businesses dealing with drug and alcohol workplace issues. Under current laws, employers can do the following:

- Require their applicants or employees to take drug tests as a condition of employment
- Prohibit the illegal use of drugs and alcohol in the workplace
- Deny employment to any current or potential employee who breaks their current drug-free workplace policy
- Cannot classify a person currently engaging in the illegal use of drugs, but who is not considered an addict, as an "individual with a disability"

In addition to these employer rights, when dealing with the abuse of alcohol, employers have these rights:

- Can classify an alcoholic as an "individual with a disability"

- Can require alcoholics to meet the same standard of employee conduct that all other employees are expected

- Can discipline or deny employment to any current or potential employee whose alcohol abuse affects their ability to perform at work

Employer Responsibilities

The Americans with Disabilities, Rehabilitation, and Family Medical Leave Acts also serve to protect employees when it comes to drug and alcohol policies in the workplace. Under current laws, employers have these responsibilities:

- Cannot discriminate against non-using drug addicts or those with a history of drug addiction

- Cannot discriminate against employees who are undergoing rehabilitation for drugs or alcohol

- Must make reasonable accommodation efforts for employees who seek help

In addition to these federal requirements, many state and local governments have regulations that affect drug-free workplace policies. In many cases these laws limit or prohibit the ability to conduct drug testing at the workplace. It is important that all employers understand the regulations required by their state and local government.

Section 47.2

Drug Testing in the Workplace

"Drug-Free Workplace Advisor: Workplace Drug Testing,"
U.S. Department of Labor (www.dol.gov/elaws/asp/drugfree),
accessed March 20, 2013.

Drug testing is one action an employer can take to determine if employees or job applicants are using drugs. It can identify evidence of recent use of alcohol, prescription drugs, and illicit drugs. Currently, drug testing does not test for impairment or whether a person's behavior is, or was, impacted by drugs. Drug testing works best when implemented based on a clear, written policy that is shared with all employees, along with employee education about the dangers of alcohol and drug abuse, supervisor training on the signs and symptoms of alcohol and drug abuse, and an Employee Assistance Program (EAP) to provide help for employees who may have an alcohol or drug problem.

Why do employers drug test?

Alcohol and drug abuse creates significant safety and health hazards and can result in decreased productivity and poor employee morale. It also can lead to additional costs in the form of health care claims, especially short-term disability claims.

Common reasons employers implement drug testing are to do the following:

- Deter employees from abusing alcohol and drugs
- Prevent hiring individuals who use illegal drugs
- Be able to identify early and appropriately refer employees who have drug and/or alcohol problems
- Provide a safe workplace for employees
- Protect the general public and instill consumer confidence that employees are working safely
- Comply with state laws or federal regulations
- Benefit from Workers' Compensation Premium Discount programs

How is drug testing conducted and how accurate is it?

Generally, most private employers have a fair amount of latitude in implementing drug testing as they see fit for their organization, unless they are subject to certain federal regulations, such as the U.S. Department of Transportation's (DOT) drug-testing rules for employees in safety-sensitive positions. However, federal agencies conducting drug testing must follow standardized procedures established by the Substance Abuse and Mental Health Services Administration (SAMHSA), part of the U.S. Department of Health and Human Services (DHHS).

While private employers are not required to follow these guidelines, doing so can help them stay on safe legal ground. Court decisions have supported following these guidelines, and as a result, many employers choose to follow them. These Mandatory Guidelines for Federal Workplace Drug Testing (also called SAMHSA's guidelines) include having a medical review officer (MRO) evaluate tests. They also identify the five substances tested for in federal drug-testing programs and require the use of drug labs certified by SAMHSA.

The most common method of drug testing, urinalysis, can be done at the workplace (at a health unit, for example), a doctor's office, or any other site selected by the employer. An employee or applicant provides a sample to be tested. Usually precautions are taken, such as putting blue dye in the toilet and turning off the water supply, to prevent adulteration or substitution of specimens so that collection can be completed in privacy without any direct visual observation by another person.

Under SAMHSA's guidelines, once a sample is provided, it is sent to a certified laboratory. The accuracy of drug tests done by certified laboratories is very high, but this certification applies only to the five substances tested for in federal drug-testing programs and alcohol.

Certain procedures required by SAMHSA's guidelines ensure accuracy and validity of the testing process:

- **Chain of custody:** A chain-of-custody form is used to document the handling and storage of a sample from the time it is collected until the time it is disposed. It links an individual to his or her sample and is written proof of all that happens to the specimen while at the collection site and the laboratory.

- **Initial screen:** The first analysis done on a sample is called an initial screen. In the event that the initial screen is positive, a second confirmatory test should be done.

- **Confirmation test:** A second, confirmation test is highly accurate and provides specificity to help rule out any false positives (mistakes) from the initial screen.

- **Split sample:** A split sample is created when an initial urine sample is split into two. One sample is used for the initial screen, and, if positive, the second sample is used for the confirmation test. If there is a positive result, the individual being tested may request the confirmation test be done at a different laboratory.

In the event that the initial screen and confirmation test are both positive, MRO, a licensed medical doctor who has special training in the area of substance abuse, then reviews the results, makes sure the chain-of-custody procedures were followed, and contacts the individual to make sure there are no medical or other reasons for the result. It is only at this point that the MRO may report a positive test result to the employer. Certain medications can sometimes cause a positive result. If this is the case, and a doctor prescribed the medicine and the employee used it in the proper amount, the test is reported as negative.

Who is allowed access to the results of a drug test?

The result of a drug test may be considered personal health information. Consequently, there may be restrictions on how and whether such information (as well as other information related to an employee's history of alcohol or drug use) can be shared with others. This is why employees who undergo a drug test generally must sign a release (usually at the time of the test) in order for their employer to receive the results. For more information about issues related to the release of health information, contact DHHS.

When are drug tests conducted?

There are a variety of circumstances under which an organization may require a drug test. Following are the most common or widespread:

Pre-employment: Pre-employment testing is conducted to prevent hiring individuals who illegally use drugs. It typically takes place after a conditional offer of employment has been made. Applicants agree to be tested as a condition of employment and are not hired if they fail to produce a negative test. However, it is possible for employees to prepare for a pre-employment test by stopping their drug use several days before they anticipate being tested. Therefore, some employers test probationary employees on an unannounced basis. Some states, however, restrict this process. Furthermore, the Americans with Disabilities Act (ADA) of 1990 prohibits the use of pre-employment testing for alcohol use.

Reasonable suspicion: Reasonable suspicion testing is similar to, and sometimes referred to as, "probable-cause" or "for-cause" testing and is conducted when supervisors document observable signs and symptoms that lead them to suspect drug use or a drug-free workplace policy violation. It is extremely important to have clear, consistent definitions of what behavior justifies drug and alcohol testing, and any suspicion should be corroborated by another supervisor or manager.

Post-accident: Since property damage or personal injury may result from accidents, testing following an accident can help determine whether drugs and/or alcohol were a factor. It is important to establish objective criteria that will trigger a post-accident test and how and by whom they will be determined and documented. Examples of criteria used by employers include: fatalities; injuries that require anyone to be removed from the scene for medical care; damage to vehicles or property above a specified monetary amount; and citations issued by the police. Although the results of a post-accident test determine drug use, a positive test result in and of itself cannot prove that drug use caused an accident. Employers also need to have guidelines to specify how soon following an accident testing must occur so results are relevant. It is usually recommended that post-accident testing be done within 12 hours.

Random: Random testing is performed on an unannounced, unpredictable basis on employees whose identifying information (e.g., social security number or employee number) has been placed in a testing pool from which a scientifically arbitrary selection is made. This selection is usually computer generated to ensure that it is indeed random and that each person of the workforce population has an equal chance of being selected for testing, regardless of whether that person was recently tested or not. Because this type of testing has no advance notice, it serves as a deterrent.

Periodic: Periodic testing is usually scheduled in advance and uniformly administered. Some employers use it on an annual basis, especially if physicals are required for the job.

Return-to-duty: Return-to-duty testing involves a one-time, announced test when an employee who has tested positive has completed the required treatment for substance abuse and is ready to return to the workplace. Some employers also use this type of testing for any employee who has been absent for an extended period of time.

Other: Other types of tests are also used by some employers. For example, follow-up testing or post-rehabilitation testing is conducted periodically after an employee returns to the workplace upon completing rehabilitation for a drug or alcohol problem. It is administered on an unannounced, unpredictable basis for a period of time specified in the drug-free workplace policy. Another type of testing, blanket testing, is similar to random testing in that it is unannounced and not based on individual suspicion; however, everyone at a worksite is tested rather than a randomly selected percentage. Other types of testing include voluntary, probationary, pre-promotion, and return-after-illness testing.

What are the different methods of drug testing?

There are a number of different bodily specimens that can be chemically tested to detect evidence of recent drug use. Although some state laws dictate which types of tests can be used, a number of options are technologically feasible. Urine is the most commonly used specimen for illicit drugs, reflecting SAMHSA's guidelines, and breath is the most common for alcohol, reflecting the Department of Transportation's guidelines.

Urine: Results of a urine test show the presence or absence of drug metabolites in a person's urine. Metabolites are drug residues that remain in the body for some time after the effects of a drug have worn off. It is important to note that a positive urine test does not necessarily mean a person was under the influence of drugs at the time of the test. Rather, it detects and measures use of a particular drug within the previous few days and has become the de facto evidence of current use.

Breath: A breath-alcohol test is the most common test for finding out how much alcohol is currently in the blood. The person being tested blows into a breath-alcohol device, and the results are given as a number, known as the blood alcohol concentration (BAC), which shows the level of alcohol in the blood at the time the test was taken. BAC levels have been correlated with impairment, and the legal limit of 0.08 for driving has been set in all states. Under DOT regulations, a BAC of 0.02 is high enough to stop someone from performing a safety-sensitive task for a specific amount of time (usually between 8 and 24 hours) and a BAC reading of 0.04 or higher is considered to be a positive drug test and requires immediate removal from safety-sensitive functions.

Blood: A blood test measures the actual amount of alcohol or other drugs in the blood at the time of the test. Blood samples provide an accurate measure of the physiologically active drug present in a person at the time the sample is drawn. Although blood samples are a better indicator of recent consumption than urine samples, there is a lack of published data correlating blood levels for drugs and impairment with the same degree of certainty that has been established for alcohol.

Hair: Analysis of hair provides a much longer "testing window," giving a more complete drug-use history going back as far as 90 days. Like urine testing, hair testing does not provide evidence of current impairment, but rather only past use of a specific drug. Hair testing cannot be used to detect for alcohol use. Hair testing is the least invasive form of drug testing, therefore privacy issues are decreased.

Oral fluids: Saliva, or oral fluids, collected from the mouth also can be used to detect traces of drugs and alcohol. Oral fluids are easy to collect (a swab of the inner cheek is the most common collection method), harder to adulterate or substitute, and may be better at detecting specific substances, including marijuana, cocaine and amphetamines/methamphetamines.

Sweat: Another type of drug test consists of a skin patch that measures drugs in sweat. The patch, which looks like a large adhesive bandage, is applied to the skin and worn for some length of time. A gas-permeable membrane on the patch protects the tested area from dirt and other contaminants. Although relatively easy to administer, this method has not been widely used in workplaces and is more often used to maintain compliance with probation and parole.

What drugs do tests detect?

Testing conducted according to SAMHSA's guidelines checks for five illicit drugs plus, in some cases, alcohol. These five illicit drugs are the following:

- Amphetamines (meth, speed, crank, ecstasy)
- THC (cannabinoids, marijuana, hash)
- Cocaine (coke, crack)
- Opiates (heroin, opium, codeine, morphine)
- Phencyclidine (PCP, angel dust)

However, most private employers are not limited in the number of substances they can test for and may include drugs that individuals legitimately and/or therapeutically take based on a physician's prescription. Although most private employers can test for any combination of drugs, there are commonly selected "panels."

The typical 8-Panel Test includes the aforementioned substances plus the following:

- Barbiturates (phenobarbital, butalbital, secobarbital, downers)

- Benzodiazepines (tranquilizers like Valium, Librium, Xanax)

- Methaqualone (Quaaludes)

The typical 10-Panel Test includes the 8-Panel Test plus these:

- Methadone (often used to treat heroin addiction)

- Propoxyphene (Darvon compounds)

Testing can also be done for the following:

- Hallucinogens (LSD, mushrooms, mescaline, peyote)

- Inhalants (paint, glue, hairspray)

- Anabolic steroids (synthesized, muscle-building hormones)

- Hydrocodone (prescription medication known as Lortab, Vicodin, oxycodone)

- MDMA (commonly known as ecstasy)

How long are drugs in one's system?

Drugs have certain "detection windows"—the amount of time after ingestion during which evidence of their use can be detected by a drug test. Though it might not be wise to publicize detection windows and invite employees who may use drugs to push their limits, when implementing drug testing, it is important to understand them. The following are estimates of the length of time that certain drugs are detectable:

- **Alcohol:** 1 ounce for 1.5 hours

- **Amphetamines:** 48 hours

- **Barbiturates:** 2–10 days

- **Benzodiazepines:** 2–3 weeks

- **Cocaine:** 2–10 days

- **Heroin metabolite:** Less than 1 day
- **Morphine:** 2–3 days
- **LSD:** 8 hours
- **Marijuana:** Casual use, 3–4 days; chronic use, several weeks
- **Methamphetamine:** 2–3 days
- **Methadone:** 2–3 days
- **Phencyclidine (PCP):** 1 week

How does a drug test determine if a person has been using substances? What are cutoff levels and what do they determine?

Aside from a breath alcohol test, drug testing does not determine impairment or current drug use. Rather, drug testing determines a specified amount or presence of a drug or its metabolite. There is a minimum measurement applied to drug testing so that only traces of a drug or its metabolite above a specified level is reported as positive. This measure is known as a "cutoff level," and it varies for each drug. Setting cutoff levels involves understanding the expected results of testing and determining the needs of the employer's drug-free workplace program. For instance, if a cutoff level is set low, test results will come back with more "false positives" as some "passive" users could test positive. (For example, a low cutoff level could cause a positive result from consuming poppy seeds.) Conversely, a high cutoff level will result in more "false negatives," and thus some users may go undetected. However, a high cutoff level lessens the likelihood of taking action against someone based on "passive" exposure, and for this reason SAMHSA's guidelines set cutoff levels on the high side.

Who pays for a drug test?

According to SAMHSA, an employer normally pays for a drug test. Also, time spent having a required drug test is generally considered hours worked (and thus compensable time) under the Fair Labor Standards Act (FLSA), a U.S. Department of Labor (DOL) regulation, for employees who are covered by the act.

Is drug testing legal?

In most cases it is legal for employers to test employees for drugs. No federal laws prohibit the practice. However, there are several states that restrict or question an employer's ability to randomly drug test employees who are not in safety-sensitive positions. Thus, it is very important that employers familiarize themselves with the various state laws that may apply to their organization before implementing a drug-testing program. Furthermore, under certain circumstances, someone with a history of alcoholism or drug addiction may be considered a qualified individual with a disability under the Americans with Disabilities Act (ADA) and other federal nondiscrimination statues. As a result, testing for alcohol without individualized suspicions (e.g. pre-employment or random) is not allowable.

How does one start a drug-testing program?

Drug testing is only one component of a comprehensive drug-free workplace program, which also includes a written policy that clearly outlines employer expectations regarding drug use; training for supervisors on the signs and symptoms of drug use and their role in enforcing the policy; education for employees about the dangers of drug use; and an EAP to provide counseling and referral to employees struggling with drug problems. DOL's online Drug-Free Workplace Advisor helps employers develop customized drug-free workplace policies (that may or may not including drug testing) by reviewing the different components of a comprehensive policy and then generating a written policy statement based on the user's responses to preset questions and statements. It is also recommended that legal consultation be sought before commencing a drug testing program.

A comprehensive drug-free workplace program contributes to a workplace free of the health, safety, and productivity hazards caused by employees' abuse of alcohol or drugs. By educating employees about the dangers of alcohol and drug abuse and encouraging individuals with related problems to seek help, employers can protect their businesses from such dangers, retain valuable employees, and help play a part in making communities safer and healthier.

Chapter 48

Federal Drug Abuse Prevention Campaigns

Chapter Contents

Section 48.1

Above the Influence

Excerpted from "Above the Influence," White House Office of National
Drug Control Policy (www.whitehouse.gov/ondcp), June 2012.

A Brand that Speaks to Teens

The Office of National Drug Control Policy (ONDCP)'s multi-tiered
"Above the Influence" (ATI) campaign provides sound information to
young people about the dangers of drug use and strengthens efforts
to prevent drug use in communities.

In 2010, the National Youth Anti-Drug Media Campaign relaunched
the ATI youth brand with broad prevention messaging at the national
level—including television, print, and internet advertising—as well
as more targeted efforts at the local level. Since the relaunch, results
from the campaign's year-round tracking study of teens consistently
show that more than 85% of teens are aware of the ATI brand, and
that more than three-quarters of teens say the ATI message speaks to
someone like them—regardless of race, gender, or ethnicity.

More important, teens who are aware of or interacted with ATI
have significantly stronger anti-drug beliefs than teens who are not
aware of or do not interact with ATI. The ATI Facebook site recently
surpassed 1.3 million "likes," making it one of the largest teen-targeted
Facebook communities among the federal government or nonprofit
youth organizations.

Engaging Communities Directly

To foster participation at the community level, the campaign partners with hundreds of youth-serving organizations in communities
across the country. It also provides technical assistance and training
to community organizations through conference workshops and webinars. ONDCP's efforts to reach out to teens and communities have
produced impressive results:

- More than 80 established local community partners are implementing the campaign.

- Nearly a thousand community organizations have received technical assistance and training through conference workshops and webinars.

- In an evaluation of the localized campaign, partners reported that "Above the Influence" activities are useful to their organization in meeting their missions to serve youth.

- 98% of partners reported they are willing to implement ATI activities again.

Campaign partners include local chapters and affiliates representing Drug Free Communities Support Program grantees, the Boys and Girls Club of America, the YMCA (or Y), Girls Inc., ASPIRA (a national organization dedicated to developing the educational and leadership capacity of Hispanic youth), Students Against Destructive Decisions (SADD), Community Anti-Drug Coalitions of America (CADCA), the National Organization for Youth Safety (NOYS), and the Partnership at Drugfree.org.

Campaign Effectiveness

Evidence for the effectiveness of the "Above the Influence" campaign has appeared in several recently published independent research studies, including an analysis published online by the peer-reviewed journal *Prevention Science*. This analysis concluded that "exposure to the ONDCP (ATI) campaign predicted reduced marijuana use."[1]

The analysis, funded through a grant by the National Institute on Drug Abuse (NIDA), showed that youth who reported exposure to the ATI campaign were less likely to begin use of marijuana than those not exposed to the campaign—a finding consistent with the campaign's own year-round Youth Ad Tracking Survey results.

A second study, published in the *American Journal of Public Health* in March 2011,[2] provides "evidence that greater exposure to the Above the Influence Campaign is significantly associated with reduced marijuana usage." Specifically, this research found lower rates of past-month and lifetime marijuana use among 8th grade girls who had greater exposure to the ATI campaign's anti-drug advertisements.[3]

A third study, published in the *Journal of Drug Education*, has also shown encouraging findings about the effectiveness of the campaign. The findings suggest that awareness of the "Above the Influence" campaign "is associated with greater anti-drug beliefs, fewer drug use intentions, and less marijuana use" among the campaign's target audience.[4]

ATI Is Valuable to Communities

Community partners have embraced the ATI campaign and use ATI activities as a new way to engage youth in a dialogue about the negative effects of substance use. ATI community partners use the ATI campaign as a valuable asset to which they can anchor their individual youth substance abuse prevention programs, thereby furthering their respective youth-serving missions.

Notes

1. Slater, et al. (2011), "Assessing Media Campaigns Linking Marijuana Non-Use with Autonomy and Aspirations: 'Be Under Your Own Influence' and ONDCP's 'Above the Influence,' " *Prevention Science*, 12(1), 12–22.

2. Carpenter and Pechmann (2011), "Exposure to the Above the Influence Antidrug Advertisements and Adolescent Marijuana Use in the United States, 2006–2008," *American Journal of Public Health*, published online.

3. Farrelly, et al. (2005), "Evidence of a Dose-Response Relationship between 'Truth' Antismoking Ads and Youth Smoking Prevalence," *American Journal of Public Health*, 95(3), 425–431.

4. Scheier, L. M., Grenard, J. L., & Holtz, K. D. (2011). "An Empirical Assessment of the 'Above the Influence' Advertising Campaign," *Journal of Drug Education*, 41(4), 431–461.

Section 48.2

Drug-Free Communities Support Program

Excerpted from "Drug Free Communities Support Program,"
White House Office of National Drug Control Policy
(www.whitehouse.gov/ondcp), 2012.

The Drug-Free Communities Support Program (DFC) is a federal grant program that provides funding to community-based coalitions that organize to prevent youth substance use. Since the passage of the DFC Act in 1997, the DFC program has funded nearly two thousand coalitions and currently mobilizes nearly nine thousand community volunteers across the country. The philosophy behind the DFC program is that local drug problems require local solutions. With a small federal investment, the DFC program doubles the amount of funding through the DFC program's match requirement to address youth substance use. Recent evaluation data indicate that where DFC dollars are invested, youth substance use is lower. Over the life of the DFC program, youth living in DFC communities have experienced reductions in alcohol, tobacco, and marijuana use.

DFC National Evaluation

In the past eight years that DFC has been evaluated, DFC-funded communities have achieved significant reductions in youth alcohol, tobacco, and marijuana use. For middle school youth living in DFC-funded communities, data from the DFC National Evaluation indicate a 16% reduction in alcohol use, 27% reduction in tobacco use, and 23% reduction in marijuana use. High school–aged youth have reduced their use of alcohol by 9%, tobacco by 16%, and marijuana by 7% in DFC-funded communities. DFC-funded coalitions are actively engaged in facilitating prescription drug take-back programs in conjunction with local law enforcement, as well as local policy change to effectively address the accessibility and available of alcohol, tobacco, and other drugs.

Recent data from the National Survey on Drug Use and Health (NSDUH) indicate increases in youth prescription drug abuse, as well as marijuana, ecstasy, and methamphetamine use. Now, more than ever, the DFC program is needed in communities across the country to help prevent drug use and reduce its consequences. Drug problems manifest in local communities and show up in our schools, churches, health centers, and homes. The DFC program helps local leaders organize to identify the youth drug issues unique to their communities and develop the infrastructures necessary to effectively prevent and respond to the disease of addiction.

The DFC program operates on a yearly grant cycle that starts with a Request for Applications (RFA) being posted in January of each year. The RFA, when open, is posted on Grants.gov and SAMSHA.gov and www.whitehouse.gov/ondcp. Community coalitions meeting all of the statutory eligibility requirements can apply during the open period for funding. DFC grants are awarded for 5 years with a maximum of 10 years. Coalitions can ask for up to $125,000 per year and must provide at least a one-to-one match (cash, in-kind, donations, but no federal funds) each year, with increases in years 8–10.

Purpose of the DFC Program

The primary purpose of the DFC program is to strengthen collaboration among community entities and reduce substance use among youth. DFC grantees are required to work toward these two goals as the primary focus of their federally funded effort. Grants awarded through the DFC program are intended to support established community-based coalitions capable of effecting community-level change. For the purposes of the DFC program, a coalition is defined as a community-based formal arrangement for cooperation and collaboration among groups or sectors of a community in which each group retains its identity, but all agree to work together toward a common goal of building a safe, healthy, and drug-free community. Coalitions receiving DFC funds are expected to work with leaders within their communities to identify and address local youth substance use problems and create sustainable community-level change through environmental strategies.

What DFC Funds

The DFC program funds one thing: community coalitions that have formed to address youth substance use. Communities often understand that local stakeholders and citizens hold the key to solving local problems. In realizing this, community-based coalitions are created every day in this country. A typical DFC budget submission includes the salary and benefits of an individual that ensures effective day-to-day operations of the coalition, training and technical assistance for the coalition, travel, and prevention efforts that place emphasis on environmental strategies. DFC funding can be considered the financial support required to further leverage funding to support the various strategies a community needs in order to solves its youth substance use problems.

The ONDCP announced $84.6 in total funding for FY 2012 Drug-Free Communities Support Program grants.

Section 48.3

Prescription Drug
Abuse Prevention Campaign

"Prescription Drug Abuse," White House Office of National Drug Control Policy (www.whitehouse.gov/ondcp), accessed March 20, 2013.

The Centers for Disease Control and Prevention has classified prescription drug abuse as an epidemic. While there has been a marked decrease in the use of some illegal drugs like cocaine, data from the National Survey on Drug Use and Health show that nearly one-third of people aged 12 and over who used drugs for the first time in 2009 began by using a prescription drug nonmedically.

Some individuals who misuse prescription drugs, particularly teens, believe these substances are safer than illicit drugs because they are prescribed by a health care professional and dispensed by a pharmacist. Addressing the prescription drug abuse epidemic is not only a top priority for public health, it will also help build stronger communities and allow those with substance abuse disorders to lead healthier, more productive lives.

ONDCP's Prescription Drug Abuse Prevention Plan

The 2011 Prescription Drug Abuse Prevention Plan expands upon the Obama administration's National Drug Control Strategy and includes action in four major areas to reduce prescription drug abuse:

- **Education:** A crucial first step in tackling the problem of prescription drug abuse is to educate parents, youth, and patients about the dangers of abusing prescription drugs, while requiring prescribers to receive education on the appropriate and safe use, and proper storage and disposal, of prescription drugs.

- **Monitoring:** Implement prescription drug monitoring programs (PDMPs) in every state to reduce "doctor shopping" and diversion, and enhance PDMPs to make sure they can share data across states and are used by healthcare providers.

- **Proper medication disposal:** Develop convenient and environmentally responsible prescription drug disposal programs to help decrease the supply of unused prescription drugs in the home.

- **Enforcement:** Provide law enforcement with the tools necessary to eliminate improper prescribing practices and stop pill mills.

Read the full plan: *Epidemic: Responding to America's Prescription Drug Abuse Crisis* (at www.whitehouse.gov/sites/default/files/ondcp/issues-content/prescription-drugs/rx_abuse_plan_0.pdf).

Research

According to the recent Monitoring the Future study—the nation's largest survey of drug use among young people—prescription drugs are the second-most abused category of drugs after marijuana. In addition, the latest National Survey on Drug Use and Health shows that over 70% of people who abused prescription pain relievers got them from friends or relatives, while approximately 5% got them from a drug dealer or over the internet. Further, opiate overdoses, once almost always due to heroin use, are now increasingly due to abuse of prescription painkillers. In our military, illicit drug use increased from 5% to 12% among active duty service members from 2005 to 2008, primarily due to nonmedical use of prescription drugs.

The number of prescriptions filled for opioid pain relievers—some of the most powerful medications available—has increased dramatically in recent years. From 1997 to 2007, the milligram-per-person use of prescription opioids in the U.S. increased from 74 milligrams to 369 milligrams, an increase of 402%. In addition, in 2000, retail pharmacies dispensed 174 million prescriptions for opioids; by 2009, 257 million prescriptions were dispensed, an increase of 48%. These increases mirror increases in prescription drug abuse.

Partner Programs

Successful substance abuse prevention programs, combined with public education and penalties for those who fail to comply with the law, will continue to receive support in the effort to reduce prescription drug abuse. Here are some programs:

- **Drug-Free Communities Support Program:** Funding hundreds of communities around the country, the DFC program helps communities identify and respond to local substance abuse issues.

- **National Youth Anti-Drug Media Campaign:** This campaign is aimed at preventing and reducing youth drug use across the country by increasing teen exposure to anti-drug messages with a highly visible national media presence and on-the-ground activities, including a number of free online resources to help prevent teen prescription and over-the-counter (OTC) drug abuse.

Part Seven

Additional Help
and Information

Chapter 49

Glossary of Terms Related to Drug Abuse

Addiction: A chronic, relapsing disease characterized by compulsive drug seeking and use and by long-lasting changes in the brain.[1]

Agonist: A chemical compound that mimics the action of a natural neurotransmitter to produce a biological response.[2]

Amphetamine: Stimulant drugs whose effects are very similar to cocaine.[3]

Analog: A chemical compound that is similar to another drug in its effects but differs slightly in its chemical structure.[2]

Anabolic effects: Drug-induced growth or thickening of the body's nonreproductive tract tissues—including skeletal muscle, bones, the larynx, and vocal cords—and decrease in body fat.[3]

Analgesics: A group of medications that reduce pain.[3]

Anesthetic: An agent that causes insensitivity to pain and is used for surgeries and other medical procedures.[3]

Antagonist: A drug that counteracts or blocks the effects of another drug.[2]

This chapter excerpted from glossaries produced by the National Institute on Drug Abuse (NIDA): http://www.drugabuse.gov/publications/marijuana-abuse/glossary, marked with a superscripted 1, http://www.drugabuse.gov/publications/research-reports/heroin-abuse-addiction/glossary, marked with a superscripted 2, and http://teens.drugabuse.gov/glossary, marked with a superscripted 3.

Basal ganglia: Structures located deep in the brain that play an important role in the initiation of movements. These clusters of neurons include the caudate nucleus, putamen, globus pallidus, and substantia nigra. It also contains the nucleus accumbens, which is the main center of reward in the brain.[1]

Buprenorphine: A mixed opiate agonist/antagonist medication for the treatment of heroin addiction.[2]

Cannabinoids and cannabinoid receptors: A family of chemicals that bind to specific (cannabinoid) receptors to influence mental and physical functions. Cannabinoids that are produced naturally by the body are referred to as endocannabinoids. They play important roles in development, memory, pain, appetite, among others. The marijuana plant (*Cannabis sativa*) contains delta-9-tetrahydrocannabinol (THC), which can disrupt these processes, if administered repeatedly and/or in high enough concentrations.[1]

Cerebellum: A large structure located in the back of the brain that helps control the coordination of movement by making connections to other parts of the central nervous system (pons, medulla, spinal cord, and thalamus). It also may be involved in aspects of motor learning.[1]

Cerebral cortex: The outermost layer of the cerebral hemispheres of the brain. It is largely responsible for conscious experience, including perception, emotion, thought, and planning.[1]

Cocaine: A highly addictive stimulant drug derived from the coca plant that produces profound feelings of pleasure.[3]

Cognitive-behavioral therapy (CBT): A form of psychotherapy that teaches people strategies to identify and correct problematic behaviors in order to enhance self-control, stop drug use, and address a range of other problems that often co-occur with them.[1]

Contingency management (CM): A therapeutic management approach based on frequent monitoring of the target behavior and the provision (or removal) of tangible, positive rewards when the target behavior occurs (or does not). CM techniques have shown to be effective for keeping people in treatment and promoting abstinence.[1]

Craving: A powerful, often uncontrollable desire for drugs.[2]

Depressants: Drugs that relieve anxiety and produce sleep. Depressants include barbiturates, benzodiazepines, and alcohol.[3]

Detoxification: A process of allowing the body to rid itself of a drug while managing the symptoms of withdrawal; often the first step in a drug treatment program.[2]

Dopamine: A brain chemical, classified as a neurotransmitter, found in regions of the brain that regulate movement, emotion, motivation, and pleasure.[3]

Ecstasy (MDMA): A chemically modified amphetamine that has hallucinogenic as well as stimulant properties.[3]

Euphoria: A feeling of well-being or elation.[3]

Fentanyl: A medically useful opioid analog that is 50 times more potent than heroin.[2]

Hallucinations: Perceptions of something (such as a visual image or a sound) that does not really exist. Hallucinations usually arise from a disorder of the nervous system or in response to drugs (such as LSD).[3]

Hormone: A chemical substance formed in glands in the body and carried in the blood to organs and tissues, where it influences function, structure, and behavior.[3]

Ingestion: The act of taking in food or other material into the body through the mouth.[3]

Inhalant: Any drug administered by breathing in its vapors. Inhalants commonly are organic solvents, such as glue and paint thinner, or anesthetic gases, such as ether and nitrous oxide.[3]

Injection: A method of administering a substance such as a drug into the skin, subcutaneous tissue, muscle, blood vessels, or body cavities, usually by means of a needle.[3]

Marijuana: A drug, usually smoked but can be eaten, that is made from the leaves of the cannabis plant. The main psychoactive ingredient is THC.[3]

Methadone: A long-acting synthetic medication shown to be effective in treating heroin addiction.[2]

Motivational enhancement therapy (MET): A systematic form of intervention designed to produce rapid, internally motivated change. MET does not attempt to treat the person, but rather mobilize his or her own internal resources for change and engagement in treatment.[1]

Neurotransmitter: A chemical produced by neurons to carry messages to other neurons.[3]

Nitrites: A special class of inhalants that act primarily to dilate blood vessels and relax the muscles. Whereas other inhalants are used to alter mood, nitrites are used primarily as sexual enhancers.[3]

Physical dependence: An adaptive physiological state that occurs with regular drug use and results in a withdrawal syndrome when drug use is stopped; usually occurs with tolerance.[3]

Psychedelic drug: A drug that distorts perception, thought, and feeling. This term is typically used to refer to drugs with actions like those of LSD.[3]

Receptor: A large molecule that recognizes specific chemicals (normally neurotransmitters, hormones, and similar endogenous substances) and transmits the message carried by the chemical into the cell on which the receptor resides.[3]

Relapse: In drug abuse, relapse is the resumption of drug use after trying to stop taking drugs. Relapse is a common occurrence in many chronic disorders, including addiction, that require behavioral adjustments to treat effectively.[3]

Reward system (or brain reward system): A brain circuit that, when activated, reinforces behaviors. The circuit includes the dopamine-containing neurons of the ventral tegmental area, the nucleus accumbens, and part of the prefrontal cortex. The activation of this circuit causes feelings of pleasure.[3]

Route of administration: The way a drug is put into the body. Drugs can enter the body by eating, drinking, inhaling, injecting, snorting, smoking, or absorbing a drug through mucous membranes.[3]

Rush: A surge of euphoric pleasure that rapidly follows administration of a drug.[3]

Stimulants: A class of drugs that elevates mood, increases feelings of well-being, and increases energy and alertness. These drugs produce euphoria and are powerfully rewarding. Stimulants include cocaine, methamphetamine, and methylphenidate (Ritalin).[3]

Tolerance: A condition in which higher doses of a drug are required to produce the same effect as during initial use; often leads to physical dependence.[2]

Withdrawal: A variety of adverse symptoms that occur after use of an addictive drug is reduced or stopped.[2]

Chapter 50

Glossary of Street Terms for Drugs of Abuse

Abyssinian Tea: Khat

Acid: LSD

Adam: Ecstasy (MDMA)

African Salad: Khat

Ah-pen-yen: Opium

Amidone: Methadone

Angel Dust: PCP

Arnolds: Steroids

Aunt Mary: Marijuana

Aunti Emma: Opium

Aunti: Opium

Barbs: Barbiturates

Batu: Methamphetamine

BC Bud: Marijuana

Beans: Ecstasy (MDMA)

Bennies: Amphetamines

Benzos: Benzodiazepines

Big H: Heroin

Big O: Opium

Bikers Coffee: Methamphetamine

Bilss: Bath salts (synthetic cathinones) or K2/"Spice"

Black Beauties: Amphetamines

Black Beauties: Methamphetamine

Black Mamba: K2/"Spice"

Black Pill: Opium

Black Tar: Heroin

Block Busters: Barbiturates

Blotter Acid: LSD

This chapter compiled from material from the Drug Enforcement Administration, U.S. Department of Justice (www.justice.gov/dea).

Blubbers: Cannabis

Blue Silk: Bath salts (synthetic cathinones)

Blue: Morphine

Blunts: Marijuana

Bombay Blue: K2/"Spice"

Boom: Marijuana

Buttons: Peyote and mescaline

Cactus: Peyote and mescaline

Cat Tranquilizer: Ketamine

Cat Valium: Ketamine

Catha: Khat

CCC: Dextromethorphan

Chalk: Methamphetamine

Chandoo: Opium

Chandu: Opium

Chat: Khat

Chicken Feed: Methamphetamine

Chinese Molasses: Opium

Chinese Tobacco: Opium

Chiva: Heroin

Chocolate Chip Cookies: Methadone

Christmas Trees: Barbiturates

Chronic: Marijuana

Circles: Rohypnol

Clarity: Ecstasy (MDMA)

Cloud Nine: Bath salts (synthetic cathinones)

Coca: Cocaine

Coke: Cocaine

Crack: Cocaine

Crank: Amphetamines or methamphetamine

Crystal: Methamphetamine

D: Hydromorphone

Dex: Dextromethorphan

Dillies: Hydromorphone

Disco Biscuit: Ecstasy (MDMA)

Dope: Marijuana

Dopium: Opium

Dots: LSD

Dover's Powder: Opium

Downers: Benzodiazepines

Dream Gun: Opium

Dream Stick: Opium

Dreamer: Morphine

Dreams: Opium

Drone: Bath salts (synthetic cathinones)

Drug: Rohypnol

Dust: Hydromorphone

DXM: Dextromethorphan

E: Ecstasy (MDMA)

Easing Powder: Opium

Easy Lay: Gamma-hydroxybutyric acid (GHB)

Embalming Fluid: PCP

Emsel: Morphine

Energy-1: Bath salts (synthetic cathinones)

Eve: Ecstasy (MDMA)

Fake Weed: K2/"Spice"

Fi-do-nie: Opium

First Line: Morphine

Fizzies: Methadone

Flake: Cocaine

Footballs: Hydromorphone

Forget Pill: Rohypnol

Forget-Me-Pill: Rohypnol

G: Gamma-hydroxybutyric acid (GHB)

Gangster: Marijuana

Ganja: Marijuana

Gee: Opium

Genie: K2/"Spice"

Georgia Home Boy: Gamma-hydroxybutyric acid (GHB)

GHB: Gamma-hydroxybutyric acid

Glass: Methamphetamine

Gluey: Inhalants

Go: Ecstasy (MDMA)

God's Drug: Morphine

God's Medicine: Opium

Go-Fast: Methamphetamine

Gondola: Opium

Goof Balls: Barbiturates

Goop: Gamma-hydroxybutyric acid (GHB)

Goric: Opium

Grass: Marijuana

Great Tobacco: Opium

Grievous Bodily Harm: Gamma-hydroxybutyric acid (GHB)

Guma: Opium

Hash: Marijuana

Hashish/Chara: Cannabis

Hell Dust: Heroin

Herb: Marijuana

Hillbilly Heroin: Oxycodone

Hiropon: Methamphetamine

Hop/hops: Opium

Horse: Heroin

Hows: Morphine

Huff: Inhalants

Hug Drug: Ecstasy (MDMA)

Hydro: Hydrocodone

Ice: Amphetamines or methamphetamine

Indo: Marijuana

Ivory Wave: Bath salts (synthetic cathinones)

Jet K: Ketamine

Jet: Ketamine

Joint: Marijuana

Joy Plant: Opium

Juice: Hydromorphone or steroids

K: Ketamine

Kat: Khat

Kicker: Oxycodone

Kif: Marijuana

Killer Weed: PCP

Kit Kat: Ketamine

La Rocha: Rohypnol

Liquid Ecstasy: Gamma-hydroxybutyric acid (GHB)

Liquid X: Gamma-hydroxybutyric acid (GHB)

Lover's Speed: Ecstasy (MDMA)

Lunar Wave: Bath salts (synthetic cathinones)

Lunch Money: Rohypnol

M.S.: Morphine

Maria Pastora: *Salvia divinorum*

Maria: Methadone

Mary Jane: Marijuana

MDMA: Ecstasy

Mellow Yellow: LSD

Meow Meow: Bath salts (synthetic cathinones)

Mesc: Peyote and mescaline

Meth: Methamphetamine

Methlies: Methamphetamine

Mexican Valium: Rohypnol

Midnight Oil: Opium

Mira: Opium

Mister: Morphine

Morf: Morphine

Morpho: Morphine

Mota: Marijuana

Negra: Heroin

Norco: Hydrocodone

O: Opium

Oa: Khat

OC: Oxycodone

Ocean Burst: Bath salts (synthetic cathinones)

O.P.: Opium

Ope: Opium

Ox: Oxycodone

Oxy: Oxycodone

Pastora: Methadone

Peace: Ecstasy (MDMA)

Pen Yan: Opium

Perc: Oxycodone

Peyoto: Peyote and mescaline

Pin Gon: Opium

Pingus: Rohypnol

Pinks: Barbiturates

Poor Man's Cocaine: Methamphetamine

Poor Man's PCP: Dextromethorphan

Pot: Marijuana

Pox: Opium

Pumpers: Steroids

Pure Ivory: Bath salts (synthetic cathinones)

Purple: Ketamine

Purple Wave: Bath salts (synthetic cathinones)

Quick: Methamphetamine

R2: Rohypnol

Red Devils: Barbiturates

Red Dove: Bath salts (synthetic cathinones)

Reds & Blues: Barbiturates

Reefer: Marijuana

Reynolds: Rohypnol

Roach: Rohypnol

Roaches: Rohypnol

Roachies: Rohypnol

Roapies: Rohypnol

Robo: Dextromethorphan

Robutal: Rohypnol

Rochas Dos: Rohypnol

Rocket Fuel: PCP

Roids: Steroids

Rojo: Dextromethorphan

Roofies: Rohypnol

Rophies: Rohypnol

Ropies: Rohypnol

Roples: Rohypnol

Row-Shay: Rohypnol

Roxy: Oxycodone

Ruffies: Rohypnol

Rush: Inhalants

Sally-D: *Salvia divinorum*

Scoop: Gamma-hydroxybutyric acid (GHB)

Shabu: Methamphetamine

Shards: Methamphetamine

Sinsemilla: Marijuana

Skee: Opium

Skittles: Dextromethorphan

Skunk: Marijuana

Smack: Heroin or hydromorphone

Smoke: Marijuana

Snow Leopard: Bath salts (synthetic cathinones)

Snow: Cocaine

Soda Cot: Cocaine

Special K: Ketamine

Special La Coke: Ketamine

Speed: Amphetamines or methamphetamine

Spice: K2

Stackers: Steroids

Stardust: Bath salts (synthetic cathinones)

Stove Top: Methamphetamine

STP: Ecstasy (MDMA)

Super Acid: Ketamine

Super K: Ketamine

Supergrass: PCP

Thunder: Heroin

Tina: Methamphetamine

Toxy: Opium

Toys: Opium

Trash: Methamphetamine

Triple C: Dextromethorphan

Tweak: Methamphetamine

Unkie: Morphine

Uppers: Amphetamines or methamphetamine

Vanilla Sky: Bath salts (synthetic cathinones)

Velvet: Dextromethorphan

Ventana: Methamphetamine

Vidrio: Methamphetamine

Vikes: Hydrocodone

Vitamin K: Ketamine

Wafer: Methadone

Weed: Marijuana

Weight Gainers: Steroids

When-shee: Opium

Whippets: Inhalants

White Dove: Bath salts (synthetic cathinones)

White Knight: Bath salts (synthetic cathinones)

White Lightening: Bath salts (synthetic cathinones)

Window Pane: LSD

Wolfies: Rohypnol

X: Ecstasy (MDMA)

XTC: Ecstasy (MDMA)

Yaba: Methamphetamine

Yellow Bam: Methamphetamine

Yellow Jackets: Barbiturates

Yerba: Marijuana

Ze: Opium

Zero: Opium

Zohai: K2/"Spice"

Chapter 51

Directory of State Substance Abuse Agencies

Alabama
Division of Mental Health and
Substance Abuse Services
Alabama Department of Mental
Health
P.O. Box 301410
Montgomery, AL 36130-1410
Toll-Free: 800-367-0955
(Hotline)
Phone: 334-242-3454
Fax: 334-242-0725
Website:
http://www.mh.alabama.gov/sa
E-mail: Alabama.DMH@
mh.alabama.gov

Alaska
Division of Behavioral Health
Alaska Department of Health
and Social Services
P.O. Box 110620
Juneau, AK 99811-0620
Phone: 907-465-5808
Toll-Free: 877-266-4357
(Hotline)
Fax: 907-465-2185
Website: http://dhss.alaska.gov/
dbh/Pages/default.aspx

Arizona
Behavioral Health Services
Arizona Department of Health
Services
150 North 18th Avenue, #200
Phoenix, AZ 85007
Phone: 602-364-4558
Fax: 602-364-4570
Website: http://www.azdhs.gov

Excerpted from "Substance Abuse Treatment Facility Locator," Substance Abuse and Mental Health Services Administration (www.samhsa.gov). All contact information was verified and updated in July 2013.

Arkansas

Division of Behavioral Health
Services
Arkansas Department of Human
Services
305 South Palm Street
Little Rock, AR 72205
Phone: 501-686-9164
TDD: 501-686-9176
Fax: 501-686-9182
Website: http://humanservices
.arkansas.gov/dbhs/Pages/
default.aspx

California

Editor's Note: Effective with the
passage of the 2013–2014
Budget Act and associated
legislation, the Department of
Alcohol and Drug Programs
(ADP) no longer exists as of July
1, 2013. All ADP programs and
staff, except the Office of Problem Gambling, transferred to the
Department of Health Care
Services (DHCS).

Colorado

Office of Behavioral Health
Department of Human Services
3824 West Princeton Circle
Denver, CO 80236-3111
Phone: 303-866-7400
Fax: 303-866-7428
Website: http://www.colorado.gov/
cs/Satellite/CDHS-Behavioral
Health/CBON/1251578892077
E-mail: cdhs.communications
@state.co.us

Connecticut

Department of Mental Health
and Addiction Services
P.O. Box 341431
Hartford, CT 06134
Toll-Free: 800-446-7348
Phone: 860-418-7000
TDD: 860-418-6707
Website:
http://www.ct.gov/dmhas

Delaware

Division of Substance
Abuse and Mental Health
Community Mental Health
and Addiction Services
1901 North DuPont Highway
Main Building
New Castle, DE 19720
Toll-Free: 800-652-
2929 (Helpline—Delaware Only)
Phone: 302-255-9399
Fax: 302-255-4427
Website: http://www.dhss.delaware
.gov/dsamh/index.html

District of Columbia

Department of Health
Addiction Prevention and
Recovery Administration (APRA)
70 N Street NE
Washington, DC 20002
Phone: 202-727-8857
Phone: 202-727-8473
(Assessment/Referral Center)
Fax: 202-727-0092
Fax: 202-727-8411
(Assessment/Referral Center)
Website: http://doh.dc.gov/apra
E-mail: doh@dc.gov

Florida

Substance Abuse Program Office
Florida Department of Children
and Families
1317 Winewood Boulevard
Building 6, Room 334
Tallahassee, FL 32399-0700
Phone: 850-487-2920
Fax: 850-414-7474
Website: http://www.myfl
families.com/service-programs/
substance-abuse

Georgia

Division of Addictive Diseases
Department of Behavioral
Health and Developmental
Disabilities
Two Peachtree Street NW
24th Floor
Atlanta, GA 30303-3171
Toll-Free: 800-715-4225
(Hotline)
Phone: 404-657-2331
Fax: 404-657-2256
Website:
http://dbhdd.georgia.gov

Hawaii

Alcohol and Drug Abuse Division
Hawaii Department of Health
601 Kamokila Boulevard
Room 360
Kapolei, HI 96707
Phone: 808-692-7506
Fax: 808-692-7521
Website: http://health.hawaii.gov/
substance-abuse
E-mail: webmail@hawaii.gov

Idaho

Division of Behavioral Health
Department of Health and
Welfare
P.O. Box 83720
Boise, ID 83720-0036
Toll-Free: 800-922-3406
(Screening/Referral)
Phone: 208-334-6997
Website:
http://www.healthandwelfare
.idaho.gov
E-mail: DPHInquiries
@dhw.idaho.gov

Illinois

Division of Alcoholism
and Addiction
Department of Human Services
100 West Randolph
Suite 5-600
Chicago, IL 60601
Toll-Free:
800-843-6154 (Help Line)
Toll-Free TTY:
800-447-6404 (Help Line)
Phone: 312-814-3840
Fax: 312-814-2419
Website: http://www.dhs.state
.il.us/page.aspx?item=29725
E-mail: DHSWebBits
@illinois.gov

Indiana

Division of Mental Health
and Addiction
Family and Social Services
Administration
P.O. Box 7083
Indianapolis, IN 46207-7083
Toll-Free: 800-901-1133
Toll-Free: 800-662-4357
(Hotline)
Phone: 317-233-4454
Fax: 317-233-4693
Website: http://www.in.gov/fssa/
dmha/index.htm

Iowa

Division of Behavioral Health
Department of Public Health
Lucas State Office Building
321 East 12th Street
Des Moines, IA 50319-0075
Toll-Free: 866-227-9878
Phone: 515-281-4417
Fax: 515-281-4535
Website: http://www.idph.state
.ia.us/bh/substance_abuse.asp

Kansas

Community Services
and Programs
Department for Aging
and Disability Services
New England State Office
Building
503 South Kansas Avenue
Topeka, KS 66603-3404
Phone: 785-296-4986
Fax: 785-296-0557
Website: http://www.dcf.ks.gov/
Pages/Default.aspx

Kentucky

Cabinet for Health and Family
Services
Department for Behavioral
Health, Developmental,
and Intellectual Disabilities
100 Fair Oaks Lane, 4E-B
Frankfort, KY 40621
Phone: 502-564-4527
TTY: 502-564-5777
Fax: 502-564-5478
Website: http://dbhdid.ky.gov/
kdbhdid/default.aspx

Louisiana

Office of Behavioral Health
Department of Health
and Hospitals
P.O. Box 629
Baton Rouge, LA 70821-0629
Phone: 225-342-9500
Fax: 225-342-5568
Website:
http://www.dhh.louisiana.gov/
index.cfm/subhome/10/n/6

Maine

Substance Abuse and Mental
Health Services
Department of Health
and Human Services
41 Anthony Avenue
#11 State House Station
Augusta, ME 04333-0011
Phone: 207-287-2595
Fax: 207-287-4334
Website: http://www.maine.gov/
dhhs/samhs/osa
E-mail: osa.ircosa@maine.gov

Maryland

Alcohol and Drug Abuse
Administration
Department of Health and
Mental Hygiene
Spring Grove Hospital Center
Vocational Rehabilitation
Building
55 Wade Avenue, Room 216
Catonsville, MD 21228
Phone: 410-402-8600
Fax: 410-402-8601
Website: http://adaa.dhmh
.maryland.gov/SitePages/
Home.aspx
E-mail: DHMH.ADAA_info
@maryland.gov

Massachusetts

Bureau of Substance
Abuse Services
Health and Human Services
250 Washington Street
Boston, MA 02108-4609
Toll-Free: 800-327-5050
(Helpline)
Toll-Free TTY: 888-448-8321
(Helpline)
Phone: 617-624-5171
Fax: 617-624-5395
Website: http://www.mass.gov/
dph/bsas

Michigan

Office of Recovery Oriented
Systems of Care
Department of Community
Health
320 South Walnut Street
Lansing, MI 48913
Phone: 517-373-4700
TTY/TTD: 517-373-3573
Fax: 517-335-2121
Website: http://www.michigan.gov/
mdch-bsaas
E-mail: MDCH-BSAAS
@michigan.gov

Minnesota

Alcohol and Drug Abuse Division
Department of Human Services
P.O. Box 64977
Saint Paul, MN 55164-0977
Toll-Free TTY/TDD:
800-627-3529
Phone: 651-431-2460
Fax: 651-431-7449
Website: http://mn.gov/dhs/
E-mail: dhs.adad@state.mn.us

Mississippi

Bureau of Alcohol and
Drug Services
Mississippi Department
of Mental Health
1101 Robert E. Lee Building
239 North Lamar Street
Jackson, MS 39201
Toll-Free: 877-210-8513
(Helpline)
Phone: 601-359-1288
TDD: 601-359-6230
Fax: 601-359-6295
Website: http://www.dmh.ms.gov/
alcohol-and-drug-services

Missouri
Division of Behavioral Health
Missouri Department of Mental
Health
P.O. Box 687
Jefferson City, MO 65102
Toll-Free: 800-575-7480
Phone: 573-751-4942
Fax: 573-751-7814
Website:
http://www.dmh.mo.gov/ada/
E-mail: dbhmail@dmh.mo.gov

Montana
Addictive and Mental Disorders
Division
Department of Public Health
and Human Services
P.O. Box 202905
Helena, MT 59620-2905
Phone: 406-444-3964
Fax: 406-444-9389
Website: http://www.dphhs.mt
.gov/amdd/
E-mail: hhsamdemail@mt.gov

Nebraska
Division of Behavioral Health
Department of Health
and Human Services
P.O. Box 95026
Lincoln, NE 68509-5026
Toll-Free: 888-866-8660
(Helpline)
Phone: 402-471-8553
Fax: 402-471-9449
Website: http://www.dhhs.ne.gov/
Behavioral_Health/
E-mail: DHHS.BehavioralHealth
Division@Nebraska.Gov

Nevada
Substance Abuse Prevention
and Treatment Agency
Department of Health
and Human Services
Division of Mental Health and
Development Services
4126 Technology Way, 2nd Floor
Carson City, NV 89706
Phone: 775-684-4190
Fax: 775-684-4185
Website: http://mhds.state.nv.us/
E-mail: MHDS@mhds.nv.gov

New Hampshire
Bureau of Drug and Alcohol
Services
Department of Health
and Human Services
105 Pleasant Street
Concord, NH 03301
Toll-Free: 800-804-0909
Phone: 603-271-6738
Fax: 603-271-6105
Website: http://www.dhhs.nh.gov/
dcbcs/bdas/index.htm

New Jersey
Division of Addiction Services
Department of Human Services
222 South Warren Street
Trenton, NJ 08625
Toll-Free: 800-238-2333
(Hotline)
Phone: 609-292-5760
Fax: 609-292-3816
Website: http://www.state.nj.us/
humanservices/das/home
E-mail: dmhas@dhs.state.nj.us

New Mexico
Behavioral Health
Services Division
Human Services Department
P.O. Box 2348
Santa Fe, NM 87504
Toll-Free: 800-362-2013
Phone: 505-476-9266
Fax: 505-476-9277
Website: http://www.hsd.state
.nm.us/bhsd/

New York
New York State Office of
Alcoholism and Substance Abuse
Services
1450 Western Avenue
Albany, NY 12203-3526
Toll-Free: 877-846-7369
(Hotline)
Phone: 518-473-3460
Fax: 518-457-5474
Website: http://www.oasas.ny.gov
E-mail: communications
@oasas.ny.gov

North Carolina
Department of Health
and Human Services
Division of Mental Health,
Developmental Disabilities,
and Substance Abuse Services
3007 Mail Service Center
Raleigh, NC 27699-3007
Toll-Free: 800-662-7030
Phone: 919-733-4670
Fax: 919-733-4556
Website: http://www.dhhs.state
.nc.us/mhddsas

North Dakota
Division of Mental Health and
Substance Abuse Services
Department of Human Services
Prairie Hills Plaza
1237 West Divide Avenue
Suite 1C
Bismarck, ND 58501-1208
Toll-Free: 800-755-2719
(North Dakota only)
Phone: 701-328-8920
Fax: 701-328-8969
Website: http://www.nd.gov/dhs/
services/mentalhealth/
E-mail: dhsmhsas@nd.gov

Ohio
Ohio Department of Mental
Health and Addiction Services
30 East Broad Street, 36th Floor
Columbus, OH 43215-3430
Toll-Free: 877-275-6364
Toll-Free TTY: 888-636-4889
Phone: 614-466-2596
TTY: 614-752-9696
Fax: 614-752-9453
Website: http://mha.ohio.gov
E-mail: askODMH@mh.ohio.gov

Oklahoma
Oklahoma Department of
Mental Health and Substance
Abuse Services
P.O. Box 53277
Oklahoma City, OK 73152-3277
Toll-Free: 800-522-9054
Phone: 405-522-3908
TDD: 405-522-3851
Fax: 405-522-3650
Website: http://ok.gov/odmhsas/

Oregon

Addictions and Mental Health
Division
Oregon Health Authority
500 Summer Street NE
Salem, OR 97301-1079
Toll-Free TTY: 800-375-2863
Phone: 503-945-5763
Fax: 503-378-8467
Website: http://www.oregon.gov/
oha/amh/Pages/index.aspx
E-mail: Amh.web@state.or.us

Pennsylvania

Department of Drug and Alcohol
Programs
Pennsylvania Department
of Health
02 Kline Plaza, Suite B
Harrisburg, PA 17104-1579
Phone: 717-783-8200
Fax: 717-787-6285
Website: http://www.health
.state.pa.us/bdap

Rhode Island

Department of Behavioral
Healthcare
Developmental Disabilities
and Hospitals
Barry Hall Building
14 Harrington Road
Cranston, RI 02920
Phone: 401-462-2339
Fax: 401-462-3204
Website: http://www.bhddh.ri
.gov/SA/

South Carolina

Department of Alcohol
and Other Drug Abuse Services
P.O. Box 8268
Columbia, SC 29202
Phone: 803-896-5555
Fax: 803-896-5557
Website: http://www.daodas.org

South Dakota

Division of Community
Behavioral Health
Department of Social Services
c/o 700 Governor's Drive
Pierre, SD 57501
Toll-Free: 800-265-9684
Phone: 605-773-3123
Fax: 605-773-7076
Website: http://dss.sd.gov/
behavioralhealthservices/
community
E-mail: infoMH@state.sd.us

Tennessee

Division of Substance
Abuse Services
Department of Mental Health
and Substance Abuse Services
601 Mainstream Drive
Nashville, TN 37243
Toll-Free: 800-560-5767
Toll-Free: 855-274-7471
(Hotline)
Phone: 615-532-6500
Website: http://www.tn.gov/
mental
E-mail: OC.TDMHSAS@tn.gov

Texas

Mental Health and Substance
Abuse Division
Department of State
Health Services
P.O. Box 149347
Austin, TX 78714-9347
Toll-Free: 866-378-8440
Phone: 512-206-5000
Fax: 512-206-5714
Website: http://www.dshs
.state.tx.us/MHSA/
E-mail: contact@dshs.state.tx.us

Utah

Division of Substance
Abuse and Mental Health
Utah Department of Human
Services
195 North 1950 West, 2nd Floor
Salt Lake City, UT 84116
Phone: 801-538-3939
Fax: 801-538-9892
Website: http://www.dsamh
.utah.gov
E-mail: dsamhwebmaster
@utah.gov

Vermont

Division of Alcohol and Drug
Abuse Programs
Department of Health
P.O. Box 70, Drawer 27
Burlington, VT 05402-0070
Phone: 802-651-1550
Fax: 802-651-1573
Website: http://healthvermont
.gov/adap/adap.aspx
E-mail: AHS.VDHADAP
@state.vt.us

Virginia

Office of Substance
Abuse Services
Department of Behavioral
Health and Developmental
Services
P.O. Box 1797
Richmond, VA 23218-1797
Phone: 804-786-3906
TDD: 804-371-8977
Fax: 804-786-9248
Website: http://www.dbhds
.virginia.gov

Washington

Division of Behavioral Health
and Recovery Services
Department of Social
and Health Services
P.O. Box 45330
Olympia, WA 98504-5330
Toll-Free: 877-301-4557
Toll-Free: 866-789-1511
(Help Line)
Toll-Free TTY: 800-833-6384
TTY: 206-461-3219 (Help Line)
Fax: 360-586-0341
Website: http://www.dshs.wa
.gov/dbhr
E-mail: DASAInformation
@dshs.wa.gov

West Virginia

Division of Alcoholism
and Drug Abuse
Bureau for Behavioral Health
and Health Facilities
Department of Health
and Human Resources
350 Capitol Street, Room 350
Charleston, WV 25304
Phone: 304-356-4811
Fax: 304-558-1008
Website: http://www.dhhr.wv.gov/
bhhf/Sections/programs/
ProgramsPartnerships/
AlcoholismandDrugAbuse/Pages/
default.aspx

Wisconsin

Department of Health Services
Bureau of Prevention,
Treatment, and Recovery
P.O. Box 7851
Madison, WI 53707-7851
Phone: 608-266-2717
Fax: 608-266-1533
Website: http://www.dhs
.wisconsin.gov/substabuse/
index.htm
E-mail:
DHSWEBMAILDMHSAS
@dhs.wisconsin.gov

Wyoming

Behavioral Health Division
Mental Health and Substance
Abuse Services
Department of Health
6101 Yellowstone Road
Suite 220
Cheyenne, WY 82002
Toll-Free: 800-535-4006
Phone: 307-777-6494
Fax: 307-777-5849
Website: http://www.health.wyo
.gov/mhsa/index.html

Chapter 52

Directory of Organizations Providing Information about Drug Abuse

Government Organizations

Centers for Disease Control and Prevention (CDC)
1600 Clifton Road
Atlanta, GA 30333
Toll-Free: 800-CDC-INFO
(800-232-4636)
Website: http://www.cdc.gov
E-mail: cdcinfo@cdc.gov

Drug Enforcement Administration (DEA)
Office of Diversion Control
8701 Morrissette Drive
Springfield, VA 22152
Toll-Free: 800-882-9539
Website: http://www.dea
diversion.usdoj.gov

Just Think Twice:
http://www.JustThinkTwice.com

Get Smart about Drugs: http://
www.GetSmartAboutDrugs.com

National Criminal Justice Reference Service (NCJRS)
P.O. Box 6000
Rockville, MD 20849-6000
Toll-Free: 800-851-3420
Phone: 301-519-5500
TTY: 301-947-8374
Fax: 301-519-5212
Website: http://www.ncjrs.gov

National Institute on Alcohol Abuse and Alcoholism (NIAAA)
Toll-Free: 888-MY-NIAAA
(888-696-4222)
Website:
http://www.niaaa.nih.gov
E-mail: niaaaweb-r
@exchange.nih.gov

Resources in this chapter were compiled from several sources deemed reliable. All contact information was verified and updated in July 2013.

National Institute on Drug Abuse (NIDA)
Office of Science Policy
and Communications
Public Information
and Liaison Branch
6001 Executive Boulevard
Room 5213, MSC 9561
Bethesda, MD 20892-9561
Phone: 301-443-1124
Website:
http://www.drugabuse.gov
NIDA for Teens:
http://teens.drugabuse.gov

New York State Office of Alcoholism and Substance Abuse Services (OASAS)
1450 Western Avenue
Albany, NY 12203-3526
Phone: 518-473-3460
Website:
http://www.oasas.ny.gov
E-mail: communications
@oasas.ny.gov

Office of National Drug Control Policy (ONDCP)
Website: http://www.whitehouse
.gov/ondcp
National Youth Anti-Drug Media Campaign:
http://www.whitehouse.gov/
ondcp/anti-drug-media
-campaign
Above the Influence:
http://abovetheinfluence.com

Substance Abuse and Mental Health Services Administration (SAMHSA)
SAMHSA's Health
Information Network
P.O. Box 2345
Rockville, MD 20847-2345
Phone: 877-SAMHSA-7
(877-726-4727)
Toll-Free TTY: 800-487-4889
Fax: 240-221-4292
Website:
http://www.samhsa.gov
E-mail:
SAMHSAInfo@samhsa.hhs.gov
SAMHSA Center for Substance
Abuse Prevention
Phone: 240-276-2420
Fax: 240-276-2430
Website: http://www.samhsa.gov/
prevention
SAMHSA Center for Substance
Abuse Treatment
Phone: 240-276-1660
Fax: 240-276-1670
Website: http://www.samhsa.gov/
treatment

U.S. Department of Education
Office of Safe and
Healthy Students
Potomac Center Plaza
550 12th Street SW, 10th Floor
Washington, DC 20202-6450
Phone: 202-245-7896
Fax: 202-485-0013
Website: http://www2.ed.gov/
about/offices/list/oese/oshs/
index.html
E-mail: OESE@ed.gov

U.S. Department of Labor
Drug-Free Workplace Advisor
Website: http://www.dol.gov/
elaws/drugfree.htm

Nongovernmental Resources

American Society of Addiction Medicine
4601 North Park Avenue
Upper Arcade, Suite 101
Chevy Chase, MD 20815-4520
Phone: 301-656-3920
Fax: 301-656-3815
Website: http://www.asam.org
E-mail: email@asam.org

Co-Anon Family Groups World Services
P.O. Box 12722
Tucson, AZ 85732-2722
Toll-Free: 800-898-9985
Phone: 520-513-5028
Website: http://www.co-anon.org
E-mail: info@co-anon.org

Cocaine Anonymous World Services
P.O. Box 492000
Los Angeles, CA 90049-8000
Phone: 310-559-5833
Fax: 310-559-2554
Website: http://www.ca.org

Community Anti-Drug Coalitions of America
625 Slaters Lane, Suite 300
Alexandria, VA 22314
Toll-Free: 800-54-CADCA
(800-542-2322)
Phone: 703-706-0560
Fax: 703-783-0318
Website: http://www.cadca.org

Narconon International
Phone: 800-775-8750
Website:
http://www.narconon.org

Narcotics Anonymous
P.O. Box 9999
Van Nuys, CA 91409
Phone: 818-773-9999
Fax: 818-700-0700
Website: http://www.na.org
E-mail: fsmail@na.org

National Center on Addiction and Substance Abuse at Columbia University
CASAColumbia
633 Third Avenue
19th Floor
New York, NY 10017-6706
Phone: 212-841-5200
Website:
http://www.casacolumbia.org

National Council on Alcoholism and Drug Dependence, Inc. (NCADD)
217 Broadway, Suite 712
New York, NY 10007
Phone: 212-269-7797
Fax: 212-269-7510
Toll-Free Hope Line:
800-NCA-CALL (800-622-2255)
Website: http://www.ncadd.org
E-mail: http://www.ncadd.org

National Families in Action
P.O. Box 133136
Atlanta, GA 30333-3136
Phone: 404-248-9676
Website:
http://www.nationalfamilies.org
E-mail:
nfia@nationalfamilies.org

National Parents Resource Institute for Drug Education (PRIDE)
PRIDE Youth Programs
707 West Main Street
Fremont, MI 49412
Toll-Free: 800-668-9277
Phone: 231-924-1662
Fax: 231-924-5663
Website: http://www
.prideyouthprograms.org
E-mail: info
@prideyouthprograms.org

Nemours Foundation
Website: http://www
.kidshealth.org

The Partnership at Drugfree.org
352 Park Avenue South
9th Floor
New York, NY 10010
Phone: 212-922-1560
Fax: 212-922-1570
Website: http://www.drugfree.org
E-mail: webmail@drugfree.org
The Parent Toolkit:
http://theparenttoolkit.org

Students Against Destructive Decisions (SADD)
SADD National
255 Main Street
Marlborough, MA 01752
Toll-Free: 877-SADD-INC
(877-723-3462)
Fax: 508-481-5759
Website: http://www.sadd.org
E-mail: info@sadd.org

Index

Index

Page numbers followed by 'n' indicate a footnote. Page numbers in *italics* indicate a table or illustration.

Health Reference Series